HANDBOOK OF (CENTRAL) AUDITORY PROCESSING DISORDER

Volume II
Comprehensive Intervention

Edited by

Gail D. Chermak, Ph.D.
Frank E. Musiek, Ph.D.

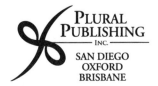

PLURAL PUBLISHING INC.

SAN DIEGO
OXFORD
BRISBANE

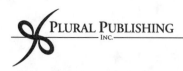
PLURAL PUBLISHING
INC.

Plural Publishing, Inc
5521 Ruffin Road
San Diego, CA 92123

e-mail: info@pluralpublishing.com
Web site: http://www.pluralpublishing.com

49 Bath Street
Abingdon, Oxfordshire OX14 1EA
United Kingdom

Typeset in 10½/13 Garamond by Flanagan's Publishing Services, Inc.
Printed in the United States of America by Bang Printing

ISBN-13: 978-1-59756-057-3
ISBN-10: 1-59756-057-X

Library of Congress Cataloging-in-Publication Data

Handbook of (central) auditory processing disorder / [edited by] Frank E. Musiek,
    Gail D. Chermak.
        v. ; cm.
    Includes bibliographical references and index.
    Contents: v. 1. Auditory neuroscience and diagnosis — v. 2. Comprehensive
intervention.
    ISBN-13: 978-1-59756-056-6 (hardcover : v. 1)
    ISBN-10: 1-59756-056-1 (hardcover : v. 1)
    ISBN-13: 978-1-59756-057-3 (hardcover : v. 2)
    ISBN-10: 1-59756-057-X (hardcover : v. 2)
    1. Word deafness. 2. Hearing disorders. 3. Language acquisition. 4. Auditory
perception.
  I. Musiek, Frank E. II. Chermak, Gail D.
    [DNLM: 1. Language Development Disorders—diagnosis.
  WL 340.2 H2353 2006]
  RC394.W63H362 2006
  617.8—dc22

                                                                    2006021068

CONTENTS

The role of central auditory processing in language and learning development and disorders has been a major focus of research for over 40 years. In 1964 Arthur Benton wrote a seminal paper that described children with specific developmental disorders of language (at that time referred to as "developmental aphasia") that appeared in the first issue of the journal *Cortex*. In this paper Benton pointed out that, in addition to severe delay in language development, these children were characterized by higher order auditory processing disorders. When I began my graduate research at Cambridge University in 1970, I was highly influenced by this paper. I decided to focus my thesis research on an empirical investigation of the higher order auditory processing abilities of children with developmental aphasia. Being in a Department of Experimental Psychology, and coming from a background in animal research, I was from the outset interested in understanding the neurobiological substrates of central auditory processing and their influence on language development and disorders. This led me to the research of Dewson and Cowey (1969) with primates and Robert Efron (1963) with adult aphasics. In both cases, there was a focus on "auditory temporal processing." Early papers by Lowe and Campbell (1965) and John Eisenson (1966, 1968) also pointed to potential theoretical as well as therapeutic implications of "temporal auditory processing" disorders in developmental aphasia. These early papers stimulated me to

develop a method (that has come to be known as the Tallal Repetition Test) that would be appropriate for assessing in young children with developmental language learning impairments (LLI) "temporal auditory processing," in a hierarchical manner, beginning with simple detection of tones differing in frequency and ending with sequencing and serial memory. My thesis studies demonstrated that these children were particularly impaired in detecting brief, rapidly successive or rapidly changing acoustic cues, both in tones sequences as well as *within* speech syllables (Tallal & Piercy, 1973, 1974). Furthermore, performance dramatically improved when the rate of acoustic change was slowed down (Tallal & Piercy, 1975). Little did I know then that the role of auditory processing disorders in developmental language-based learning disabilities (including dyslexia) would come to dominate research and debate concerning etiology as well as remediation into the 21st century.

During these same years, major advances were being made in our understanding at the cellular level of how the central nervous system is shaped by experience-dependent learning (neuroplasticity), resulting in the exquisite "mapping" of the sensory systems of the brain. Of particular relevance to temporal auditory processing was the finding that one of the most fundamental physiological functions of the neocortex is prediction and sequence learning (Rao & Sejnowski, 2003). At the cellular level, spike-timing-dependent-learning, or what

Donald Hebb (1949) called "temporally asymmetric learning," captures the influence of relative timing between input and output spikes in a neuron. Specifically, an input synapse to a given neuron that is activated slightly before a neuron fires is strengthened (also known as long term potentiation or LTP) whereas a synapse activated slightly after is weakened (long-term depression or LTD). This window of plasticity typically ranges from -40 to $+40$ milliseconds (ms). I have proposed (Tallal, 2004) that Hebb's fundamental neural learning rule may underlie essential aspects of acoustic/phonetic perception and language learning. Such a mechanism would cause multiple neurons in the primary auditory cortex that fire nearly simultaneously in time to bind together. Not only could such temporally contiguous, frequent patterns of activation build cell assemblies *representing* discrete phonemes, but such activity in one cortical circuit could, through converging projections, activate other cortical areas, leading to a sequence of activations that Hebb called a "phase sequence." Such a mechanism could account not only for the development and sharpening of neural representations for distinct phonemes that occur repeatedly in specific orders within a language, but also for the elimination through regressive and inhibitory processes of phonemes and sequential patterns that do not occur in an infant's native language. It is provocative that the critical time window for LTP and LTD is approximately 40 ms, as this is also the critical time window for the rapid temporospectral acoustic changes in formant transitions that are essential for tracking temporal order across ongoing speech (Dorman, Cutting, & Raphael, 1975) and also the time window shown to be most impaired in children with LLI (Tallal, 2004) as well as aging adults (Frisina et al., 2001).

As described in this volume, these major advances both in our understanding of central auditory processing disorder as well as in the neurobiology of the auditory system (and specifically how these are both affected by experience-dependent learning) have been integrated into novel intervention strategies for children as well as aging adults with auditory processing disorders. The finding that the neural mechanisms underlying neuroplasticity extend throughout life (Reconzone, Schreiner, & Merzenich, 1993) not only provided new hope that central auditory processing deficits can be significantly remediated at any age, but also described explicitly the most effective methods for doing so (Battin & Young, 2000; Merzenich et al, 1996; Schopmeyer, Mellon, Dobaj, Grant, & Niparko, 2000; Tallal et al., 1996; Temple et al., 2003; Tremblay & Kraus, 2002). Fortuitously, advances in computer technology, including the widespread use of the Internet, provide the final essential ingredient for developing truly research-based therapeutic interventions—the means for translating and scaling up these laboratory research advances for widespread use in clinics and educational settings.

Paula Tallal, Ph.D

References

Battin, R. R., & Young, M. (2000). Use of Fast ForWord in remediation of central auditory processing disorders. *Audiology Today, 12*(2).

Benton, A. L. (1964). Developmental aphasia and brain damage. *Cortex, 1*(1), 40-52.

Dewson, J. H., & Cowey, A. (1969). Discrimination of auditory sequences by monkeys. *Nature, 222*, 695-697.

Dorman, M. F., Cutting, J. E., & Raphael, L. J. (1975). Perception of temporal order in vowel sequences with and without formant transitions. *Journal of Experimental Psychology: Human Perception and Performance, 104*(2), 121-129.

Efron, R. (1963). Temporal perception, aphasia and deja vu. *Brain, 86*(3), 403-424.

Eisenson, J. (1966). Perceptual disturbances in children with central nervous system dysfunction and implications for language development. *British Journal of Communication, 1*(1), 21-32.

Eisenson, J. (1968) Developmental aphasia: a speculative view with therapeutic implications. *Journal of Speech and Hearing Disorders, 33*(1), 3-13.

Frisina, D. R., Frisina, R. D, Jr., Snell, K. B., Burkard, R., Walton, J. P, & Ison, J. R. (2001). Auditory temporal processing during aging. In P. R. Hoff & C. V Mobbs (Eds.), *Functional neurobiology of aging* (pp. 565-579). San Diego: Academic Press.

Hebb, D. O. (1949). *The organization of behavior: A neuropsychological theory.* New York: Wiley.

Lowe, A. D., & Campbell, R. A. (1965) Temporal discrimination in aphasoid and normal children. *Journal of Speech and Hearing Research, 8*, 313-314.

Merzenich, M., Jenkins, W. M., Johnston, P., Schreiner, C., Miller, S. L., & Tallal, P. (1996). Temporal processing deficits of language learning impaired children ameliorated by training. *Science, 271*, 77-81.

Rao, R. P. N., & Sejnowski, T. (2003). Self-organizing neural systems based on predictive learning. *Philosophical Transactions of the Royal Society of London, 361*, 1149-1175.

Recanzone, G. H., Schreiner, C. E., & Merzenich, M. M. (1993). Plasticity in the frequency representation of primary auditory cortex following discrimination training in adult owl monkeys. *Journal of Neuroscience, 13*, 87-104.

Schopmeyer, B, Mellon, N., Dobaj, H., Grant, G., & Niparko, J. K. (2000). Use of Fast ForWord to enhance language development in children with cochlear implants. *Annals of Otolaryngology, Rhinology, and Laryngology, 109*(12:2), 95-98.

Tallal, P. (2004). Improving language and literacy is a matter of time. *Nature Reviews Neuroscience, 5*, 721-728.

Tallal, P., Miller, S. L., Bedi, G., Byma, G., Wang, X., Nagaragan, S. S., Schreiner, C., Jenkins, W. M., & Merzenich, M. M. (1996). Language comprehension in language-learning impaired children improved with acoustically modified speech. *Science, 271*, 81-84.

Tallal, P., & Piercy, M. (1973). Defects of nonverbal auditory perception in children with developmental aphasia. *Nature, 241*, 468-469.

Tallal, P., & Piercy, M. (1974). Developmental aphasia: Rate of auditory processing and selective impairment of consonant perception. *Neuropsychologia, 12*, 83-93.

Tallal, P., & Piercy, M. (1975). Developmental aphasia: The perception of brief vowels and extended stop consonants. *Neuropsychologia, 13*, 69-74.

Temple., E. Deutsch, G. K., Poldrack, R. A., Miller, S. L., Tallal., P, Merzenich, M. M., & Gabrieli, J. D. E. (2003). Neural deficits in children with dyslexia ameliorated by behavioral remediation: Evidence from functional MRI. *Proceedings of the National Academy of Sciences, 100*, 2860-2865.

Tremblay, K. L., & Kraus, N. (2002). Auditory training induces asymmetrical changes in cortical neural activity. *Journal Speech, Language, and Hearing Research, 45*, 564-572.

ABOUT THE EDITORS

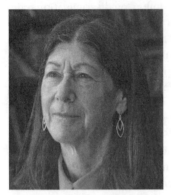

Gail D. Chermak, Ph.D.

Dr. Chermak is Professor and Chair of the Department of Speech and Hearing Sciences at Washington State University. She held the Washington State University College of Liberal Arts Edward R. Meyer Distinguished Professorship in 1999–2002 and received the College's Distinguished Faculty Award in 2002. She holds the Certificate of Clinical Competence in Audiology and is a Fellow of the American Academy of Audiology (AAA) and the American Speech-Language-Hearing Association (ASHA). Funded by the Kellogg Foundation, the World Institute on Disability, and the Fulbright American Republics Research Program, she has traveled extensively, consulting with public and private agencies in the area of rehabilitation service delivery. She has chaired and served on a number of national professional committees and task forces, including the ASHA Work Group on Central Auditory Processing Disorder (CAPD), which recently completed a technical report and position statement. Presently, she serves on the AAA's CAPD Task Force. She is an assistant editor for the *Journal of the American Academy of Audiology* and serves as editorial consultant for several other professional and scientific journals. She has published extensively and delivered numerous workshops, nationally and internationally, on differential diagnosis, assessment and rehabilitation of CAPD. Her coauthored articles and letters to the editor on CAPD and attention deficit hyperactivity disorder were named by her peers as among the best in diagnostic audiology in four of the last five consecutive years. Her 1997 book, *Central Auditory Processing Disorders: New Perspectives*, co-authored with Frank Musiek, has become a landmark volume in the field.

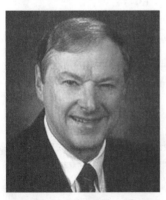

Frank E. Musiek, Ph.D.

Dr. Musiek is Professor and Director of Auditory Research in the Department of Communications Sciences and Professor of Otolaryngology, School of Medicine, University of Connecticut. He has published more than 160 articles and book chapters in the areas of auditory evoked potentials, central auditory disorders, auditory neuroanatomy, and auditory pathophysiology. He has developed the dichotic digits, frequency and duration patterns and gaps in noise (GIN) tests as well as the dichotic interaural intensity difference (DIID) auditory training procedure. He has also authored or edited six books and three monographs.

PREFACE

Central auditory processing disorder ([C]APD) is a deficit in neural processing of auditory stimuli that is not due to higher order language, cognitive, or related factors, yet (C)APD may lead to or be associated with difficulties in higher order language, learning, cognitive, and communication functions. The comorbidity of (C)APD with a range of language, learning, and communication disorders is the result of brain organization, about which we have learned much in recent years. The perspectives contained in this two-volume Handbook reflect major advances in auditory neuroscience and cognitive science, particularly over the last two decades since then-President George H. Bush proclaimed the 1990s the "Decade of the Brain." Since that proclamation, we have witnessed great strides in basic and clinical research in neuroscience and cognitive science with considerable impact on the diagnosis and treatment of (C)APD. The multidisciplinary efforts of thousands of scientists and health care professionals have led to greater insights regarding the nature of (C)APD, brain organization and function, and directions for more efficient diagnosis (or diagnostic procedures) and efficacious interventions. With the recognition that neuroplastic changes in the brain underlie learning and rehabilitation, there is every reason to embrace an aggressive and optimistic approach to intervention knowing that behavioral interventions that appropriately stimulate plastic neural tissues should lead to positive change.

The Handbook provides comprehensive coverage of the field (C)APD in children, adults, and older adults, involving the range of developmental (i.e., neurobiological) and acquired (i.e., aging and neurological diseases, disorders, and insults, including neurodegenerative diseases) origins. Volume I focuses on auditory neuroscience foundations, diagnostic principles and procedures, and multidisciplinary assessment. Volume II concentrates on rehabilitation and professional issues. The complexity and heterogeneity of (C)APD, combined with the heterogeneity of learning and related disorders, challenge scientists and clinicians as they attempt to understand and differentially diagnose individuals with listening deficits, language comprehension problems, attention deficits, learning disabilities, and other related behavioral, emotional, and social difficulties. This Handbook offers up-to-date, comprehensive coverage of auditory neuroscience and clinical science needed to accurately diagnose, assess, and treat the auditory and related deficits of individuals with (C)APD.

The Handbook is intended to serve three primary audiences. First, the contributing authors have written a comprehensive set of manuals for clinicians, primarily audiologists, speech-language pathologists, and psychologists, and for other related health care professionals as well. The Handbook also should serve as a reference source for a range of clinical scientists engaged in research related to audition and speech perception. Finally, but not any less a focus of our efforts are graduate students, for whom we hope the Handbook can serve as a textbook(s) for use in the classroom and in support of their clinical experiences.

The approaches and recommendations offered in this Handbook are not intended to serve as a sole source of guidance for the differential diagnosis and intervention of individuals with (C)APD. Rather, the views and methods of the 33 authors contributing to the Handbook are designed to assist the clinician by providing a framework for decision making and implementing diagnostic and treatment strategies. They are not intended to replace clinical judgment or to establish a protocol for all individuals with (C)APD. Individual differences and circumstances, including the presence of comorbid conditions, require flexibility and adaptation.

Notwithstanding considerable scientific, technological, and clinical strides forward, we still have much more to learn. Continued research is needed to fully answer some of the longstanding questions, as well as answer the new questions that arise continually as new knowledge begets new questions. Collaboration between clinicians and scientists—combining the clinician's firsthand knowledge of clinical needs with the researcher's expertise in the scientific method—provides a powerful approach to asking the right questions and obtaining enduring answers. Indeed, the contributing authors to the Handbook reflect this very collaboration between scientists and clinicians. Only through continued collaboration can we truly generate creative and innovative approaches to questions and problems, and accelerate the pace of discovery. In so doing, we will continue to advance our understanding of the central auditory nervous system and its intersections with cognitive and language domains that lead to the complex and heterogeneous clinical profiles of (C)APD. It is imperative that we take advantage of the momentum that has taken us to our current level of understanding and clinical practice, as described in the Handbook.

In closing, we hope that the knowledge shared in the Handbook leads to improved health and well-being of individuals with (C)APD, their families, and their communities.

Gail D. Chermak
Frank E. Musiek

CONTRIBUTORS

Jane A. Baran, Ph.D.
Professor
Department of Communication
　Disorders
University of Massachusetts Amherst
Amherst, Massachusetts
Chapter 9

Teri James Bellis, Ph.D.
Associate Professor and Chair
Department of Communication
　Disorders
The University of South Dakota
Vermillion, South Dakota
Chapter 1

Gail D. Chermak, Ph.D.
Professor and Chair
Department of Speech and Hearing
　Sciences
Washington State University
Pullman, Washington
Chapters 1, 4, 5, and 13

Jeanane M. Ferre, Ph.D.
Audiologist
Private Practice
Oak Park, Illinois
Chapters 8 and 10

Carol Flexer, Ph.D.
Distinguished Professor of Audiology
School of Speech-Language Pathology
　and Audiology
The University of Akron
Northeast Ohio Au.D. Consortium
　(NOAC)
Chapter 7

Ella Inglebret, Ph.D.
Assistant Professor
Department of Speech and Hearing
　Sciences
Washington State University
Pullman, Washington
Chapter 2

Warren D. Keller, Ph.D.
Independent Practice
East Amherst Psychology Group
East Amherst, New York
Chapter 12

Frank E. Musiek, Ph.D.
Professor and Director of Auditory
　Research
Department of Communication Sciences
Professor of Otolaryngology
School of Medicine, University of
　Connecticut
Storrs, Connecticut
Chapters 1, 4, and 13

Jane T. Pimentel, Ph.D.
Associate Professor
Department of Communication
　Disorders
Eastern Washington University
Spokane, WA
Chapter 2

Gail J. Richard, Ph.D.
Professor and Chair
Communication Disorders and Sciences
Eastern Illinois University
Charleston, Illinois
Chapter 11

Jacek Smurzynski, Ph.D.
Associate Professor
Department of Communicative
   Disorders
East Tennessee State University
Johnson City, Tennessee
Chapter 3

Linda M. Thibodeau, Ph.D.
Professor
Program in Communication Disorders
University of Texas at Dallas
Dallas, Texas
Chapter 6

Kim L. Tillery, Ph.D.
Associate Professor and Chair
Department of Speech Pathology and
   Audiology
SUNY at Fredonia
Fredonia, New York
Chapter 12

Jeffrey Weihing, M.A.
Doctoral student
Neuroaudiology Lab
University of Connecticut
Storrs, Connecticut
Chapter 4

SECTION I

Foundations

CHAPTER 1

NEUROBIOLOGY, COGNITIVE SCIENCE, AND INTERVENTION

GAIL D. CHERMAK, TERI JAMES BELLIS, AND FRANK E. MUSIEK

A new understanding of how the brain is organized and how neuroplastic changes in the brain underlie learning has emerged over the last two decades. In this chapter, we highlight the implications of major findings in neuroscience and cognitive science for intervention. These findings help to explain the frequent comorbidity of (C)APD and related attention, language, and learning deficits, they undergird intervention methods and strategies that harness the brain's potential to *remodel* itself through learning, and they provide a framework for the development of subtypes or subprofiles of (C)APD based upon patterns or clusters of functional symptoms, central auditory test findings, and associated neurophysiologic bases. These subprofiles lead to more customized, deficit-focused, and therefore more effective intervention.

Definition and Nature of (Central) Auditory Processing Disorder

(Central) auditory processing disorder ([C]APD) is a deficit in the perceptual (i.e., neural) processing of acoustic stimuli and the neurobiologic activity that underlies those processes and gives rise to the auditory evoked potentials (ASHA, 2005a, 2005b). By definition, these perceptual deficits may co-occur with, but are *not the result of*, dysfunction in other modalities (ASHA, 2005a, 2005b). (C)APD manifests as poor performance in one or more of the following auditory behaviors: localization/lateralization, auditory discrimination, auditory pattern recognition, temporal processing (e.g., temporal integration, temporal discrimination, temporal ordering, and temporal masking), and performance with competing or degraded acoustic signals (ASHA, 2005a, 2005b). Although these processing difficulties are not attributed to higher order language, cognitive, or related supramodal (i.e., pansensory) dysfunction, (C)APD may lead to or be associated with difficulties in higher order language, learning, and communication function (ASHA, 2005a, 2005b; Bellis, 2003; Bellis & Ferre, 1999; Chermak & Musiek, 1997). A number of abilities, including phonologic awareness, attention to and memory for auditory information, auditory synthesis, and auditory comprehension and interpretation, likely are dependent on or associated with intact central auditory function; however, these abilities are considered higher order cognitive/communicative and/or language-related functions and, therefore, are not included in the definition of (C)APD (ASHA, 2005a).

Notwithstanding the potential for modulation of auditory perceptual input by concurrent stimulation from other sensory modalities and/or top-down influences (Bellis, 2002a, 2003; Cacace & McFarland, 2005; Chermak & Musiek, 1997), (C)APD is considered a *primarily* modality-specific perceptual dysfunction that cannot be attributed to peripheral hearing loss or to higher-order, global cognitive, supramodal attention, or memory, language-based, or related disorders (Musiek, Bellis, & Chermak, 2005). The nonmodular organization of the brain (discussed below) precludes defining (C)APD as an *exclusively* modality-specific perceptual dysfunction. Indeed, it would be inappropriate to apply the label of (C)APD to listening difficulties exhibited by individuals with higher-order, global, multimodal, or supramodal disorders *unless* a comorbid deficit in the central

auditory nervous system (CANS) can be demonstrated (Musiek et al., 2005). Through the use of diagnostic tests that have been shown to be sensitive to CANS dysfunction, along with additional multidisciplinary information, (C)APD is distinguishable from the frequently presented comorbid language, learning, and supramodal attention deficits (ASHA, 2005a; Bellis, 2002a, 2003; Bellis & Ferre, 1999; Chermak & Musiek, 1997; Musiek et al., 2005). The reader is referred to Volume I of this Handbook for discussion of differential diagnosis of (C)APD.

Prevalence and Etiology

Prevalence estimates of (C)APD in school-aged children range from 2 to 5% (Bamiou, Musiek, & Luxon, 2001; Chermak & Musiek, 1997). Estimates of (C)APD in older adults range from 23% to 76% (Cooper & Gates, 1991; Golding, Carter, Mitchell, & Hood, 2004; Stach, Spretnjak, & Jerger, 1990).

In the majority of children with (C)APD, the underlying etiology of the disorder cannot be determined definitively; however, it is suspected that abnormal neurophysiologic representation of auditory stimuli is to blame. Depending upon the individual, this may involve inefficient interhemispheric transfer of auditory information and/or lack of appropriate hemispheric lateralization, atypical hemispheric asymmetries, imprecise synchrony of neural firing, or a host of other factors (Jerger et al., 2002; Kraus, McGee, Carrell, Zecker, Nicol, & Koch, 1996; Moncrieff, Jerger, Wambacq, Greenwald, & Black, 2004). Much less frequently, a neurologic disorder, insult, or abnormality underlies

(C)APD in children (Musiek, Baran, & Pinheiro, 1994).

The central auditory processing deficits of adults may be acquired or may reflect unresolved central auditory dysfunction that was present, but perhaps undiagnosed, since childhood. These deficits may result from accumulated damage or deterioration to the CANS due to neurologic (including neurodegenerative) diseases, disorders, or insults, and they may or may not involve fairly circumscribed and identifiable lesions of the CANS (Baran & Musiek, 1991; Musiek & Gollegly, 1988; Musiek, Gollegly, Lamb, & Lamb, 1990). Central auditory deficits also may arise from the aging process itself, leading to poorer neural synchrony and time-locking, slower refractory periods, decreased central inhibition, atypical interhemispheric asymmetry, and interhemispheric transfer deficits (Bellis, Nicol, & Kraus, 2000; Bellis & Wilber, 2001; Jerger, Moncrieff, Greenwald, Wambacq, & Seipel, 2000; Pichora-Fuller & Souza, 2003; Tremblay, Piskosz, & Souza, 2003; Willott, 1999; Woods & Clayworth, 1986). Approximately 1 in 3 older adults 65 years of age and older present with peripheral hearing loss (Ries, 1994) which, in itself, may lead to neuroplastic alterations in central auditory function and interact multiplicatively with age-related central auditory deficits (Kim, Morest, & Bohne, 1997; Morest, Kim, Potashner, & Bohne, 1998; Willott, 1996).

Neuroplasticity

Recent research suggests that the central nervous system (CNS) is plastic, that is, capable of cortical reorganization by experience, for some time prior to stabilization of neural function (Aoki & Siekevitz, 1988). Although brain plasticity may be greatest and most obvious during development, accumulating data further suggest that the brain remains malleable throughout the life span and that significant neural reorganization can occur in response to injury or learning even in mature nervous systems (Edeline & Weinberger, 1991; Irvine, Rajan, & Robertson, 1992; Kolb, 1995; Moore, 1993; Singer, 1995). Plasticity may account for the maintenance of cognitive control across many decades despite the slow but sustained loss of neurons seen beginning in adolescence and continuing throughout the aging process (Kolb, 1995).

Long-term potentiation, the long-lasting increase in synaptic transmission induced by intense and repeated synaptic activity (Brown, Chapman, Kairiss, & Keenan, 1988) may be the physiologic mechanism underlying a variety of plastic processes in the nervous system (Pascual-Leone, Grafman, & Hallett, 1994; Schuman & Madison, 1994). Studies of long-term potentiation suggest significant opportunity to induce cognitive change through stimulation (Gustafsson & Wigstrom, 1988).

Neuroplasticity is induced through experience and stimulation and leads to reorganization (i.e., remapping) of the cortex, improved synaptic efficiency, increased neural density, and associated cognitive and behavioral change (Elbert, Pantev, Wienbruch, Rockstroh, & Taub, 1995; Merzenich, Schreiner, Jenkins, & Wang, 1993; Moore, 1993; Recanzone, Schreiner, & Merzenich, 1993; Robertson & Irvine, 1989; Weinberger & Diamond, 1987; Willott, Aitken, & McFadden, 1993). Activity-dependent plasticity is thought to underlie learning and memory as the brain changes in response to use and the needs and experiences of the individual (Elbert et al., 1995; Weinberger & Diamond, 1987). The cortical changes induced by stimulation (i.e., experience and practice) appear to be widespread and long-lasting (Merzenich & Jenkins, 1995) and include at least four different types of cortical reorganization: (1) map expansion, or the enlargement of a region dedicated to a given function; (2) compensatory allocation, or novel allocation of a particular process to another brain region; (3) crossmodal reassignment involving regions of the brain accepting input from a new sensory modality; and (4) homologous area adaptation in which the same area of the opposite hemisphere assumes responsibility for processing input that, typically, would have been lateralized to the other hemisphere (Grafman & Litvan, 1999). In addition, activation of previously inactive neuronal tissue may occur secondary to stimulation, as may the development of more efficient synaptic connections within the brain (Kaas, 1995). Recent findings suggest that cortical reorganization may be far more extensive than originally thought, and may extend into areas quite distant from the region of insult or injury (Dancause et al., 2005).

A substantial body of literature demonstrates that systematic auditory stimulation or lack thereof affects the physiologic function of the auditory system. For example, Hassmannova, Myslivecek, and Novakova (1981) observed decreased evoked potential latencies and greater ribonucleic acid (RNA) concentrations in the auditory cortex of rat pups following a two-week period of auditory stimulation. Knudsen (1988) reported changes in the spatial tuning underlying the localization function of the auditory neurons of barn owls following unilateral plugging and unplugging of the owls' ears.

Following a frequency discrimination task, Recanzone et al. (1993) demonstrated increased cortical representation and improved frequency discrimination of the trained frequencies in owl monkeys. Edeline and Weinberger (1991) reported changes in the tuning of the auditory cortex neurons of guinea pigs following frequency discrimination training. Weinberger and Bakin (1998) demonstrated receptive field changes in the auditory cortex in animals performing various types of discrimination tasks. In his excellent review, Syka (2002) provides a variety of examples of auditory plasticity related to training in both damaged and healthy auditory systems.

Documenting a remarkable example of auditory system plasticity in the human brain, Allen, Cranford, and Pay (1996) reported normal central auditory processing in an adult with congenital absence of the left temporal lobe. In fact, a rapidly accumulating body of literature provides definitive evidence of the impact of auditory stimulation in effecting behavoral change in humans, as well as in animals (Hayes, Warrier, Nicol, Zecker, & Kraus, 2003; Kraus, McGee, Carrell, King, Tremblay, & Nicol, 1995; Musiek, Baran, & Shinn, 2004; Russo, Nicol, Zecker, Hayes, & Kraus, 2005; Tremblay & Kraus, 2002; Tremblay, Kraus, Carrell, & McGee, 1997; Tremblay et al., 1998; Tremblay, Kraus, McGee, Ponton, & Otis, 2001; Warrier, Johnson, Hayes, Nicol, & Kraus, 2004). Speech discrimination training resulted in significant improvements in adults' behavioral discrimination and changes in the duration and magnitude of cortical evoked potentials (e.g., the mismatch negativity response, or MMN) (Kraus et al., 1995). Tremblay and Kraus (2002) reported that auditory training induced changes in cortical P1-P2 amplitude and improved phoneme (i.e. voice-onset time) perception in normal hearing adults. Furthermore, the changes in the neurophysiologic representation of these stimuli preceded the behavioral improvement in discrimination of the phoneme contrasts, providing insight into the time course of CANS plasticity secondary to stimulation and training. Demonstrating auditory system plasticity in children, Tallal et al. (1996) reported that progressive, adaptive, and intensive auditory training improves temporal processing and certain language skills. Musiek and Schochat (1998) and Musiek (1999) reported improvement in auditory processing and academic and communication performance of children diagnosed with (C)APD following informal auditory training. Following auditory training, children diagnosed with learning disabilities and/or attention deficit hyperactivity disorder showed improved auditory closure and sound blending skills, as well as changes in cortical potentials in quiet and in noise (Hayes et al., 2003). Russo et al. (2005) observed improvement in auditory brainstem potentials triggered by abbreviated speech stimuli after consistent use of a commercial auditory training program. These brainstem responses which were measured over a 40-msec time period yielded enhanced amplitude to a 40-msec /da/ stimulus for both positive and negative peaks over this time period. Their findings provide some evidence for plasticity at the brainstem level.

Implications of Neuroplasticity for Rehabilitation

The foregoing studies have demonstrated the brain's capacity to remap or reorganize itself to best meet auditory processing demands (Moore, 1993; Recanzone et al., 1993; Robertson & Irvine, 1989;

Willott, Aitken, & McFadden, 1993). The inherent plasticity of the CNS has provided a foundation for renewed interest in various treatment and management approaches, including auditory training (see Chapter 4). Plasticity enables the CNS to accommodate and offers speech-language pathologists and audiologists the opportunity to improve central auditory processing (Chermak & Musiek, 1992, 1997). The array of neuroplastic changes underlying different cortical reorganization strategies (as discussed above) bodes well for successful outcomes when intervention is undertaken comprehensively and broadly, engaging and exploiting the multimodal, cross-modal, and supramodal neural interfaces that support auditory performance. Stimulation enables plasticity and may extend the brain's so-called sensitive or critical periods for learning particular behaviors, thereby maximizing the potential for successful rehabilitative efforts (Hassmannova et al., 1981). In fact, continued practice results in overlearning that leads to automaticity wherein auditory skills can be accomplished with less metacognitive control (i.e., reduced self-allocation of attention or memory resources), thereby releasing internal resources for deployment to other tasks (Chermak & Musiek, 1997; Merzenich & Jenkins, 1995).

Because plasticity is dependent on activity and stimulation, neural plasticity affords opportunity for functional change only insofar as intervention is initiated in a timely manner (Aoki & Siekevitz, 1988; Bolshakov & Siegelbaum, 1995; Hassmannova et al., 1981). Intervention efforts should be aggressive and implemented as early as possible following either confirmed diagnosis or the time the individual, particularly the child, is identified as at-risk for (C)APD (Chermak & Musiek, 1992, 1997). However, because the absolute time course of the critical or sensitive periods prior to which time neural function begins to stabilize has not yet been established and may extend into adulthood (Merzenich et al., 1984), intervention efforts should never be viewed as too late. Presumably, children and adults with (C)APD present normal cortical plasticity and capability to learn. Therefore, with training and practice, these individuals should be able to resolve auditory events and information to a degree that is more compatible with the demands inherent to spoken language processing.

Change is facilitated by presenting stimulation in an organized manner that progressively challenges the client with the proper gradation of difficulty level and by integrating that stimulation into everyday activities (Rumbaugh & Washburn, 1996). Furthermore, active participation in the training on the part of the patient, along with inclusion of immediate feedback, salient reinforcement, and activities that work at or near the patient's skill threshold maximize neuroplasticity (Ahissar et al., 1992; Beninger & Miller, 1998; Blake, Strata, Churchland, & Merzenich, 2002; Holroyd, Larson, & Cohen, 2004). Because the remapping of the brain underlying improvements in auditory function probably requires some as yet unknown period of time that most likely varies widely among individuals and as a function of task demands, clinicians must demonstrate patience and counsel the client similarly, giving the intervention program ample opportunity to activate the neural processes of plasticity that will lead to change (Chermak & Musiek, 1997). Intensive training seems to accelerate the remapping and relearning process (Merzenich et al., 1996; Tallal et al., 1996). Our inability to quantify the requisite time period for remapping complicates clinical decisions to maintain or modify a particular therapeutic course based on progress to date. Ultimately, neurophysiologic markers of cortical reorganization, which may in fact precede behavioral markers of learning (Tremblay et al., 1998), may inform these clinical decisions. The present uncertainty surrounding the time required to induce and to stabilize cortical reorganization and learning underscores the importance of appropriately selected outcome measures, as discussed below.

CANS plasticity compels us to provide direct treatment (i.e., auditory training) to improve central auditory processes and skills (see Chapter 4). However, the array of neuroplastic changes that may occur (e.g., compensatory allocation, crossmodal assignment) augments and broadens the potential for successful efforts undertaken to strengthen related systems through central resources training. As discussed in Chapter 5, central resources training engages supramodal systems that interface with the CANS and can, through those interactions, increase treatment effectiveness by reducing the functional impact of (C)APD and enhancing listening, communication, social and learning outcomes. (The reader is referred to Chapter 1 of Volume I of this Handbook for additional discussion of neuroplasticity.)

Auditory Deprivation

As stimulation can induce change, so too can auditory deprivation induce cortical reorganization. In a plastic CNS, lack of effective practice can stabilize deficits and reinforce defective brain function. The observation of altered cortical tonotopicity secondary to partial cochlear hearing loss in guinea pigs underscores this possibility (Robertson & Irvine, 1989). In contrast, studies of children with histories of chronic otitis media confirm the resilience of the auditory system in rebounding from at least mild degrees of auditory deprivation. Following myringotomy and intubation, masking level differences of children with histories of chronic otitis media returned to normal suggesting recovery of binaural function (Hall, Grose, & Pillsbury, 1995). Similarly, Schwaber, Garraghty, and Kaas (1993) found extensive reorganization of adult macaque monkeys' auditory cortex following induced cochlear hearing loss. The deprived region of the auditory cortex became responsive to frequencies of an adjacent auditory region to ensure the viability of the neural tissue. Findings of cortical changes in adult monkeys suggest that auditory training may be successful regardless of the subject's age or duration of auditory deprivation, including deprivation caused by an auditory processing deficit.

Brain Organization, Nonmodularity of the Central Nervous System, and Comorbidity

The neural activity of the brain is temporally coupled across the cortex, modalities, and hemispheres; therefore, dysfunction, especially deficient timing, can impose limitations that spread or ripple across brain regions and modalities (Merzenich et al., 1993). These cascading effects may reduce the degree of neural synchronization and connectivity among brain regions, leading to the frequently observed range

of comorbid conditions (e.g., [C]APD and attention deficit disorder, language impairment, learning disability, etc.).

Recent studies demonstrate a great deal of interaction among even those areas that were considered previously to be sensory specific. The auditory system is large and overlaps with the neural substrate and networks of other sensory, cognitive, executive, and motor control systems (Poremba et al., 2003; Salvi et al., 2002). The assumption of spatially segregated cortical areas subserving attention, memory, and individual sensory systems has been replaced by the recognition that widespread cortical networks span across cortical areas (Gaffan, 2005; Merzenich et al., 1993; Thiebaut de Schotten et al., 2005). Auditory tasks (e.g., listening in noise) activate auditory and nonauditory areas of the brain, including areas involved in attention, executive control, working memory, language processing, and motor planning (Salvi et al., 2002). Moreover, there is growing evidence of the involvement of cognitive processes in basic perceptual events. For example, working memory has been shown to be integral to numerous auditory processes, including localization, temporal resolution, and pattern recognition (Marler, Champlin, Gillam, 2002; Martinkauppi, Rama, Aronen, Korvenoja, & Carolson, 2002; Zattore, 2001). Consistent with a network model, emphasizing the distributed nature of information processing within the nervous system, perceptual responses to sensory stimuli are mediated across a large number of brain regions involving multiple serial, parallel, and dispersed neural networks (ASHA, 1996; Masterton, 1992; Ungerleider, 1995).

That (C)APD co-occurs with other disorders is expected given the complexity, as well as the geographic proximity of *auditory areas* to polymodal association areas (Musiek et al., 2005). Dysfunction in or insult to (primarily) auditory regions is likely to spread beyond the artificial boundary of the so-called *auditory-specific* area (Musiek et al., 2005). Although some brain regions have been characterized as *auditory-specific*, neurons in these areas respond primarily, though not exclusively, to auditory stimuli (Cacace & McFarland, 2005; Musiek et al., 2005). An accumulating body of literature demonstrates the absence of complete modality specificity. For example, Sams et al. (1991) demonstrated that neuronal activity in even the primary auditory cortex is modified by visual input. Similarly, Calvert et al. (1997) demonstrated that areas formerly thought to be sensitive only to auditory stimuli are activated during solely visual tasks. Using functional magnetic resonance imaging, Wright, Pelphrey, Allison, McKeowin, and McCarthy (2003) characterized the superior temporal sulcus as a polysensory area, observing that the response to bimodal stimuli in this area was greater than that to either modality alone. Poremba et al. (2003) observed that bimodal stimulation enhances neuronal response from areas of overlap. Behavioral responses to multimodal inputs presented in close spatial and temporal proximity are faster and more accurate than responses to unimodal stimuli (Stein & Meredith, 1993). Booth et al. (2002) observed *both* modality-specific and polysensory activations during judgments of semantic relatedness of words presented in the visual and auditory modalities. In fact, auditory neurons in the cerebrum exhibit interconnectedness with a variety of neurons in other nonauditory areas of the brain. In reviewing this topic, Streitfeld (1980) emphasized the interconnections between specific brain regions and other areas with totally different functions. For example, she noted that the auditory cortex in primates has direct and indirect connections to the limbic system, cingulate gyrus, hippocampus, and frontal lobe. Bamiou, Musiek, and Luxon (2003) reported the presence of considerable auditory activity in the insula—a structure not usually considered an auditory region. Additional areas of the brain not generally considered as auditory regions that have been identified as auditory responsive include the amygdala, striatum, and frontal lobe, among others (e.g., Poremba et al., 2003; Salvi et al., 2002).

Taken together, a considerable corpus of research questions the ecologic validity of modality-exclusive brain regions and demonstrates clearly that polysensory regions are located within so-called modality-specific regions, raising serious questions regarding the likelihood a disorder will affect one small, possibly modular area, leaving a polysensory area a micron away unaffected. It seems clear that *complete* modality specificity is neurophysiologically untenable and that the organization of the brain underlies comorbidity (ASHA, 2005a; Bellis, 2002a; 2003; Musiek et al., 2005).

Implications of Brain Organization for (C)APD Intervention

Individuals are referred for central auditory processing evaluation because of listening problems that typically are impacting communication, learning, language processing, attention, and related areas. The nonmodularity and nonexclusively segregated organization of the brain underlies the heterogeneous nature of

(C)APD and the comorbidity frequently observed between (C)APD and communication, language, learning, attention, and social deficits (Musiek et al., 2005). Individuals often present central auditory dysfunction comorbidly with other valid diagnoses such as dyslexia, specific language impairment, attention deficit, and learning disability (e.g., Cunningham, Nicol, Zecker, Bradlow, & Kraus, 2001; Gomez & Condon, 1999; Kraus et al., 1996; Moncrieff. & Musiek, 2002; Pillsbury, Grose, Coleman, Conners, & Hall, 1995; Purdy, Kelly, & Davies, 2002; Riccio, Hynd, Cohen, Hall, & Molt, 1994; Tillery, Katz, & Keller, 2000; Warrier et al., 2004; Wible, Nicol, & Kraus, 2002, 2005; Wright et al., 1997). Although links between inefficient auditory processing and language or learning problems have been documented both behaviorally and electrophysiologically (e.g., Bellis & Ferre, 1999; Kraus et al., 1996; Moncrieff & Musiek, 2002; Wible, Nicol, & Kraus, 2005), (C)APD should not be viewed as a direct cause of all or even most cases of academic failure, learning disability, reading disability, or related disabilities. Nonetheless, as is true of many disorders, (C)APD certainly can exacerbate academic challenge (e.g., listening in noisy classroom environments) even when direct causation is unlikely. In cases of comorbidity, the (C)APD must be diagnosed fully and accurately and an intervention program must be developed and implemented by a team of professionals to address all significant functional deficits.

Based on the neurophysiologic foundations elaborated above, the framework underlying the conceptualization, diagnosis, assessment, and intervention for (C)APD incorporates multidisciplinary and multimodal perspectives (ASHA, 2005a, 2005b; Bellis, 2002a; Bellis, 2003; Bellis & Ferre, 1999; Chermak & Musiek,

1997; Musiek et al., 2005). The complexity and interactive organization of the brain, comprised of interfacing sensory, cognitive, and linguistic networks underlies comorbidity of disorders and often exacerbates the functional impact of (C)APD, resulting in associated difficulties in related areas, including language, learning, and social function. At the same time, however, these same interactions offer opportunities for more far-reaching and effective intervention for (C)APD (Chermak & Musiek, 1997). A comprehensive approach to intervention capitalizes on the complex organization of the brain and its neuroplasticity. Cognitive, metacognitive, and language resources (i.e., central resources) can be engaged to buttress central auditory processing and complement direct auditory skills training, thereby minimizing the functional consequences of (C)APD (Chermak & Musiek, 1997).

Auditory and Cognitive Neuroscience Foundations and Training Principles

A comprehensive approach to (C)APD intervention is based upon the accumulated auditory and cognitive neuroscience literature that demonstrates: (1) the plasticity of the auditory system, (2) the role of experience in reorganizing the cortex and shaping auditory behavior, (3) that stimulation induces cognitive and behavioral change, and (4) that stimulation enables plasticity and may extend the time course of sensitive or critical periods, thereby maximizing the potential for successful rehabilitative efforts (Aoki & Siekevitz, 1988; Gustafsson & Wigstrom, 1988; Hassmannova, Myslivecek, & Novakova, 1981; Kolb, 1995). These findings translate into three principles that guide intervention (Merzenich & Jenkins, 1995). First, training should be *intensive* to exploit plasticity and cortical reorganization. The brain is malleable; however, change requires considerable practice as well as significant challenge by working near the patient's skill threshold (Blake et al., 2002; Hayes et al., 2003; Musiek et al., 2004; Russo et al., 2005; Tallal et al., 1996). Second, training should be *extensive* to maximize generalization and reduce functional deficits. Training should incorporate various stimuli (nonverbal and verbal) and stimulus parameters, in multiple contexts, involving tasks that deploy cognitive, metacognitive and language resources (Chermak & Musiek, 1997; Chermak & Musiek, 2002). Third, active participation and salient reinforcement must be incorporated into the training process to engage motivation and maximize learning (Ahissar et al., 1992; Holroyd et al., 2004). This third principle also is derived from learning theory (Swanson & Cooney, 1991).

Integrating Learning Theory

In designing intervention programs, clinicians should integrate the third neuroscience-based training principle (i.e., active participation and salient) with other longstanding tenets of learning theory (Swanson & Cooney, 1991). Following the principles of neuroscience as well as learning theory leads the clinician to recognize the importance of both the quality and the quantity (or intensiveness) of intervention. Learning theory emphasizes the efficiency of distributing practice over time rather than compressing the same amount of practice into a short period of time (Spence

& Norris, 1950; Starch, 1912). Moreover, both the neuroscience-based training principles and the tenets of learning theory direct clinicians to sequence tasks to provide opportunities for correct performance and positive reinforcement (Ausubel & Robinson, 1969; Clifford, 1978; Hegde, 1993). Also supported by learning theory, skills and strategies should be overlearned to the level of mastery and automaticity to increase retention (Krueger, 1929).

Treatment Effectiveness, Efficacy, and Evidence-Based Practice

The efficacy and effectiveness of efforts to improve central auditory processing and strategy learning ultimately depend on the plasticity of the CNS, adherence to neuroscience-based training principles, and early and aggressive intervention. Efficacy refers to the extent to which a specific treatment has been shown to be beneficial under ideal (experimentally controlled) conditions (Office of Technology Assessment, 1978; Robey & Schulz, 1998). In contrast, effectiveness refers to the extent to which a specific treatment has been shown to be beneficial under typical (real-life) conditions (Office of Technology Assessment, 1978; Robey & Schulz, 1998). Clearly, treatment effectiveness is the goal to be achieved with each client.

Effective intervention is beneficial to the client, efficient, persists in time, and generalizes beyond the training parameters and settings (Chermak & Musiek, 1997). Effective behavioral treatments depend on motivated and assertive clients. Treatment variables, however, determine the ultimate success of intervention efforts, including the use of the best available clinical strategies/interventions, intensive practice using engaging tasks of graded difficulty, generous feedback, and opportunities to generalize (Chermak & Musiek, 1997). Determining which treatments are the "best available" requires reliance on evidence-based practice.

Related to efficacy and effectiveness is the growing interest in evidence-based practice (EBP). As defined by Sackett, Straus, Richardson, Rosenberg, and Haynes (2000), EBP is the "the integration of best research evidence with clinical expertise and patient values" (p. 1). EBP encourages clinicians to adopt treatment recommendations on the basis of a client's needs and values in concert with the best available data regarding the most effective methods for use in one's clinical practice. A five-step process, EBP encourages clinicians to undertake a systematic review of the literature to identify high levels of evidence that establish the scientific validity of clinic practices. The clinician begins the process by generating a focused question. Next, databases must be searched to find the best available evidence to answer the question. After collecting the evidence, the clinician must evaluate the evidence (e.g., is the evidence of high quality—derived from a double-blinded, prospective, randomized clinical trials or from a less rigorous observational study, case study, or retrospective study). The clinician must then integrate the evidence with the client's profile and needs, make recommendations for intervention, and finally evaluate the results and identify ways to improve the outcomes (Sackett et al., 2000). (See Chapter 2 and Cox [2005] for an in-depth discussion of evidence-based practice and treatment efficacy.)

Although studies with high levels of evidence (e.g., randomized controlled trials; meta-analysis of randomized controlled trials) are lacking for specific intervention programs for a variety of disorders, including (C)APD (Abrams, McArdle, & Chisolm, 2005), a solid base of research documents improved psychophysical performance, neurophysiologic representation of acoustic stimuli, and listening and related function in children and adults following targeted auditory training (e.g., Hayes et al., 2003; Jirsa, 1992; Kraus & Disterhoft, 1982; Kraus et al., 1995; Merzenich, Grajski, Jenkins, Recanzone, & Peterson, 1991; Merzenich et al., 1996; Musiek, Baran, & Pinheiro, 1994; Musiek et al., 2004; Russo et al., 2005; Tallal et al., 1996; Tremblay & Kraus, 2002; Tremblay et al., 1997; Tremblay et al., 1998; Tremblay et al., 2001; Warrier et al., 2004).

Outcome Measures

Various outcome measures can be used to demonstrate the effectiveness of therapy. Outcome measures are dependent variables that measure aspects of benefit provided by intervention. Measures can incorporate quantitative or qualitative data and include physical, physiologic, and behavioral measures obtained through observations, interviews, self-report, or direct measurement. Post-therapy changes on central auditory tests, psychoacoustic measures, and electrophysiologic procedures can be used to document the effectiveness of (C)APD intervention directed toward improving central auditory processes.

To demonstrate treatment outcomes in a more ecologically relevant context, one should measure changes in listening (comprehension) or spoken language processing. For example, speech recognition for time-compressed speech or speech recognition in interrupted noise provides ecologically appropriate outcome measures to supplement pitch or duration patterns, gap detection, or masking level differences used to assess changes in temporal processing. Similarly, one can measure auditory discrimination by measuring difference thresholds for intensity, frequency, or duration, or one might assess auditory discrimination in a more functional context of phonemic analysis or synthesis.

One must exercise caution, however, in selecting ecologic (i.e., functional) outcome measures. Even though improvements in language processing, academics, and social areas may be seen in some cases following intervention for central auditory deficits, many other variables, some of which are far removed from the auditory domain, also contribute to learning and socialization (Musiek et al., 2005). As such, the effectiveness (and efficacy) of (C)APD intervention should not be gauged primarily by academic outcomes or social skills, but rather by improvements in auditory function which, then, may support improvements in those domains that are dependent upon audition (Musiek et al., 2005).

Collaboration Promotes Treatment Effectiveness/Efficacy

The potential adverse impact of (C)APD on language, academic performance, and employment underscores the importance of multidisciplinary collaboration among professionals and with families (Bellis, 2003; Bellis & Ferre, 1999; Chermak & Musiek, 1997). As emphasized by Rumbaugh and Washburn (1996), optimizing brain plasticity in support of change requires that stimulation be integrated into one's everyday activities and lifestyle. Collaboration among professionals, clients, and families facilitates this integration.

Collaboration involves mutual deliberation in which participants collectively establish or clarify goals and values for the purpose of problem solving (Chermak, 1993). Engaging clients, families, and other professionals in planning, decision-making, and program implementation maximizes problem resolution and successful therapeutic outcomes (Coufal, Hixson, & Stick, 1990; Crais, 1991, Luterman, 1990). Collaboration does not begin, however, with intervention. As discussed in Volume I of this Handbook, the diagnosis of (C)APD is made on the basis of performance deficits demonstrated on valid tests of central auditory processing; however, other measures, particularly, speech-language measures and psychoeducational measures, provide needed information about language ability and communicative function, and academic achievement, respectively, which contribute to the differential diagnosis of (C)APD, and illuminate functional deficits requiring intervention (ASHA, 2005a, 2005b). Hence, both audiologists and speech-language pathologists (SLPs) should assume lead roles in implementing comprehensive intervention for (C)APD (see Chapter 11 for the role of the SLP). Typically, the audiologist leads the effort to improve signal quality by enhancing the acoustic signal and improving the listening environment. In serving patients with (C)APD, SLPs focus on enhancing the scope and use of language and other central resources. Auditory training should be undertaken by both professionals, as described in Chapter 4. Other professionals, including psychologists and/or neuropsychologists, regular and special educators, and others also are integral to the overall intervention program.

Collaborative consultation should lead to improved diagnostic and treatment strategies, more practical goals for intervention, and increased probability of successfully implementing diagnostic and treatment strategies (Coufal et al., 1990; Crais, 1991). Given family involvement in developing goals and designing strategies, and their subsequent motivation to implement treatment activities in the home and other natural environments, collaboration should maximize the transfer of skills (i.e., generalization) from treatment to daily routines (Crais, 1991). Because collaboration promotes the client's self-efficacy by emphasizing an active, metacognitive approach to problem-solving and encouraging self-regulation, it is a particularly valuable component of central resources training and the comprehensive intervention approach (Chermak & Musiek, 1997). The reader is referred to Chermak (1993) and Chermak and Musiek (1997) for in-depth discussion of the especially important role of collaboration in building partnerships that are both consistent with cultural paradigms and appropriate to the treatment needs of the client when working with culturally diverse individuals and families. The reader is referred to other chapters in this volume, including Chapters 8, 9, 10, 11, and 12 for additional perspectives on the role of collaboration for effective intervention.

Foundations of Comprehensive Intervention

All auditory tasks, from pure tone detection to spoken language processing, are influenced by higher-order, nonmodality-specific systems such as attention and memory, as well as motivation and decision processes, and the underlying multimodal, crossmodal, and supramodal neural interfaces supporting performance of complex behaviors (Chermak & Musiek, 1997; Musiek et al., 2005). Conversely, and as elaborated above, successful spoken language comprehension requires the listener to coordinate various knowledge bases and skills, including auditory vigilance, auditory discrimination, and temporal processing to discern and organize basic acoustic features; segmentation skills to parse the continuous sound stream into constituent phonetic units; language knowledge; general knowledge; and metacognitive knowledge and executive control (Abbs & Sussman, 1971; ASHA, 1996; Chermak & Musiek, 1992, 1997; Danks & End, 1987; Fant, 1967; Kintsch, 1977; Massaro, 1975a, 1975b; Ronald & Roskelly, 1985; Samuels, 1987). Effective listeners employ various self-regulation strategies to guide extraction of information and synthesis of the spoken message (Chermak & Musiek, 1997). Throughout the process, they must reflect continually on the processes and products of their listening. Experience, expectation, and motivation influence both the allocation of resources and the particular meaning derived from the acoustic signal. Given the number and range of skills and knowledge bases demanding coordination in service of central auditory processing and spoken language understanding, comprehensive intervention programs for (C)APD must integrate specific skills development, general problem solving strategies, and self-regulation of strategy use (Chermak & Musiek, 1997).

Because listening takes place within the multiple contexts of the acoustic, phonetic, linguistic, and social domains, simultaneous and integrated orchestration of multiple knowledge bases and skills is required for spoken language comprehension (Chermak & Musiek, 1997). Moreover, the complex organization of the brain and the resulting interdependence of sensory, cognitive, and language networks necessitate a comprehensive intervention program that includes intensive training via *bottom-up*, auditory training, signal enhancement, and environmental modifications, coupled with extensive *top-down* training focused on central resources knowledge, skills, and strategy training (ASHA, 2005a, 2005b; Bellis, 2002b, 2003; Chermak & Musiek, 1997). Bottom-up approaches include specific auditory training techniques, assistive listening systems, and clear speech. Top-down approaches include language and metalanguage strategies, cognitive strategies, metacognitive strategies, classroom, instructional, and learning strategies, and workplace, recreational, and home accommodations. Combined, these bottom-up and top-down approaches exploit the interactions supported by supramodal, multimodal, and crossmodal interfaces in addressing the range of functional deficits that characterize (C)APD and the often occurring comorbid disorders. Together, these approaches offer tremendous potential to mitigate listening difficulties stemming from (C)APD.

Customizing Intervention

Central auditory diagnostic data are pivotal to intervention planning; however, comprehensive intervention cannot be designed on the basis of central auditory test results alone. Understanding the processes underlying successful task performance helps to bridge the gap between data collection and intervention strategies and techniques (Chermak & Musiek, 1992). Information from multidisciplinary evaluations combined with central auditory test outcomes reveal the full range of functional deficits and areas of concern relevant to intervention program planning (Bellis, 2002b, 2003; Bellis & Ferre, 1999). In fact, the practical relevance of data to intervention programming varies considerably across tests. For example, although both masking level differences (MLDs) and tests involving auditory performance with competing messages both provide useful diagnostic insights regarding site or level of CANS dysfunction and compromised central auditory processes, the abstract nature of the MLD paradigm and the absence of an everyday listening analog renders MLDs less useful for counseling purposes. Both tests, however, provide valuable information regarding appropriate foci for auditory training (i.e., reduced MLDs indicate binaural interaction training; depressed auditory performance with competing messages suggest binaural integration and binaural separation training) (Chermak, 1996; Musiek & Chermak, 1994; Musiek & Chermak, 1995).

The heterogeneity of (C)APD and its occurrence across the life span, as well as the imperative to intervene efficiently as well as effectively, leads to several questions regarding the distinctiveness of intervention. First, can we truly customize intervention to the specific auditory profile? Second, can distinctive intervention strategies be formulated to manage (C)APD within a constellation of comorbid language or cognitive deficits? Third, should management strategies differ as a function of the client's age?

Auditory Profiling

With a firm understanding of (C)APD gained from auditory and cognitive neuroscience, it now may be possible to develop functional deficit profiles that reflect patterns of central auditory deficits and functional cognitive, language, learning, and communication sequelae (Bellis, 2002a, 2002b, 2003; Bellis & Ferre, 1999). These deficit profiles, which should conform to well-established neuroscience tenets that demonstrate the presence of brain-behavior relationships across a wide variety of functional areas, can be used to guide development of comprehensive intervention programs that address the cluster of central auditory and functional symptoms. Consider, for example, the difference in emphases for individuals diagnosed with (C)APD who present similar auditory performance decrements with competing signals, but dissimilar temporal processing abilities. Both individuals would probably benefit from auditory training focused on degraded signal processing (e.g., filtered speech recognition, speech recognition in noise, reverberation, and competing messages), signal enhancement strategies (e.g., FM technology and preferential seating), and linguistic strategies that emphasize use of context to resolve messages (i.e., closure skills). The individual experiencing temporal processing diffi-

culties, however, might also benefit from auditory training focused on temporal discrimination (e.g., gap detection) and time-compressed speech recognition exercises, as well as activities directed toward the use of prosody to predict degraded messages and recommendations that partners speak more slowly, pause more often, and emphasize key words.

Assumptions of Deficit-Specific Intervention

The utility of deficit-specific intervention derives from four assumptions, at least one of which may be of questionable veracity (Bellis, 2002b). The first assumption, that auditory processes and skills actually support listening, language use, and learning is fairly well documented (see Bellis, 2003, and Chermak & Musiek, 1997 for reviews). The second assumption, that central auditory diagnostic tests can identify deficient auditory processes is questionable. In fact, several studies employing factor analyses concluded that commonly used central auditory tests load on the same factor and do not adequately assess individual auditory processes (Domitz & Schow, 2000; Schow & Chermak, 1999; Schow, Seikel, Chermak, & Berent, 2000). Indeed, successful performance on behavioral tests typically is dependent on several auditory and related processes, as illustrated by pitch pattern tests which require pitch discrimination and sequencing (temporal processing), contour (pattern) recognition, linguistic labeling, working memory, and interhemispheric transfer (Musiek & Chermak, 1995; Musiek, Pinheiro, & Wilson, 1980). A considerable body of research substantiates the third and fourth assumptions that posit that available treatments can target deficient auditory processes and that intervention improves auditory processes and reduces functional deficits (see Neuroplasticity above, and Chapters 4 and 5).

Effectiveness of Deficit-Specific Intervention

(C)APD profiling is based on theoretical constructs and relates test findings to observed day-to-day behaviors; however, they have not yet been fully validated empirically (ASHA, 2005a; Bellis, 2002b). The effectiveness of deficit-specific auditory intervention should be gauged, primarily, by improvements seen on central auditory tests, as well as concomitant improvement in functional listening skills. Nonetheless, given the neurophysiologic interdependencies across sensory, cognitive, and language networks, improvements in academic and social arenas may be anticipated, especially when the comprehensive approach is fully implemented.

Customized Deficit-Specific Intervention

It should be emphasized that the use of function-deficit profiling for purposes of devising deficit-specific and individualized intervention programs should not be construed to be a *cookie-cutter* approach to (C)APD intervention. The unique confluence of bottom-up and top-down abilities present in a given individual, along with his or her functional difficulties and complaints, will necessarily dictate the components of the intervention program that will be most appropriate in any given situation. With this caveat in mind, however, the

following example illustrates the application of (C)APD profiling and customized intervention.

The likelihood of an interhemispheric transfer deficit is inferred from findings of a significant left-ear deficit on dichotic tests and poor performance on temporal patterning tests in the linguistic labeling report condition. These test data are consistent with the child's functional deficit profile, which includes difficulty listening in noisy environments, little or no benefit seen from bimodal summation (i.e., looking and listening), some bipedal and bimanual (motor coordination) difficulties, and reading and spelling difficulties despite normal language levels. The customized intervention program derived from multidisciplinary assessment focuses on: (1) dichotic listening training; (2) interhemispheric transfer exercises; (3) classroom modifications, including the use of an FM system; (4) acoustic enhancements; (5) central resource compensatory strategies, including active listening, attribution training, and cognitive problem-solving; and (6) continued reading and spelling resource services. Post-therapy improvements are observed in left-ear performance on the central auditory test battery, ability to listen in noise, ability to handle concurrently presented multimodality cues, as well as some improvement in reading and spelling.

Accommodating Comorbidity in Customizing Intervention

To formulate distinctive intervention strategies, the relative contribution of the constellation of concomitant auditory, language, cognitive, and learning deficits must be determined. Accurate differential diagnosis must precede efforts to customize therapy; however, notwithstanding careful assessment using an efficient, comprehensive, and multidisciplinary test battery, the relative contributions of auditory, language, and cognitive processes to spoken language comprehension problems may remain uncertain (ASHA, 1996). For example, several explanations can be offered to account for the fairly typical case of a child who presents with difficulty understanding spoken language in the presence of competing noise. The child may lack control over language resources, which prevents him or her from using language knowledge to compensate for the degraded acoustic signal. Alternatively, the nature and severity of the child's (C)APD may contravene his or her ability to separate signal from noise, despite full use of normal language knowledge (Chermak & Musiek, 1997). In addition, the child may exhibit an attention-based deficit which interferes with his or her ability to selectively attend to auditory stimuli in the presence of distractors, despite intact language and central auditory function. Similarly, it is often difficult to determine the relative contribution of cognitive, linguistic, and (central) auditory processing deficits for the language comprehension problems experienced by an adult with cognitive/linguistic disorders (e.g., aphasia) (ASHA, 1996). In fact, it is likely that spoken language comprehension problems in aphasia result from some combination of processing deficits. With information gleaned from a robust central auditory test battery interpreted in the context of a multidisciplinary test battery, clinicians can begin to disentangle the relative contributions of sensory, cognitive, and language processing deficits to a spoken language comprehension deficit and implement intervention directed toward improving the individual's functional abilities in appropriate contexts. (The reader is referred to Volume I of this Handbook for discussion of diagnosis, differential diagnosis, and multidisciplinary assessment.)

Life Span Considerations

Children with (C)APD frequently present with comorbid cognitive, language, and learning deficits. Older adults frequently present with both peripheral and central auditory disorders, as well as a range of age-related decline in cognitive abilities (e.g., working memory and speed of processing) and language processes that compound spoken language understanding difficulties, especially when there is reverberation and the competing signal is speech (Hickson & Worrall, 2003; McCoy et al., 2005; Pichora-Fuller, 2003; Pichora-Fuller & Souza, 2003). Individual differences are expected, given the normal variation in brain organization and age-related change across individuals coupled with the variable manifestations of central auditory pathologies (Phillips, 1995, 2002). Only comprehensive assessment can determine the ultimate relative role of these factors in explaining the spoken language difficulties experienced by the older adult (Chermak & Musiek, 1997).

Although many of the strategies and techniques described in this volume are likely to benefit the great majority of clients with (C)APD across the life span, specific emphases will vary depending on the nature of the processing deficits identified, the functional consequences of these deficits, the presence of comorbid conditions, and the client's age. For example, given the inherent neural plasticity of the developing CNS, intervention for children with (C)APD should emphasize direct auditory training and acoustic signal enhancement. Given the frequent comorbid constellation of attention, language, and learning issues, however, central resources training also is recommended and should be integrated with the academic curriculum (Bellis, 2002b, 2003; Chermak & Musiek, 1997).

Intervention goals and approaches with older adults with (C)APD must take into account neurophysiologic changes, co-morbid conditions, and the lifestyle and attendant demands of the older adult. The diminished plasticity of the older nervous system implies that management strategies in adults and older adults might necessarily be directed more toward compensation (i.e., assistive listening system, central resources training) rather than recovery of function (ASHA, 1996), although spontaneous and/or stimulus-induced recovery of function following acute brain injury may suggest a role for direct treatment (i.e., auditory training) approaches as well (e.g., Bellis, in press; Sweetow & Henderson-Sabes, in press). Opportunities to infuse multidisciplinary treatment and management strategies to address comorbid conditions in older adults (e.g., aphasia) should not be overlooked (Chermak & Musiek, 1997).

Intervention Strategies Appropriate Across Profiles

Notwithstanding the value of customizing intervention to achieve effective and efficient outcomes of the greatest functional significance, a number of intervention principles and strategies should be applied across clinical deficit profiles.

Common principles guiding intervention across clinical populations include an emphasis on collaboration, self-regulation, and an ecologic- and strategy-based orientation (Chermak & Musiek, 1997). Intervention strategies common across profiles include implementation of active listening techniques, use of *clear speech* to enhance acoustic cues, and coupling of auditory training with central resources (compensatory strategies) training. In many cases, trial of assistive listening systems (e.g., FM, infrared systems) may be indicated, as well. In producing clear speech, speakers attempt to produce every word and phrase in a precise and clear fashion, without exaggerating. Speakers are directed to speak clearly (e.g., as if speaking to someone with hearing loss or from a different language background), to focus on a slower and louder rate of speech, and to enunciate, emphasize key words, and pause more frequently and for longer durations. Acoustically, clear speech results in increased power of the consonants relative to vowels, wider pitch range, expanded vowel spaces, and more varied intonation and more prominent stress markers (Bradlow, Kraus, & Hayes, 2003; Pichney, Durlach, & Braida, 1985, 1986, 1989).

Summary

A clearer understanding of the brain's complex organization and plasticity carries considerable implications for intervention. The accumulated literature in auditory and cognitive neuroscience elucidates the nature of (C)APD and helps explain the frequent comorbid presentation with related attention, language, and learning deficits. The new understanding translates into training principles grounded in neuroscience and learning theory. The overlapping and widespread distribution of sensory, cognitive, and language networks undergird auditory training and central resource intervention methods and strategies that harness the brain's potential to *remodel* itself through learning. The emerging understanding also provides a framework to begin subtyping (C)APD around clusters of symptoms and associated neurophysiologic bases to implement effective intervention directed to those functional deficit clusters.

References

Abbs, J. H., & Sussman, H. M. (1971). Neurophysiological feature detectors and speech perception: A discussion of theoretical implications. *Journal of Speech and Hearing Research, 14,* 23–36.

Abrams, H. B., McArdle, R., & Chisolm, T. H. (2005). From outcomes to evidence: Establishing best practices for audiologists. *Seminars in Hearing, 26*(3), 157–169.

Ahissar, E., Vaadia, E., Ahissar, M., Bergman, H., Arieli, A., & Abeles, M. (1992). Dependence of cortical plasticity on correlated activity of single neurons and on behavioral context. *Science, 257,* 1412–1415.

Allen, R. L., Cranford, J. L., & Pay, N. (1996). Central auditory processing in an adult with congenital absence of left temporal lobe. *Journal of the American Academy of Audiology, 7*(4), 282–288.

American Speech-Language-Hearing Association Task Force on Central Auditory Processing Consensus Development. (1996). Central auditory processing: Current status of research and implications for clinical practice. *American Journal of Audiology, 5*(2), 41–54.

American Speech-Language-Hearing Association. (2005a). (Central) auditory processing disorders. Available at http://www.asha.org/members/deskref-journals/deskref/default.

American Speech-Language-Hearing Association. (2005b). (Central) auditory processing disorders—the role of the audiologist [Position statement]. Available at http://www.asha.org/members/deskref-journals/deskref/default

Aoki, C., & Siekevitz, P. (1988). Plasticity in brain development. *Scientific American, 259*(6), 56–64.

Ausubel, D. P., & Robinson, F. C. (1969). *School learning.* New York: Holt, Rinehart, and Winston.

Bamiou, D. E., Musiek, F. E., & Luxon, L. M. (2001). Aetiology and clinical presentation of auditory processing disorders—a review. *Archives of Disease in Childhood, 85,* 361–365.

Bamiou, D. E., Musiek, F. E., & Luxon, L. M. (2003). The insula (island of Reil) and its role in auditory processing: Literature review. *Brain Research Reviews, 42,* 143–154.

Baran, J. A., & Musiek, F. E. (1991). Behavioral assessment of the central auditory nervous system. In W. F. Rintelmann (Ed.), *Hearing assessment* (pp. 549–602). Austin, TX: Pro-Ed.

Bellis, T. J. (2002a). Considerations in diagnosing auditory processing disorders in school-aged children. *American Speech-Language-Hearing Association Special Interest Division Perspectives on Hearing and Hearing Disorders in Children, 12,* 3–9.

Bellis, T. J. (2002b). Developing deficit-specific intervention plans for individuals with auditory processing disorders. *Seminars in Hearing, 23*(4), 287–295.

Bellis, T. J. (2003). *Assessment and management of central auditory processing disorders in the educational setting: From science to practice* (2nd ed.). Clifton Park, NY: Thomson Learning.

Bellis, T. J. (in press). Treatment options for patients with (central) auditory processing disorders. In M. Valente, H. Hosford-Dunn, & R. Roeser (Eds.), *Audiology: Treatment* (2nd ed.). New York: Thieme.

Bellis, T. J., & Ferre, J. M. (1999). Multidimensional approach to the differential diagnosis of central auditory processing disorders in children. *Journal of the American Academy of Audiology, 10*, 319-328.

Bellis, T. J., Nicol, T., & Kraus, N. (2000). Aging affects hemispheric asymmetry in the neural representation of speech sounds. *Journal of Neuroscience, 20*, 791-797.

Bellis, T. J., & Wilber, L.A. (2001). Effects of aging and gender on interhemispheric function. *Journal of Speech, Language, and Hearing Research, 44*, 246-263.

Beninger, R. J., & Miller, R. (1998). Dopamine D1-like receptors and reward-related incentive learning. *Neuroscience and Biobehavior Review, 22*(2), 335-345.

Blake, D. T., Strata, E., Churchland, A. K., & Merzenich, M. M. (2002). Neural correlates of instrumental learning in primary auditory cortex. *Proceedings of the National Academy of Sciences USA, 99*(15), 10114-10119.

Bolshakov, V. Y., & Siegelbaum, S. A. (1995). Regulation of hippocampal transmitter release during development and long-term potentiation. *Science, 269*, 1730-1733.

Booth, J. R., Burman, D. D., Meyer, J. R., Gitelman, D. R., Parrish, T. B., & Mesulam, M. M. (2002). Modality independence of word comprehension. *Human Brain Mapping, 16*, 251-261.

Bradlow, A.R., Kraus, N., & Hayes, E. (2003). Speaking clearly for children with learning disabilities: Sentence perception in noise. *Journal of Speech, Language, and Hearing Research, 46*, 80-97.

Brown, T. H., Chapman, P. F. E., Kairiss, W., & Keenan, C. L. (1988). Long-term synaptic potentiation. *Science, 242*, 724-728.

Cacace, A., & McFarland, D. (2005). The importance of modality specificity in diagnosing central auditory processing disorder (CAPD). *American Journal of Audiology, 14*(2), 112-123.

Calvert, G. A., Bullmore, E. T., Brammer, M. J., Campbell, R., Williams, S. C. R., McGuire, P. K., Woodruff, P. W. R., Iverson, S. D., & David, A. S. (1997). Activation of auditory cortex during silent lipreading. *Science, 276*, 593-596.

Chermak, G. D. (1993). Dynamics of collaborative consultation with families. *American Journal of Audiology, 2*(3), 38-43.

Chermak, G. D. (1996). Central testing. In S. E. Gerber (Ed.), *Handbook of pediatric audiology*, (pp. 206-253). Washington, DC: Gallaudet University Press.

Chermak, G. D., & Musiek, F. E. (1992). Managing central auditory processing disorders in children and youth. *American Journal of Audiology, 1*(3), 61-65.

Chermak, G. D. & Musiek, F. E. (1997). *Central auditory processing disorders: New perspectives.* San Diego, CA: Singular Publishing Group.

Chermak, G. D., & Musiek, F. E. (2002). Auditory training: Principles and approaches for remediating and managing auditory processing disorders. *Seminars in Hearing, 23*(4), 297-308.

Clifford, M. M. (1978). Have we underestimated the facilitative effects of failure? *Canadian Journal of Behavioral Science, 10*, 308-316.

Cooper, J. C., Jr., & Gates, G. A. (1991). Hearing in the elderly—The Framingham Cohort, 1983-1985: Part II. Prevalence of central auditory processing disorders. *Ear and Hearing, 12*, 304-311.

Coufal, K. L., Hixson, P. K., & Stick, S. L. (1990, November). *Collaborative consultation —an alternative treatment: Efficacy data and policy issues.* Paper presented at the annual Convention of the American Speech-Language-Hearing Association, Seattle, WA.

Cox, R. (2005). Evidence-based practice in provision of amplification. *Journal of the American Academy of Audiology, 16*, 419-438.

Crais, E. R. (1991). Moving from "parent involvement" to family-centered services.

American Journal of Speech-Language Pathology, 1(1), 5–8.

Cunningham, J., Nicol, T., Zecker, S. G., Bradlow, A., & Kraus, N. (2001). Neurobiologic responses to speech in noise in children with learning problems: Deficits and strategies for improvement. *Clinical Neurophysiology, 112,* 758–767.

Dancause, N., Barbay, S., Frost, S.B., Plautz, E. J., Chen, D., Zoubina, E. V., Stowe, A. M., & Nudo, R. J. (2005). Extensive cortical rewiring after brain injury. *Journal of Neuroscience, 25*(44), 10167–10179.

Danks, J. H., & End, L. J. (1987). Processing strategies for reading and listening. In R. Horowitz & S. J. Samuels (Eds.), *Comprehending oral and written language* (pp. 271–294). San Diego, CA: Academic Press.

Domitz, D., & Schow, R. (2000). A new CAPD battery—multiple auditory processing assessment (MAPA): Factor analysis and comparisons with the SCAN. *American Journal of Audiology, 9,* 101–111.

Edeline, J. M., & Weinberger, N. M. (1991). Thalamic short-term plasticity in the auditory system: Associative retuning of receptive fields in the ventral medial geniculate body. *Behavioral Neuroscience, 105,* 618–639.

Elbert, T., Pantev, C., Wienbruch, C., Rockstroh, B. & Taub, E. (1995). Increased cortical representation of the fingers of the left hand in string players. *Science, 270,* 305–306.

Fant, G. (1967). Auditory patterns of speech. In W. Wathen-Dunn (Ed.), *Models for the perception of speech and visual form* (pp. 111–125). Cambridge, MA: MIT Press.

Gaffan, D. (2005). Widespread cortical networks underlie memory and attention. *Science, 309,* 2172–2173.

Golding, M., Carter, N., Mitchell, P., & Hood, L. (2004). Prevalence of central auditory processing (CAP) abnormality in an older Australian population: The Blue Mountains hearing study. *Journal of the American Academy of Audiology, 15,* 633–642.

Gomez, R., & Condon, M. (1999). Central auditory processing ability in children with ADHD with and without learning disabilities. *Journal of Learning Disabilities, 32*(2), 150–158.

Grafman, J., & Litvan, I. (1999). Evidence for four forms of neuroplasticity. In J. Grafman & Y. Christen (Eds.) *Neuronal plasticity: Building a bridge from the laboratory to the clinic* (pp. 131–139). New York: Springer-Verlag.

Gustafsson, B., & Wigstrom, H. (1988). Physiologic mechanisms underlying long term potentiation. *Trends in Neuroscience, 11*(4), 156–162.

Hall, J. W., Grose, J. H., & Pillsbury, H.C. (1995). Long-term effects of chronic otitis media on binaural hearing in children. *Archives of Otolaryngology-Head and Neck Surgery, 121,* 847–852.

Hassamannova, J., Myslivecek, J., & Novakova, V. (1981). Effects of early auditory stimulation on cortical areas. In J. Syka & L. Aitkin (Eds.), *Neuronal mechanisms of hearing* (pp. 355–359). New York: Plenum Press.

Hayes, E. A., Warrier, C. M., Nichol, T. G., Zecker, S. G., & Kraus, N. (2003). Neural plasticity following auditory training in children with learning problems. *Clinical Neurophysiology, 114,* 673–684.

Hegde, M. N. (1993). *Treatment procedures in communicative disorders.* Austin, TX: Pro-Ed.

Hickson, L., & Worrall, L. (2003). Beyond hearing aid fitting: Improving communication for older adults. *International Journal of Audiology, 42*(Suppl 2), S84–S91.

Holroyd, C. B., Larsen, J. T., & Cohen, J. D. (2004). Context dependence of the event-related brain potential associated with reward and punishment. *Psychophysiology, 41*(2), 245–253.

Irvine, D. R. F., Rajan, R., & Robertson, D. (1992). Plasticity in auditory cortex of adult mammals with restricted cochlear lesions. In R. Naresh Singh (Ed.), *Nervous systems: Principles of design and function* (pp. 319–350). New Delhi: Wiley-Eastern Ltd.

Jerger, J., Moncrieff, D., Greenwald, R., Wambacq, I., & Seipel, A. (2000). Effect of age on interaural asymmetry of event-related potentials in a dichotic listening task. *Journal of the American Academy of Audiology, 11*, 383-389.

Jerger, J., Thibodeau, L., Martin, J., Mehta, J., Tillman, G., Greenwald, R., Britt, L., Scott, J., & Overson, G. (2002). Behavioral and electrophysiologic evidence of auditory processing disorder: A twin study. *Journal of the American Academy of Audiology, 13*, 438-460.

Jirsa, R. E. (1992). The clinical utility of the P3 AERP in children with auditory processing disorders. *Journal of Speech and Hearing Research, 35*, 903-912.

Kaas, J. H. (1995). Neurobiology. How cortex reorganizes. *Nature, 375*(6534), 735-736.

Kim, J., Morest, D. K., & Bohne, B. A. (1997). Degeneration of axons in the brain stem of the chinchilla after auditory overstimulation. *Hearing Research, 103*, 169-191.

Kintsch, W. (1977). On comprehending stories. In M. A. Just & P. A. Carpenter (Eds.), *Cognitive processes in comprehension* (pp. 33-62). Hillsdale, NJ: Lawrence Erlbaum.

Knudsen, E. I. (1988). Experience shapes sound localization and auditory unit properties during development in the barn owl. In G. Edelman, W. Gall, & W. Kowan (Eds.), *Auditory function: Neurobiological basis of hearing* (pp. 137-152). New York: John Wiley.

Kolb, B. (1995). *Brain plasticity and behavior*. Mahwah, NJ: Lawrence Erlbaum.

Kraus, N., & Disterhoff, J. F. (1982). Response plasticity of single neurons in rabbit auditory association cortex during tone-signalled learning. *Brain Research, 246*(2), 205-215.

Kraus, N., McGee, T., Carrell, T., King, C., Tremblay, K., & Nicol, T. (1995). Central auditory system plasticity associated with speech discrimination training. *Journal of Cognitive Neuroscience, 7*(1), 25-32.

Kraus, N., McGee, T., Carrell, T., Zecker, S., Nicol, T., & Koch, D. (1996). Auditory neurophysiologic responses and discrimination deficits in children with learning problems. *Science, 273*, 971-973.

Krueger, W. C. F. (1929). The effect of overlearning on retention. *Journal of Experimental Psychology, 12*, 71-78.

Luterman, D. M. (1990). Audiological counseling and the diagnostic process. *American Speech-Language-Hearing Association, 32*(4), 35-37.

Marler, J. A., Champlin, C. A., & Gillam, R. B. (2002). Auditory memory for backward masking signals in children with language impairment. *Psychophysiology, 39*(6), 767-780.

Martinkauppi, S., Rama, P., Aronen, H. J., Korvenoja, A., & Carolson, S. (2002). Working memory of auditory localization. *Cerebral Cortex, 10*, 889-898.

Massaro, D. W. (1975a). Language and information processing. In D. W. Massaro (Ed.), *Understanding language: An information-processing analysis of speech perception, reading, and psycholinguistics* (pp. 3-28). New York: Academic Press.

Massaro, D. W. (1975b). *Understanding language: An information-processing analysis of speech perception, reading, and psycholinguistics*. New York: Academic Press.

Masterton, R. B. (1992). Role of the central auditory system in hearing: The new direction. *Trends in Neuroscience, 15*, 280-285.

McCoy, S. L., Tun, P. A., Cox, L. C., Colangelo, M., Stewart, R. A., & Wingfield, A. (2005). Hearing loss and perceptual effort: Downstream effects on older adults' memory for speech. *Journal of Experimental Psychology, 58*(1), 22-33.

Merzenich, M. M., Grajski, K., Jenkins, W., Recanzone, G., & Peterson, B. (1991). Functional cortical plasticity: Cortical network origins of representations changes. *Cold Spring Harbor Symposium on Quantitative Biology, 55*, 873-887.

Merzenich, M., & Jenkins, W. (1995). Cortical plasticity, learning and learning dysfunction. In B. Julesz & I. Kovacs (Eds.) *Maturational Windows and Adult Cortical Plasticity: SFI Studies in the Sciences of*

Complexity, Vol. XXIII (pp. 247–272). Reading, PA: Addison-Wesley.

Merzenich, M., Jenkins, W. M., Johnston, P., Schreiner, C., Miller, S. L., & Tallal, P. (1996). Temporal processing deficits of language-learning impaired children ameliorated by training. *Science, 271*, 77–80.

Merzenich, M., Nelson, R. J., Stryker, M. P., Cynader, M. S., Schoppmann, A., & Zook, J. M. (1984). Somatosensory cortical map changes following digit amputation in adult monkeys. *Journal of Comparative Neurology, 224*(4), 591–605.

Merzenich, M., Schreiner, C., Jenkins, W., & Wang, X. (1993). Neural mechanisms underlying temporal integration, segmentation, and input sequence representations: Some implications for the origin of learning disabilities. *Annals of the New York Academy of Science, 682*, 1–22.

Moncrieff, D., Jerger, J., Wambacq, I., Greenwald, R., & Black, J. (2004). ERP evidence of a dichotic left-ear deficit in some dyslexic children. *Journal of the American Academy of Audiology, 15*, 518–534.

Moncrieff, D., & Musiek, F. (2002). Interaural asymmetries revealed by dichotic listening tests in normal and dyslexic children. *Journal of the American Academy of Audiology, 13*, 428–437.

Moore, D. R. (1993). Plasticity of binaural hearing and some possible mechanisms following late-onset deprivation. *Journal of the American Academy of Audiology, 4*(5), 227–283.

Morest, D. K., Kim, J., Potashner, S. J., & Bohne, B. A. (1998). Long-term degeneration in the cochlear nerve and cochlear nucleus of the adult chinchilla following acoustic overstimulation. *Microscopy Research and Technique, 41*, 205–216.

Musiek, F. E. (1999). Habilitation and management of auditory processing disorders: Overview of selected procedures. *Journal of the American Academy of Audiology, 10*, 329–342.

Musiek, F. E., Baran, J. A., & Pinheiro, M. L. (1994). *Neuroaudiology case studies*. San Diego, CA: Singular Publishing Group.

Musiek, F. E., Baran, J. A., & Shinn, J. (2004). Assessment and remediation of an auditory processing disorder associated with head trauma. *Journal of the American Academy of Audiology, 15*(2), 117–132.

Musiek, F. E., Bellis, T. J., & Chermak, G. D. (2005). Nonmodularity of the CANS: Implications for (central) auditory processing disorder. *American Journal of Audiology, 14*(2), 128–138.

Musiek, F. E., & Chermak, G. D. (1994). Three commonly asked questions about central auditory processing disorders: Assessment. *American Journal of Audiology, 3*(3), 23–27.

Musiek, F. E., & Chermak, G. D. (1995). Three commonly asked questions about central auditory processing disorders: Management. *American Journal of Audiology, 4*(1), 15–18.

Musiek, F. E., & Gollegly, K. (1988). Maturational considerations in the neuroauditory evaluation of children. In F. Bess (Ed.), *Hearing impairment in children* (pp. 231–252). Parkton, MD: York Press.

Musiek, F. E., Gollegly, K., Lamb, L., & Lamb, P. (1990). Selected issues in screening for central auditory processing of dysfunction. *Seminars in Hearing, 11*, 372–384.

Musiek, F. E., Lenz, S., & Gollegly, K. M. (1991). Neuroaudiologic correlates to anatomical changes of the brain. *American Journal of Audiology, 1*(1), 19–24.

Musiek, F. E., Pinheiro, M. L., & Wilson, D. (1980). Auditory pattern perception in split-brain patients. *Archives of Otolaryngology, 106*, 610–612.

Musiek, F. E., & Schochat, E. (1998). Auditory training and central auditory processing disorders. *Seminars in Hearing, 19*, 357–365.

Office of Technology Assessment. (1978). *Assessing the efficacy and safety of medical technologies*. OTA-H-75. Washington, DC: US Government Printing Office.

Pascual-Leone, A., Grafman, J., & Hallett, M. (1994). Modulation of cortical motor output maps during development of implicit and explicit knowledge. *Science, 263*, 1287–1292.

Phillips, D.P. (1995). Central auditory processing: A view from auditory neuroscience. *The American Journal of Otology, 16*(3), 338-352.

Phillips, D. P. (2002). Central auditory system and central auditory processing disorders: Some conceptual issues. *Seminars in Hearing, 23*(4), 251-261.

Pichney, M. A., Durlach, N. I., & Braida, L. D. (1985). Speaking clearly for the hard of hearing. I: Intelligibility differences between clear and conversational speech. *Journal of Speech and Hearing Research, 28*, 96-103.

Pichney, M. A., Durlach, N. I., & Braida, L. D. (1986). Speaking clearly for the hard of hearing. II: Acoustic characteristics of clear and conversational speech. *Journal of Speech and Hearing Research, 29*, 434-446.

Picheny, M. A., Durlach, N. I., & Braida, L. D. (1989). Speaking clearly for the hard of hearing: III. An attempt to determine the contribution of speaking rates to differences in intelligibility between clear and conversational speech. *Journal of Speech and Hearing Research, 32*, 600-603.

Pichora-Fuller, M. K. (2003). Cognitive aging and auditory information processing. *International Journal of Audiology, 42*(2), 26-32.

Pichora-Fuller, M., & Souza, P. (2003). Effects of aging on auditory processing of speech. *International Journal of Audiology, 42*(2), 2S11-2S16.

Pillsbury, H. C., Grose, J. H., Coleman, W. L., Conners, C. K., & Hall, J. W. (1995). Binaural function in children with attention-deficit hyperactivity disorder. *Archives of Otolaryngology-Head and Neck Surgery, 121*, 1345-1350.

Poremba, A., Saunders, R. C., Crane, A. M., Cook, M., Sokoloff, L., & Mishkin, M. (2003). Functional mapping of the primate auditory system. *Science, 299*, 568-571.

Purdy, S., Kelly, A., & Davies, M. (2002). Auditory brainstem response, middle latency response, and late cortical evoked potentials in children with learning disabilities. *Journal of the American Academy of Audiology, 13*, 367-382.

Recanzone, G. H., Schreiner, C. E., & Merzenich, M. M. (1993). Plasticity in the frequency representation of primary auditory cortex following discrimination training in adult owl monkeys. *Journal of Neuroscience, 13*, 87-103.

Riccio, C. A., Hynd, G. W., Cohen, M. J., Hall, J., Molt, L. (1994). Comorbidity of central auditory processing disorder and attention-deficit hyperactivity disorder. *Journal of the American Academy of Child and Adolescent Psychiatry, 33*(6), 849-857.

Ries, P. W. (1994). Prevalence and characteristics of persons with hearing trouble: United States. National Center for Health Statistics. *Vital Statistics, 24*, 188.

Robertson, D., & Irvine, D. R. F. (1989). Plasticity of frequency organization in auditory cortex of guinea pigs with partial unilateral deafness. *Journal of Comparative Neurology, 282*, 456-471.

Robey, R., & Schulz, M. (1998). A model for conducting clinical-outcome research: An adaptation of the standard protocol for use in aphasiology. *Aphasiology, 12*, 787-810.

Ronald, K., & Roskelly, H. (1985, March). *Listening as an act of composing.* Paper presented at the Annual Meeting of the Conference on College Composition and Communication, Minneapolis, MN.

Rumbaugh, D. M., & Washburn, D. A. (1996). Attention and memory in relation to learning: A comparative adaptation perspective. In G. R. Lyon & N. A. Krasnegor (Eds.), *Attention, memory, and executive function* (pp. 199-220). Baltimore: Paul H. Brookes.

Russo, N., Nicol, T., Zecker, S., Hayes, E., & Kraus, N. (2005). Auditory training improves neural timing in the human brainstem. *Behavioural Brain Research, 156*, 95-103.

Sackett, D., Straus, S., Richardson, W.S., Rosenberg, W., & Haynes, B. (2000). *Evidence-based medicine: How to practice and teach EBM*. Edinburgh: Churchill Livingstone.

Salvi, R. J., Lockwood, A. H., Frisina, R. D., Coad, M. L., Wack, D. S., & Frisina, D. R. (2002). PET imaging of the normal human auditory system: Responses to speech in quiet and in background noise. *Hearing Research, 170*, 96-106.

Sams, M., Aulanko, R., Hamalainen, M., Hari, R., Lounasmaa, O. V., Lu, S. T., & Simola, J. (1991). Seeing speech: Visual information from lip movements modifies activity in the human auditory cortex. *Neuroscience Letters, 127*, 141-145.

Samuels, S. J. (1987). Factors that influence listening and reading comprehension. In R. Horowitz & S. J. Samuels (Eds.), *Comprehending oral and written language* (pp. 295-325). San Diego: Academic Press.

Schow, R. L., & Chermak, G. D. (1999). Implications from factor analysis for central auditory processing disorders. *American Journal of Audiology, 8*, 137-142.

Schow, R. L., Seikel, J. A., Chermak, G. D., & Berent, M. (2000). Central auditory processes and test measures: ASHA 1996 revisited. *American Journal of Audiology, 9*, 63-68.

Schuman, E. M., & Madison, D. V. (1994). Locally distributed synaptic potentiation in the hippocampus. *Science, 263*, 532-536.

Schwaber, M. K., Garraghty, P. E., & Kaas, J. H. (1993). Neuroplasticity of the adult primate auditory cortex following cochlear hearing loss. *American Journal of Otology, 14*(3), 252-258.

Singer, W. (1995). Development and plasticity of cortical processing architectures. *Science, 270*, 758-764.

Spence, K. W., & Norris, E. B. (1950). Eyelid conditioning as a function of the intertrial interval. *Journal of Experimental Psychology, 40*, 716-720.

Stach, B. A., Spretnjak, M. L., & Jerger, J. (1990). The prevalence of central presbycusis in a clinical population. *Journal of the American Academy of Audiology, 1*(2), 109-115.

Starch, D. (1912). Periods of work in learning. *Journal of Educational Psychology, 3*, 209-213.

Stein, B. E., & Meredith, M. A. (1993). *The merging of the senses*. Cambridge, MA: MIT Press.

Streitfeld, B. (1980). The fiber connections of the temporal lobe with emphasis on Rhesus monkey. *International Journal of Neuroscience, 11*, 51-71.

Swanson, H. L., & Cooney, J. B. (1991). Learning disabilities and memory. In B. Y. L. Wong (Ed.), *Learning about learning disabilities* (pp. 104-127). San Diego: Academic Press.

Sweetow, R. W., & Henderson-Sabes, J. H. (in press). The need for and development of an adaptive listening and communication (LACE™) Program. *Journal of the American Academy of Audiology.*

Syka, J. (2002). Plastic changes in the central auditory system after hearing loss, restoration of function and during learning, *Physiology Review, 82*, 601-636

Tallal, P., Miller, S., Bedi, G., Byma, G., Wang, X., Nagarajan, S. S., Schreiner, C., Jenkins, W. M., & Merzenich, M. M. (1996). Language comprehension in language-learning impaired children improved with acoustically modified speech. *Science, 271*, 81-84.

Thiebaut de Schotten, M., Urbanski, M., Duffau, H., Volle, E., Levy, R., Dubois, B., & Bartolomeo, P. (2005). Direct evidence for a parietal frontal pathway subserving spatial awareness in humans. *Science, 309*, 2226-2228.

Tillery, K. L., Katz, J., & Keller, W. D. (2000). Effects of methylphenidate (Ritalin) on auditory performance in children with attention and auditory processing disorders. *Journal of Speech, Language, and Hearing Research, 43*, 893-901.

Tremblay, K., & Kraus, N. (2002). Auditory training induces asymmetrical changes in cortical neural activity. *Journal of Speech, Language, and Hearing Research, 45*, 564-572.

Tremblay, K., Kraus, N., Carrell, T., & McGee, T. (1997). Central auditory system plasticity:

Generalization to novel stimulation following listening training. *Journal of the Acoustical Society of America, 102,* 3762–3773.

Tremblay, K., Kraus, N., & McGee, T. (1998). The time course of auditory perceptual learning: Neurophysiological changes during speech-sound training. *NeuroReport, 9,* 3557–3560.

Tremblay, K., Kraus, N., McGee, T., Ponton, C., & Otis, B. (2001). Central auditory plasticity: Changes in the N1-P2 complex after speech-sound training. *Ear and Hearing, 22*(2), 79–90.

Tremblay, K., Piskosz, M., & Souza, P. (2003). Effects of age and age-related hearing loss on the neural representation of speech cues. *Clinical Neurophysiology, 114,* 1332–1343.

Ungerleider, L. G. (1995). Functional brain imaging studies of cortical mechanisms for memory. *Science, 270,* 769–775.

Warrier, C. M., Johnson, K. L., Hayes, E. A., Nicol, T., & Kraus, N. (2004). Learning impaired children exhibit timing deficits and training-related improvements in auditory cortical responses to speech in noise. *Experimental Brain Research, 157,* 431–441.

Weinberger, N., & Bakin, J. (1998) Learning induced physiological memory in the adult primary auditory cortex: Receptive field plasticity, model and mechanisms. *Audiology and Neuro-otology, 3,* 145–167.

Weinberger, N. M., & Diamond, D. M. (1987). Physiological plasticity in auditory cortex: Rapid induction by learning. *Progress in Neurobiology, 29,* 1–55.

Wible, B., Nicol, T., & Kraus, N. (2002). Abnormal neural encoding of repeated speech stimuli in noise in children with learning problems. *Clinical Neurophysiology, 113,* 485–494.

Wible, B., Nicol, T., & Kraus, N. (2005). Correlation between brainstem and cortical auditory processes in normal and language-impaired children. *Brain, 128,* 417–423.

Willott, J. F. (1996). Physiological plasticity in the auditory system and its possible relevance to hearing aid use, deprivation effects, and acclimatization. *Ear and Hearing, 17*(3, Suppl.), 66S–77S.

Willott, J. F. (1999). *Neurogerontology: Aging and the nervous system.* New York: Springer.

Willott, J. F., Aitken, L. M., & McFadden, S. L. (1993). Plasticity of auditory cortex associated with sensorineural hearing loss in adult mice. *Journal of Comparative Neurology, 329*(3), 402–411.

Woods, D. L., & Clayworth, C. C. (1986). Age-related changes in human middle latency auditory evoked potentials. *Electroencephalography and Clinical Neurophysiology, 65,* 297–303.

Wright, B. A., Lombardino, L. J., King, W. N., Puranik, C. S., Leonard, C. M., & Merzenich, M. M. (1997). Deficits in auditory temporal and spectral resolution in language-impaired children. *Nature, 387,* 176–178.

Wright, T. M., Pelphrey, K. A., Allison, T., McKeown, M. J., & McCarthy, G. (2003). Polysensory interactions along lateral temporal regions evoked by audiovisual speech. *Cerebral Cortex, 13,* 1034–1043.

Zatorre, R. J. (2001). Neural specialization for tonal processing. *Annals of the New York Academy of Sciences, 930,* 193–210.

CHAPTER 2

EVIDENCE-BASED PRACTICE AND TREATMENT EFFICACY

JANE T. PIMENTEL AND ELLA INGLEBRET

Clinical decision making for audiologists and speech-language pathologists has been oriented historically toward providing the best quality service possible to meet the individual needs of specific clients. To ensure optimal service delivery, clinicians have built their professional expertise through both formal and informal education, as well as through experience. Educational programs in communication disorders equip clinicians with strong foundational knowledge in their respective fields (i.e., audiology; speech-language pathology), with exposure to a variety of clients to begin building their experiential base, and with a beginning knowledge regarding experts in a given topic area such as (central) auditory processing disorder ([C]APD). Professionals traditionally take this foundation, pair it with continuing education

opportunities, and build their clinical expertise through informal observations of client's performance to influence future clinical decision making (Cox, 2005). Although very important, this approach alone no longer suffices. Rather, each clinician is responsible for determining the best course of action for a client based on this traditional approach in combination with the best available, systematically generated evidence along with client/family values (American Speech-Language-Hearing Association [ASHA], 2005c).

Today's work environment has placed additional demands on professionals in both educational and medical settings to provide empirical evidence that the approaches used in service delivery result in the intended outcomes. To address the demands for increased accountability set forth by legal mandates, such as the No

Child Left Behind Act (NCLB) and the Individuals with Disabilities Education Act (IDEA), as well as those of third-party payers, evidence-based practice (EBP) has become the cornerstone for decision making regarding client care. ASHA (2004c) especially highlights the need to apply principles of EBP to complex diagnostic categories like (C)APD where heterogeneous clinical profiles and frequent comorbidity (e.g., attention deficit hyperactivity disorder, language impairment, and learning disability) render differential diagnosis crucial to effective and efficient intervention.

This chapter provides the background and principles of EBP in relation to (C)APD. Examples illustrate how clinicians can utilize EBP in their clinical work. This chapter also elucidates the differences between treatment outcomes, treatment efficacy, treatment effectiveness, and treatment efficiency so the clinician can better determine the level of evidence available for a specific treatment approach. The reader is referred to other chapters in this series for comprehensive reviews of the evidence in specific topic areas regarding (C)APD. Finally, the importance of the clinician evaluating the treatment approach based on best evidence is emphasized.

Principles of Evidence-Based Practice

The most widely cited definition of evidence-based medicine (of which EBP has its origins) is that by Sackett, Richardson, and Rosenberg (1997): "Evidence based medicine is the conscientious, explicit and judicious use of current best evidence in making decisions about the care of individual patients" (p. 2). This definition implies a tripartite focus. First, the practitioner's clinical judgment comes into play with "conscientious, explicit and judicious" selection and use of particular practices. Second, "best evidence" suggests that practice is supported by high-quality, scientific research and, third, the "individual" patient's needs are considered. The American Speech-Language-Hearing Association (ASHA) has reframed these three components into a triad of clinical expertise, current best evidence, and client/family values. ASHA's position is that all three components converge for the best clinical decision making (ASHA, 2005c; Sackett, Straus, Richardson, Rosenberg, & Haynes, 2000). Each of these three components will now be further described.

Consideration of client/family values, perspectives, and needs forms one leg of the EBP triad. The ultimate goal of service delivery is "improving the lives of individuals with communication disorders in terms of sense-of-wellness and functional health through high-quality services which they consider important and valuable" (ASHA, 2004b, p. 7). This is best accomplished when the clinician carefully considers the disorder as it is framed by the background of the client and his or her family. The International Classification of Functioning, Disability, and Health (ICF) (World Health Organization, 2001), which has been integrated into ASHA's Scope of Practice for Audiology (2004a) and Speech-Language Pathology (2001), provides a useful framework to ensure that the client's situation is examined comprehensively and on multiple levels. Using the first component of the ICF, the clinician examines body functions and structures (e.g., central auditory processing in a formal testing situation) and gathers information regarding the client's activity and participation in daily life (e.g., responding to verbal directions given by a parent at home or teacher in the classroom). The second component of the ICF involves examination of contextual factors, including those of either an environmental or personal nature. Environmental variables might include acoustic characteristics of a classroom space or availability of technologic supports; whereas personal factors include cultural and linguistic background, age, gender, and lifestyle. Underlying the ICF framework is the intent to identify both barriers and facilitators that can be addressed to achieve specific targeted outcomes.

Although all aspects of the ICF model are equally important to consider, personal factors related to cultural and linguistic diversity are highlighted here. Due to rapid shifts in demographics (U.S. Bureau of the Census, 2000), audiologists and speech-language pathologists are faced with greater cultural and linguistic diversity (CLD) in their clientele than ever before. ASHA (2004d) advocates that professionals use approaches that respond to cultural diversity inclusive of "ethnicity, religious beliefs, sexual orientation, socioeconomic levels, regionalisms, age-based peer groups, educational background, and mental/physical disability" (p. 152), as well as to linguistic variations associated with English language learners or dialectal variations. Consideration of these personal factors is very important in the context of (C)APD, as it is possible to mistake characteristics associated with CLD for symptoms often associated with (C)APD. For example, an English language learner may misunderstand messages or respond inconsistently to verbal directions, particularly when background noise is present, as a normal part of second language acquisition. These charac-

teristics are also common to (C)APD (ASHA, 2005a). As an another example, individuals from some cultural backgrounds may pause for an extended period before responding to a communication partner's statement or question (Wallace, Inglebret, & Friedlander, 1997), another behavior often observed in individuals with (C)APD (ASHA, 2005a) Consequently, IDEA's mandate to identify disorders using multiple measures in multiple contexts becomes particularly important for accurate diagnosis of (C)APD for members of CLD populations.

Cultural and linguistic diversity carries additional implications for intervention. Inherent in the diverse values, beliefs, and norms associated with cultural background are variations in attitudes and preferences regarding particular treatment practices. Therefore, it is of paramount importance to actively involve each client and appropriate family members in determining which evidence-based practices will be included in the therapy plan. The client and family should continually have an active voice in evaluating the ongoing course of treatment to ensure that a "sense-of-wellness and functional health" (ASHA, 2004b, p. 7) for the individual with (C)APD is consistently facilitated. To this end, it may also be appropriate to access a cultural informant who can assist with identifying culturally relevant materials and techniques that can be meaningfully integrated into functional situations (ASHA, 2004d; Davis, Gentry, & Hubbard-Wiley, 2002). As an additional consideration, the clinician will need to determine the appropriate language(s) for intervention with English language learners.

Expertise of the clinical service provider forms the second leg of ASHA's evidence-based practice triad. Clinical expertise is dependent on the type of experience a clinician has with a certain clinical population such as individuals with (C)APD. Multiple variables factor into a clinician's experience, including years of experience, number of cases treated, and knowledge and skills from advanced training and self-study. For beginning clinicians, as well as those more experienced, it is imperative to have a theoretical model on which to base a treatment approach. For example, in the area of (C)APD, a clinician may be interested in using a cognitive approach to assist a child to develop problem-solving skills and monitor and self-regulate message comprehension (Keith, 1999). This approach may be supported by a "top-down" theory which builds on the assumption that a child's language abilities and general knowledge can assist a disordered auditory system. The approach based on this theory is considered metalinguistic or metacognitive in orientation (Chermak & Musiek, 1997). It is the responsibility of the clinician to understand the theory and determine if it supports a particular approach for treatment and make decisions accordingly. For example, the above treatment approach may be applicable to clients showing evidence of (C)APD regardless of the hypothesized etiology for the disorder, a breakdown at the perceptual level for speech (i.e., speech-specific hypothesis), or a more general auditory impairment (i.e., general auditory hypothesis; Friel-Patti, 1999).

Independent of the treatment approach chosen, the prudent clinician also collects data to generate evidence pertaining to specific interventions. Professional education programs provide clinicians with data collection skills that are a valuable resource in clinical practice. A typical starting point is to collect data prior to initiation of an intervention, which serves as a baseline measure of targeted behavior. Data pertaining to the target behavior then continue to be collected regularly throughout intervention, culminating in collection of postintervention data. Evidence-based practice takes the clinician beyond this minimal data collection to document increases in target behavior in a manner allowing the clinician to determine if the increase was due to the intervention itself or to other outside variables, such as maturation. One means to accomplish this is through collection of multiple baseline data (Bain & Dollaghan, 1991). Rather than collecting data that only pertain to the target behavior, the clinician also collects data for one or more behaviors in need of remediation but not targeted in intervention. These latter data then serve as control data. If similar increases are observed for both the target and control behaviors, then the evidence suggests that gains were not due specifically to the intervention. However, if the target data show more gains than the control data, the clinician can be more confident in saying that evidence exists indicating the increase was due to the intervention for that client.

The manner in which multiple baseline data are gathered can take on several forms; the above example represents one of a variety of single subject research designs that are available to the clinical service provider (Hayes, Barlow, & Nelson-Gray, 1999; Richards, Taylor, Ramasamy, & Richards, 1999). Practitioners may interject elements of systematic control into data collection by examining behaviors under intervention across settings, time periods, and individual subjects. Treatment may also be periodically withdrawn so that comparisons can be made between behaviors during intervention and nonintervention periods. It should be noted that all these approaches involve collection and analysis of descriptive data for only one client. As the calculation of parametric statistics is inappropriate, the results do not allow for generalization of the findings to other clients. Thus, it will be necessary for the clinician to apply the principles of single subject design to each client served.

Representing a particular strength, single-subject research designs provide a powerful tool for practitioners interested in examining functional outcomes associated with the ICF model (World Health Organization, 2001). For example, data can be gathered to examine outcomes of intervention involving socially important behaviors at home or in the community (e.g., participation in daily life activities). Data to document meaningful treatment outcomes may also include measures of generalization to activities critical to the client's success, such as academic performance in the classroom (Horner et al., 2005). By adopting multiple baseline data collection or other single-subject designs, clinicians compile their own evidence, enriching their experience, and hence, this leg of the evidence-based triad. This method of systematic data collection provides a means of documenting treatment outcomes for a particular client but does not determine if a treatment is efficacious.

When Is Treatment Efficacious?

A lack of agreed-on terminology in and across professions regarding efficacious treatment has resulted in some confusion and possible misinterpretation of evidence supporting treatments. Wertz and Katz (2004) wisely advise some "rules to live by" in regard to more precise definitions and uniform methods to conduct research and to evaluate the scientific literature. The terms most confusing are these: treatment outcome, treatment efficacy, treatment effectiveness, and treatment efficiency. First and foremost, these terms are not interchangeable as they are not synonyms. Second, the definitions provided by Robey and Schultz (1998), largely based on those proposed by the Office of Technology Assessment (OTA; 1978) provide consistency and mutual exclusivity of terms. In general, an *outcome* refers to any measurable change between two points in time; this can be positive or negative. For example, to measure an environmental modification outcome one might select a sample of school-aged children diagnosed with (C)APD, document their classroom performance before treatment (i.e., pretreatment) with an outcome measure (e.g., listening behavior rating scale), apply the treatment (i.e., modifications), and re-evaluate performance post-treatment with the same outcome measure. If listening behavior improved in the classroom for the group, then a positive outcome has occurred. This outcome, however, does not document efficacy, effectiveness, or efficiency. This outcome indicates only that treatment is "active"; that is, something happened when the treatment was applied that resulted in the children's performance improving on the measurement. Based on the design of this sample study, improvement cannot be attributed exclusively to the treatment because there are no controls. If a similar study were conducted with methodologic rigor and ideal conditions and the same positive outcomes were documented then that would support the treatment as *efficacious.*

Demonstration of treatment *efficacy* requires that multiple conditions be met.

The treatment protocol being tested must be clearly specified to allow for replication. Likewise, the population being examined must be clearly defined and the study subjects must represent that population; this allows for generalization of the findings to the population. Lastly, the conditions under which the study occurs are optimal (OTA, 1978). These ideal conditions include "ideal treatment candidates, ideally trained therapists, ideal dosage (intensity and duration of treatment), and ideal outcome measures" (Wertz & Katz, 2004, p. 231). As the treatment literature is reviewed in the area of (C)APD, it quickly becomes apparent that very few studies meet these ideal criteria. Thus, treatment efficacy studies conducted with this rigor are necessary to inform the profession regarding whether a treatment can work. It is important to stress that, given the ideal conditions required, efficacy studies do not indicate if a treatment does work under routine conditions (Robey & Schultz, 1998).

Treatment *effectiveness* indicates that treatment works under typical conditions (e.g., typical caseload, typical duration and intensity) (Wertz & Katz, 2004). Studies of treatment effectiveness must occur after efficacy has been demonstrated for a given treatment. If a study demonstrates positive outcomes following a treatment applied in typical conditions but that same treatment is not yet established as efficacious, then the study can only say the treatment is active and cannot say the treatment is effective. Of course, this scientific literature is still valuable and serves to provide preliminary data for future studies.

Treatment *efficiency* is another term that is used when referring to treatment outcomes. Basically, the study of treatment efficiency constructs research ques-

tions around the cost/benefit of a particular treatment. Wertz and Irwin (2001) define efficiency as, "acting or producing effectively with a minimum of waste, expense, or unnecessary effort, essentially, exhibiting a high ratio of output to input" (p. 236). Efficiency studies regarding a particular treatment occur after efficacy and effectiveness have been established. Commonly, issues of treatment "dosage" (intensity and/or duration) will be investigated to determine how much treatment is required to achieve the desired outcome.

Treatment, then, is efficacious when high-quality studies, with adequate control, have documented positive outcomes. It should be clear that the terms efficacy, effectiveness, and efficiency should not be used casually when referring to the treatment literature in (C)APD. Understanding the appropriate use of the outcome terminology allows improved interpretation of the literature and professional communication.

Selection and Interpretation of the Literature

Perhaps the most thought about leg of ASHA's EBP triad is the use of scientific literature available regarding the assessment and intervention for a particular clinical population. Searching for the most pertinent literature and interpreting its relevance for a given case can present a daunting task to a clinician, especially one with a large caseload. Developing an appropriate clinical question and having a method for determining the quality of the literature will make this task more efficient and clinically applicable.

Figure 2–1 illustrates the steps involved in such a search. Each of these steps is discussed in the following sections.

Guiding the Scientific Literature Quest

In order to seek the evidence specifically related to a given client and intervention, it is first necessary to frame a specific question to guide the search. According to ASHA (2005d), PICO is one accepted approach to developing a question. PICO stands for "population, intervention, comparison, and outcome." A relevant example follows: the population is children with (C)APD; the intervention of interest is auditory training/acoustic signal

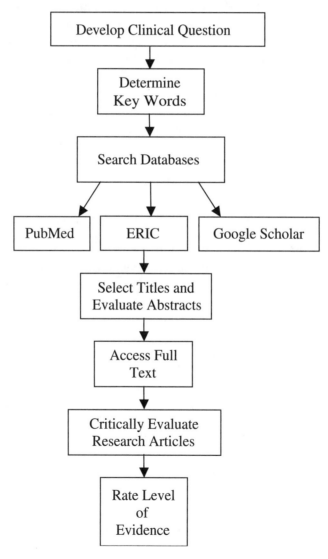

Figure 2–1. A flowchart depicting the steps involved with finding and evaluating literature for evidence-based practice.

enhancement; the comparison approach is auditory integration training; and the intended outcome would be improved auditory processing skills as measured through behavioral and electrophysiologic tests. Therefore, the clinical question may read: "Does auditory training result in better auditory processing skills as compared to auditory integration training for children with (C)APD?"

It is recognized that the question developed largely depends on the level of functioning targeted with a client and that, indeed, often a combination of treatment approaches may be utilized and multiple levels of functioning may be targeted and outcomes measured concurrently. This would simply result in guiding separate literature searches with different clinical questions. In the example above, the clinical question guides the clinician in finding the literature regarding outcomes when the auditory impairment itself is targeted. Certainly it would also be appropriate to search literature regarding interventions targeting the functional activities of the child (e.g., use of FM systems to increase academic performance in the classroom) and the environment itself (e.g., acoustic considerations in the classroom). These considerations are consistent with the International Classification of Functioning, Disability, and Health framework (ICF; WHO, 2001).

Searching for the Evidence

Clinicians are being pressed to critically evaluate the scientific literature to determine both the quality of the experimental design (Robey & Schultz, 1998) and the cumulative level of evidence (Cox, 2005; Reilly, Douglas, & Oates, 2004)

available to support their assessment and treatment decisions. The first challenge for the clinician in all service delivery settings is to access this literature in an efficient and meaningful manner to determine best practices. Understandably, clinicians may be concerned regarding additional burdens placed on an already stressed caseload. Barriers to clinicians include limited time to search for the evidence, limited search skills, and limited access to the experimental evidence (Choi, 2005; Reilly, Douglas, & Oates, 2004; Worrall & Bennett, 2001; Zipoli & Kennedy, 2005). Despite these challenges, the astute clinician knows that by equipping oneself with knowledge regarding the most valid and reliable assessment tools and the interventions most likely to work will ultimately aid all involved through better intervention efforts.

Finding the Relevant Literature

A number of search engines and databases are available to search from any Internet connection. Google Scholar, for example, (http://scholar.google.com/) provides easy access to multiple types of scholarly publications; however, critical content may be omitted and searches reveal inconsistent results (Jacso, 2005). Internet search engines such as Google and Yahoo! access about one billion documents. Although that sounds like a huge amount, consider that the part of the "Web" that Internet search engines do not access has nearly 550 billion documents —this is termed the "Invisible Web" (Devine & Effer-Sider, 2004; Pimentel & Munson, 2004). Two of the reasons Internet search engines cannot get to the Invisible Web is (a) login authorization is required or (b) the information is in databases.

Two public domain databases most pertinent to speech-language pathology and audiology are PubMed and ERIC. PubMed is provided free of charge from the National Library of Medicine. It provides access to bibliographic information in the fields of medicine, nursing, dentistry, veterinary medicine, the health care system, and the preclinical sciences. Bibliographic citations and author abstracts are drawn from more than 4,800 peer-reviewed biomedical journals published in the United States and abroad. PubMed (http://www.nlm.nih.gov) contains links for a few free full-text journal articles. ERIC (http://www.eric.ed.gov) is provided free from The Education Resources Information Center, which is sponsored by the U.S. Department of Education. This database includes journal and nonjournal education literature of more than 1.1 million citations going back to 1966. For example, a search on ERIC revealed an "ERIC Digest" which provides an overview of a relevant educational topic, in this case on Auditory Processing Disorders dated 2002. Both PubMed and ERIC databases are relevant to the area of (C)APD as pertinent literature is housed both in medically oriented research and educational research.

Professional organizations, which require login authorization, also provide a quick means to search available literature in their sponsored journals. The American Speech-Language-Hearing Association's (http://www.asha.org/default.htm) entire Web site is searchable for documents that can guide the clinician in utilizing best practices. For example, two relevant and recent documents are the position statement (ASHA, 2005b) and accompanying technical report on (C)APD (ASHA, 2005a). The position statement clearly defines (C)APD, the primary role of the audiologist as the diagnostician, and the interdisciplinary nature of intervention utilizing the skills of the speech-language pathologist. The technical report provides a valuable resource for the clinician regarding appropriate terminology to use in a search for evidence. It also provides a theoretical framework for the disorder and guides the clinician in selecting assessment and intervention approaches. Reports such as these serve to inform and update the clinician regarding best practices. From these types of documents, then, the clinician can better develop a clinical question.

Similarly, the American Academy of Audiology (AAA) provides members with search capability on their Internet site. Documents and positions of the association can be accessed. In addition, the PubMed database can be easily accessed from the AAA site to search for relevant articles indexed from the *Journal of the American Academy of Audiology (JAAA)*.

Another benefit of belonging to professional organizations is the ability to easily access the full text of the most prestigious journals in the field. ASHA provides on-line access dating back to 1990 for the *Journal of Speech-Language-Hearing Research (JSLHR), American Journal of Audiology (AJA), American Journal of Speech-Language Pathology (AJSLP)*, and *Language, Speech, and Hearing Services in the Schools (LSHSS)*. Given the interdisciplinary nature of (C)APD, searching all of these journals for pertinent literature is appropriate. Specific to audiologists, the American Academy of Audiology (AAA) offers a similar benefit, again back to 1990, to access the full text of its journal *(JAAA)*.

Developing and adding to a list of key words to use in database searching facilitates an efficient search. The clinical question and the clinician's expertise about (C)APD direct key word selection. Key words in the area of (C)APD may include: central auditory processing, central auditory nervous system, aural rehabilitation, auditory processing, auditory evoked potentials, auditory perceptual disorders, auditory training, acoustic signal enhancement, and metacognitive, cognitive, and language strategies. As literature searches become routine to support best practices, key word lists should be kept, expanded, and drawn upon for future searches. It is also important to note what key words did not aid a search for a particular database (Garrard, 1999). In addition, noting the database search dates (e.g., 1999–2005) will allow for a more narrow, repeated search in the future as more scientific literature becomes available.

Regardless of the database searched and the key words used, it is important to employ search strategies to aid efficiency. These strategies include the appropriate use of Boolean operators and knowing the database terminology. Boolean operators allow the searcher to combine words or phrases in specific ways by the appropriate use of the words AND, OR, and NOT. "AND" should be used to narrow your search as AND requires that all words be present in the retrieved articles (e.g., metacognitive AND metalinguistic). Alternatively, OR is used to broaden a search because it allows any of the words to be present in the article; this is especially helpful in the case of synonyms (e.g., central auditory processing disorder OR auditory processing disorder). The use of the term NOT allows the searcher to exclude terms; that is, NOT requires that the chosen word is not present in any of the retrieved articles (e.g., NOT auditory integration). It is suggested that NOT be used cautiously as it can eliminate relevant articles from the search.

Phrase searching and truncation are two other useful strategies to enlist. Phrase searching keeps words together as a phrase via the use of quotation marks around the phrase (e.g., "best practices"). If a phrase is used without quotations most databases will assume the Boolean "and" between words; thus, an article may be retrieved that has all the words in your phrase but not necessarily together. Truncation allows a search for words beginning with specific characters. Many databases use an asterisk (*) to truncate. For example, practic* retrieves practice, practices, practicing, and so forth (Pimentel & Munson, 2004). Truncating can be helpful to speed up your search; however, it is not advisable to truncate short words as too many possibilities exist and your search will become unwieldy. For example, hear* retrieves hear, hearing, heart, hearse, heard, and so forth.

As mentioned previously, each database has its specific terminology. The terms for PubMed may well differ from the terms used to search ERIC. The appropriate key words for a given database can be determined via a key word search. Also, try searching a thesaurus or the MeSH headings index (PubMed) for better words or phrases or use a different combination of words. Lastly, correct spelling does matter as databases do not spell check; thus, you could end up with no results due to a misspelled word! Quite a bit of literature is available on (C)APD regarding description and assessment; however, the same is not true of the intervention literature. Because of this, during a search key terms and phrases often need to be expanded beyond the original clinical question to find the relevant literature. One helpful means of expanding the search is to move beyond the target population. For example, children with attention deficit hyperactivity disorder (ADHD) may also exhibit (C)APD (Chermak, Hall, & Musiek, 1999; Jerger & Musiek, 2000); therefore, expanding the search to include ADHD results in more literature to review.

As the search is underway, the databases will provide article abstracts to review. Abstracts provide windows to peek at the article and determine if it is relevant to your clinical question. Searching the Internet, the databases, and the professional organizations, results in a number of abstracts regarding possibly relevant literature. It is important to take the time to read the abstracts prior to accessing the full text, as titles can be misleading. For example, a search of PubMed revealed an article entitled "The clinical management of perceptual skills disorders in a primary care practice" (Rosner & Rosner, 1986). When examining the abstract it was clear that this article pertained to visual and not auditory perception.

Once the selection of relevant articles has been made they need to be accessed. Some relevant papers and journal articles are available in full text via the Internet search. As mentioned previously, this is the case with ASHA and AAA journals accessed from the organizations' Web sites. PubMed and ERIC occasionally provide free access to full text for their references. Otherwise, clinicians can (a) request articles through their employer, as many hospitals and school districts maintain library services, (b) utilize area community colleges and universities, as many institutes of higher education are open to the public for on-site use, and (c) pur-

chase full-text articles through on-line resources such as http://www.ingenta connect.com/.

As previously discussed, the EBP triad includes not only the scientific literature but also clinician expertise and client/ family values. In searching for the evidence, it is wise to consult professional writings by experts in the field typically in the form of textbooks and clinical tutorials in periodicals such as *Seminars in Hearing* (2002). This body of professional literature is extremely helpful in building the clinician's expertise, in pointing out relevant research literature, and in providing references. However, a caution is in order in that non-peer-reviewed texts should not be used as the sole basis for clinical decision making (ASHA, 2004c) and clinical tutorials, although helpful in learning how to do the job of providing services better (Cox, 2005), do not evaluate a treatment approach for efficacy or effectiveness.

Evaluating the Evidence

Not all literature is created equal in that the quality of the assessment tools (e.g., reliability and validity) and quality of the research design are variable. Therefore, once the clinician has accessed the relevant literature, judgments must be made regarding the value of the literature (ASHA, 2005c). Professional literature, in most cases, is trustworthy based on the peer-review process and code of ethics that guides our professions. Nonetheless, even quality literature will deserve various rankings of worthiness dependent on a number of factors.

ASHA (2004c) presents five explicit criteria to use when evaluating the quality of the available evidence in making a clinical decision. These criteria include: (1) independent confirmation and converging evidence, (2) experimental control, (3) avoidance of subjectivity and bias, (4) effect size and confidence intervals, and (5) relevance and feasibility.

Independent Confirmation and Converging Evidence

A specific assessment and/or intervention approach requires multiple studies done by different researchers to establish the strength of a specific approach. As a search is completed, it is the cumulative evidence regarding the clinical question that bears weight. The best example of this is the case where a meta-analysis or a systematic review is available on a given topic for a population (e.g., (C)APD treatment studies in school-aged children). This level of information is emerging in the (C)APD literature. For example, Sweetow and Palmer recently completed a systematic review of the evidence supporting auditory training in adults (2005). When such a review is not available, the individual studies found regarding a clinical question require examination to determine if there is an independent and converging body of evidence coming together regarding a specific treatment. One example of this in the (C)APD literature is the positive outcomes being reported in the use of auditory training in adults and children as measured by psychophysical performance and neurophysiologic responses to acoustic stimuli (e.g., Kraus et al., 1995; Musiek, Baran, & Pinheiro, 1990; Russo, Nicol, Zecker, Hayes, & Kraus, 2005; Tallal et al., 1996, Tremblay & Kraus, 2002). Clearly, there is an initial convergence of evidence in this area from more than one research lab; this begins to demonstrate independent confirmation.

Experimental Control

The quality of the research design is largely dictated by the control demonstrated in the experiment. Experimental control refers to the ability to attribute the effects of an intervention to the intervention itself and not to other factors. The best method to obtain control is via random assignment of subjects to treatment and no treatment groups. Obviously, not all, or even many, treatment studies in the fields of audiology and speech-language pathology are randomized controlled trials (RCT). Nonetheless, when RCTs are available and of high quality they denote a high level of evidence.

A variety of research designs are utilized in order to answer different types of research questions. Robey and Schultz (1998) describe a five-phase model of clinical outcome research applicable to aphasiology; Robey (2004) later extends this model to multiple treatment domains. Case studies, single-subject designs, and small sample size studies are appropriate for Phase I and Phase II in this five-phase model. Phase I studies are largely exploratory in nature where researchers are seeking to determine if a treatment is active; that is, if there is any therapeutic effect and, if there is, the magnitude of the effect (Robey, 2004). Phase I studies can also provide clinical insights leading to valuable hypotheses for research to move into Phase II and beyond (Cox, 2005). Phase II studies build on the previous findings by further establishing treatment protocols as well as reliability and validity of measurements, by finalizing operational definitions, confirming the therapeutic effect and the amount of therapy required (optimal intensity and duration). When these research parameters are well defined and the treatment protocols are well established then Phase III research is conducted. Phase III research is the randomized clinical trial. Only at Phase III are the terms "trial" and "efficacy" used appropriately (Robey, 2004).

A clinical trial is characterized by large sample sizes and, through the control of variables, answers treatment efficacy questions. Robey and Schultz (1998) refer to treatment efficacy as defined by the Office of Technology Assessment (OTA, 1978) as "the probability of benefit to individuals in a defined population from a medical technology applied for a given medical problem under ideal conditions of use" (p. 16). The ideal condition implies control and is not meant to be mistaken for what clinicians can accomplish in their everyday, real-world settings. Nonetheless, it can be argued that if efficacy cannot be demonstrated for a treatment in ideal conditions (e.g., well-established and followed treatment protocols, reliable and valid measures, adequate treatment time, high-quality treatment materials) then this same treatment cannot be expected to work in less than ideal conditions. Although not randomized, Russo and colleagues (2005) conducted a clinical trial to investigate the effects of computer-based auditory perceptual training on the auditory brainstem responses of children with a language-based learning problem. They found that treatment resulted in improved brainstem responses to complex sounds; furthermore, they documented improvement in perceptual, academic, and cognitive measures.

Phase IV and V studies seek to expand the therapeutic effect found in ideal conditions to day-to-day clinical practice (Robey, 2004). Phase IV studies have the goal to document treatment effectiveness. Treatment effectiveness is defined by the Office of Technology Assessment (1978) as "the probability of benefit to individuals in a defined population from a medical technology applied for a given medical problem under average conditions of use" (p. 16). As indicated earlier, when using this model, efficacy must first be established prior to conducting effectiveness research. Lastly, Phase V studies seek to validate the treatments via cost/benefit analyses and expand the questions asked to those affecting regulations and policy. The methodologic rigor appropriate for these different phases will, to a large extent, dictate the level of evidence supported by a given study.

Avoidance of Subjectivity and Bias

As the literature is reviewed for the quality of evidence, experimenter subjectivity and possible bias should be considered. Ideally, subjectivity is avoided by conducting "blind" studies in that all involved with the study including the subjects themselves are unaware of information that could bias the results (ASHA, 2004c). Understandably, it is difficult if not impossible to conduct behavioral studies with complete blinding, but steps can be taken to minimize the tendency toward bias and studies should be evaluated regarding their rigor in controlling this variable. As clinicians read research articles, they should note who measured the treatment effects, as it should be someone without knowledge of treatment assignments. In group studies, all participants initially enrolled in the study should be included in the analyses; this also indicates stronger research quality.

Effect Sizes and Confidence Intervals

The practitioner is ultimately concerned with the clinical significance of research results. Bain and Dollaghan (1991) have operationalized the concept of clinical significance to include three aspects of observed change: (a) it results from clinical services and not from extraneous variables, (b) it is real, reliable, and not random, and (c) it is important and not trivial. As was pointed out previously, researchers use experimental control to reduce the effects of extraneous variables, so the focus of this section will be on the second two components of clinical significance: determining whether research findings represent real phenomena, versus random occurrences, and measuring the importance of the results to clinical practice.

To measure whether or not observed change is real, scientific research papers have traditionally reported results of data analysis in relation to their statistical significance (Goldstein, 2005). Measures of statistical significance allow the researcher to determine whether or not the original null hypothesis can be rejected and, thus, rule out the possibility that the results were due to chance. Statistical procedures used will vary depending on whether or not basic criteria regarding the target population(s) are met. When it can be assumed that a normal distribution exists, interval or ratio data are involved, and the sample size is large, parametric statistics can be calculated. When these assumptions cannot be met, nonparametric statistics are often calculated (Schiavetti & Metz, 2002). Meline (2005) points out that the relevance of statistical analysis to actual clinical practice can be limited, as statistical significance is largely influenced by sample size. Statistically significant differences between groups may also be found when the observed behavior for both groups falls within a normal range. For example, Gunnarson and Finitzo (1991) observed a significant difference for auditory brainstem response latency when comparing responses of groups of children with and without histories of early otitis media. In spite of this difference, latencies for the children exhibiting early otitis media still fell within a normal latency range, making this difference clinically insignificant. Limitations in applicability of statistical significance to clinical practice, such as these, have led the fields of audiology and speech-language pathology, as well as other health and education-related fields, to look for other means to systematically identify patterns in data pertaining to service delivery outcomes (Meline & Wang, 2004). As a result, measures of practical significance are now more commonly reported in research articles.

Practical significance reflects the importance or meaningfulness of research findings to clinical outcomes (Meline & Paradiso, 2003; Meline & Schmitt, 1997). Effect sizes are the calculated measures used to determine the extent of practical significance for particular results. An effect size represents the magnitude of difference or correlation between data sets independent of the sample size (Cohen, 1988). Various metrics are used to calculate effect sizes depending on the research design used (Meline & Wang, 2004). Practitioners should expect effect sizes to be reported in research articles and should also look for interpretation of the effect sizes (Goldstein, 2005). For example, general guidelines do exist for interpreting effect size (ES) for one type of metric, Cohen's d (i.e., ES greater than or equal to 0.67 is meaningful, ES equal to 0.50 may be meaningful, ES less than or equal to 0.30 is not meaningful) is based on Lipsey and Wilson's (1993) results of 302 meta-analyses in psychological, educational, and behavioral treatments. However, Cohen cautions that degree of magnitude of effect sizes will be discipline-specific. Because the fields of audiology and speech-language pathology have only recently begun including calculation of effect sizes as a part of research reporting, discipline-specific interpretation standards have not yet been developed (Goldstein, 2005).

Practitioners should also expect to find the confidence intervals for the effect sizes reported in research articles (ASHA, 2004c). Confidence intervals represent a range of values in both positive and negative directions within which the true effect size is likely to occur (Guyatt & Rennie, 2002; Sackett et al., 2000). Focusing on a range of possible values allows the researcher to address possible measurement error (Meline & Schmitt, 1997). A commonly used confidence interval is 95%. This means that in 95 out of 100 instances the true effect size will fall within the specified range of values. Examination of confidence intervals aids the practitioner in determining the strength of the difference between outcomes for treatment types or for treatment versus control groups. For example, when the confidence interval surrounding the calculated effect size is small, it is considered a more precise representation of the true effect size so that a stronger argument can be made for applicability of the clinical practice to a broader population.

At the same time it should be considered that calculation of effect sizes and confidence intervals is dependent on agreement as to what constitutes normal versus pathologic behavior. The field of (C)APD is still establishing electrophysiologic and other behavioral patterns (e.g., performance on speech recognition or gap detection tasks) that are associated with pathology. Without these data, judgments about practical significance of findings as reflected in effect size and confidence intervals may be misleading. For instance, Musiek et al. (1989) found that what might be considered a negative result, unilateral high percentage scores on the Dichotic Rhyme Test, were actually abnormal. Individuals with normal central auditory nervous systems typically score at 50%. Until normative data are settled upon by the field, care should be taken in the interpretation of research results.

Relevance and Feasibility

The literature under review also requires evaluation in regard to the applicability and meaningfulness of the findings to EBP (Kazdin, 1999). Returning to the concepts mentioned above, Kazdin differentiated between statistical significance and, what he termed, clinical significance defined as "the practical or applied value or importance of the effect of the intervention—that is, whether the intervention makes any real (e.g., genuine, palpable, practical, noticeable) difference in everyday life to the clients or to others with whom the client interacts" (p. 332). Noting the relevance of a study's findings to the particular clinical situation is important. The closer the subjects studied are to the characteristics of the clients being served the more relevant the evidence. In addition to relevance, the practical implications of applying the research findings to clinical practice need to be addressed.

Feasibility refers to the practicality of applying what is learned from the evidence to the service delivery setting. This applicability is considered to be high when the activity being investigated (i.e., screening, diagnostic, or treatment) can be implemented by clinicians in the real-world setting (ASHA, 2004c). Hence, phase IV research that addresses treatment effectiveness would most naturally generalize to the clinician's work environment. Meline (2005) also points out the practical challenges of making changes to a clinical practice. These challenges include issues of expense, public policy, ethical codes, and legal implications. Lastly, as highlighted earlier, Meline indicates that any change in service delivery practice must be acceptable to the clients and family. Nonetheless, it is imperative that clinicians strive to incorporate change when the evidence indicates better outcomes. This includes educating clients and family regarding the benefits of utilizing best practices.

What About "Expert" Opinion?

Conducting a search will often yield expert reports and links to other resources, such as monographs, rather than high-quality peer-reviewed documents. These resources are helpful given the paucity of research evidence to support many of our treatment practices. When utilizing these resources, the clinician must determine how expert the "expert" is in order to pass judgment on the worthiness (i.e., validity) of the information. The individual clinician's acquired foundational knowledge is relevant here as both students and clinicians can utilize information from respected authorities from texts, from exposure via continuing education, and from relying on respected colleagues in their fields for insight. An example of an "expert opinion" of high quality is the report from 14 senior scientists and clinicians regarding the appropriate diagnosis of auditory pro-

cessing disorders in school-aged children (Jerger & Musiek, 2000). In this case, the "expert" opinion came from a reputable source, the *Journal of the American Academy of Audiology*, which assists in the evaluation of quality. In addition, as the literature in (C)APD becomes familiar so, too, will the names of the respected authorities writing in the area.

Levels of Evidence

There are a multitude of hierarchies available to assign levels of evidence. The evidence table presented by ASHA (2004c) as modified from the Scottish Intercollegiate Guidelines Network is presented here (see Table 2–1). The hierarchy expressed in Table 2–1 has four levels with subcomponents to level I. Evaluating the literature for evidence follows from understanding the quality of the research design and the judgment made based on clinician expertise. Meta-analyses deserve the highest ranking (Ia) followed by randomized controlled (Ib) trials (RCT). Currently, most of the literature in (C)APD will be rated at level II and below. In order to warrant a ranking at levels Ia to II the study must be determined to be well-designed; thus, as individual studies are evaluated in regard to the phase of research (Robey, 2004), the weaknesses and strengths of each study should also be noted.

A number of resources are available to aid the clinician in evaluating the literature, especially in regard to research articles. For example, Law et al. (1998) developed protocols to aid in the critical review of both quantitative and qualitative research articles. The protocols present a series of questions addressing the study's purpose, rationale, design, subjects, outcome measures, intervention, results, and

Table 2–1. Level of Evidence Hierarchy

Level	Sources of Evidence
Ia	meta-analysis including more than one randomized clinical trial
Ib	randomized controlled study
II	non-randomized controlled (quasi-experimental) study
III	non-experimental study (e.g., case studies with controls, observational studies with controls, retrospective studies, cohort studies with controls)
IV	expert reports (committees, consensus conference); clinical experience of respected authorities; case, observational, and cohort studies without controls

conclusion to guide the clinician in the evaluation. These protocols, and accompanying guidelines, are available on-line at http://www.fhs.mcmaster.ca/rehab/ebp/. Minimally, treatment research should be evaluated by answering the following for each article reviewed: (1) how well were the subjects described? (2) how well was the treatment described? (3) what measures of control were imposed in the study? and (4) were the consequences of the intervention well described? (Chambless & Hollon, 1998).

Finally, the literature reviewed for the specific clinical question is cumulatively summed to receive a "grade" of worthiness dependent on the number of studies supporting the various levels of evidence. Cox (2005) presents a system to grade studies resulting in a recommendation for a treatment approach ranging from "A" (Level I and Level II studies with consistent conclusions) to "D" (this would be Level IV evidence only, or inconclusive studies, or low-quality studies at any level).

The clinician then returns to the client/family to present the evidence regarding treatment options to ensure the best practice for a particular client. In this way, clients with (C)APD and their families are active participants in selecting from best practices in choosing the optimal course of action (ASHA, 2004b). Returning to the triad, the client and family values as well as clinician expertise are considered along with the evidence available to make the best treatment decision.

The clinician finally applies the evidence to his or her assessment and/or treatment plan based on the above factors. Importantly, it is the clinician's duty to evaluate the outcomes achieved in clinical work in light of the evidence found. This is considered the evaluation phase or follow-up component of evidence-based practice (Cox, 2005). In evaluating the evidence-based practice approach, especially in the area of intervention, the clinician can apply a number of methodologies from single-subject design to addressing social validation by gaining input from the clients themselves or significant others regarding the results of the treatment efforts (Schlosser & Raghavendra, 2004). Degree of success of the assessment/treatment plan is then reviewed and interpreted to either (1) stay the course and apply the findings to future cases or (2) make modifications to the assessment or treatment plan to achieve greater success. Either way, the clinician learns about the clinical applicability of the evidence and builds a knowledge base for future application.

Summary

This chapter has presented information to take the clinician from a traditional approach regarding assessment and intervention to the more current approach of incorporating the available literature and client/family values along with clinical expertise in practicing evidence-based clinical decision making. The clinician can build expertise through critical evaluation of the literature followed up by changes in his or her practice based on the evidence. This follow through includes documenting change through data collection methods to determine if the evidence supporting a given assessment and/or intervention is realized in the service delivery setting. In this way, the clinician makes sound judgments regarding the value of the evidence for an individual client.

Evidence-based practice requires a profession to become more deliberate and systematic in provision of the best assessment and treatment practices both in research and in clinical work. No doubt, applying the methodology of evidence-based practice will take some effort, but it will be effort well expended on behalf of all clients with (C)APD as clinicians become better informed, better equipped, and better at serving their clientele.

References

American Speech-Language-Hearing Association. (2001). *Scope of practice in speech-language pathology*. Rockville, MD: Author.

American Speech-Language-Hearing Association. (2004a). *Scope of practice in audiology*. Rockville, MD: Author.

American Speech-Language-Hearing Association. (2004b). *Report of the Joint Coordinating Committee on Evidence-Based Practice*. Rockville, MD: Author.

American Speech-Language-Hearing Association. (2004c). *Evidence-based practice in communication disorders: An introduction* [Technical report]. Available at: http://www.ash.org/members/deskref-journals/deskref/default.

American Speech-Language-Hearing Association. (2004d). Knowledge and skills needed by speech-language pathologists and audiologists to provide culturally and linguistically appropriate services. *ASHA Supplement, 24*, 152–158.

American Speech-Language-Hearing Association. (2005a). *(Central) auditory processing disorders*. Available at http://www.asha.org/members/deskref-journals/deskref/default.

American Speech-Language-Hearing Association. (2005b). *(Central) auditory processing disorders—The role of the audiologist* [Position statement]. Available at http://www.asha.org/members/deskref-journals/deskref/default.

American Speech-Language-Hearing Association. (2005c). *Evidence-based practice in communication disorders* [Position statement]. Available at http://www.asha.org/members/deskref-journals/deskref/default.

American Speech-Language-Hearing Association. (2005d, October 28). *Introduction to evidence-based practice*. Retrieved December 21, 2005 from the World Wide Web: http://www.asha.org/members/ebp/.

Bain, B. A., & Dollaghan, C. A. (1991). The notion of clinically significant change. *Language, Speech, and Hearing Services in Schools, 22*, 264-270.

Berard, G. (1993). *Hearing equals behavior.* New Canaan, CT: Keats Publishing.

Chambless, D. L., & Hollon, S. D. (1998). Defining empirically supported therapies. *Journal of Consulting and Clinical Psychology, 66*, 7-18.

Chermak, G. D., Hall, J. W., & Musiek, F. E. (1999). Differential diagnosis and management of central auditory processing disorder and attention deficit hyperactivity disorder. *Journal of the American Academy of Audiology, 10*, 289-303.

Chermak, G. D., & Musiek, F. E. (1997). *Central auditory processing disorders: New perspectives.* San Diego, CA: Singular.

Choi, D. M. (2005). *Evidence-based practice in speech-language pathology: Dysphagia treatment approaches.* Unpublished master's research project, Washington State University, Spokane, WA.

Cohen, J. (1988). *Statistical power analysis for the behavioral sciences* (2nd ed.). Hillsdale, NJ: Erlbaum.

Cox, R. M. (2005). Evidence-based practice in provision of amplification. *Journal of the American Academy of Audiology, 16*, 419-438.

Davis, P. N., Gentry, B., & Hubbard-Wiley, P. (2002). Clinical practice issues. In D. E. Battle (Ed.), *Communication disorders in multicultural populations* (pp. 461-486). Boston: Butterworth-Heinemann.

Devine, J., & Egger-Sider (2004). Beyond Google: The invisible web in the academic library. *The Journal of Academic Librarianship, 30*(4), 265-269.

Friel-Patti, S. (1999). Clinical decision-making in the assessment and intervention of central auditory processing disorders. *Language, Speech, and Hearing Services in Schools, 30*, 345-352.

Garrard, J. (1999). *Health sciences literature made easy: The matrix method.* Gaithersburg, MD: Aspen Publishing.

Goldstein, B. A. (2005). From the editor. *Language, Speech, and Hearing Services in Schools, 36*(2), 91.

Gunnarson, A. D., & Finitzo, T. (1991). Conductive hearing loss during infancy: Effects on later auditory brain stem electrophysiology. *Journal of Speech and Hearing Research, 34*(5), 1207-1215.

Guyatt, G., & Rennie, D. (2002). *Users' guide to the medical literature: Essentials of evidence-based practice.* Chicago: American Medical Association.

Hayes, S. C., Barlow, D. H., & Nelson-Gray, R. O. (1999). *The scientist practitioner: Research and accountability in the age of managed care.* Boston: Allyn & Bacon.

Horner, R. H., Carr, E. G., Halle, J., McGee, G., Odom, S., & Wolery, M. (2005). The use of single-subject research to identify evidence-based practice in special education. *Exceptional Children, 71*(2), 165-179.

Jacso, P. (2005). Google scholar: The pros and the cons. *Online Information Review, 29*(2), 208-214.

Jerger, J., & Musiek, F. (2000). Report of the consensus conference on the diagnosis of auditory processing disorders in school-aged children. *Journal of the American Academy of Audiology, 11*, 467-474.

Kazdin, A. E. (1999). The meanings and measurement of clinical significance. *Journal of Consulting and Clinical Psychology, 67*, 332-339.

Keith, R. W. (1999). Clinical issues in central auditory processing disorders. *Language, Speech, and Hearing Services in Schools, 30*, 339-344.

Kraus, N., McGee, T., Carrell, T., King, C., Tremblay, K., & Nicol, T. (1995). Central auditory system plasticity associated with speech discrimination training. *Journal of Cognitive Neuroscience, 7*(1), 25-32.

Law, M., Stewart, D., Pollock, N., Letts, L., Bosch, J., & Westmorland, M. (1998). *Critical review form—Quantitative studies.* Retrieved December 29, 2005 from http://www.fhs.mcmaster.ca/rehab/ebp.

Lipsey, M. W., & Wilson, D. B. (1993). The efficacy of psychological, educational, and behavioral treatment: Confirmation from meta-analysis. *American Psychologist, 48,* 1181–1209.

Meline, T. (2005, November). Statistics for evidence-based practice (EBP): *Statistics and their relevance for evidence-based speech-language pathology.* Seminar presented at the Annual Convention of the American Speech-Language-Hearing Association, San Diego, CA.

Meline, T., & Paradiso, T. (2003). Evidence-based practice in schools: Evaluating research and reducing barriers. *Language, Speech, and Hearing Services in the Schools, 34,* 273–283.

Meline, T., & Schmitt, J. F. (1997). Case studies for evaluating significance in group designs. *American Journal of Speech-Language Pathology, 6,* 33–41.

Meline, T., & Wang, B. (2004). Effect-size reporting practices in AJSLP and other AHSA journals, 1999–2003. *American Journal of Speech-Language Pathology, 13*(3), 202–207.

Musiek, F. E., Baran, J. A., & Pinheiro, M. L. (1990). Duration pattern recognition in normal subjects and in patients with cerebral and cochlear lesions. *Audiology, 29,* 304–313.

Musiek, F. E., Kurdziel-Schwan, S., Kibbe, K. S., Gollegly, K. M., Baran, J. A., & Rintelmann, W. F. (1989). The dichotic rhyme task: Results in split-brain patients. *Ear and Hearing, 10*(1), 33–39.

Office of Technology Assessment. (1978, September). *Assessing the efficacy and safety of medical technologies.* OTA-H-75. Washington, DC: Government Printing Office.

Pimentel, J., & Munson, D. (2004, October). *Searching for evidence: Supporting best practices.* Paper presented at the Annual Washington State Speech and Hearing Convention. Spokane, WA

Reilly, S., Douglas, J., & Oates, J. (2004). *Evidence Based Practice in Speech Pathology.* London: Whurr Publishers.

Richards, S. B., Taylor, R. L., Ramasamy, R., & Richards, R. Y. (1999). *Single subject research: Applications in educational and clinical settings.* San Diego, CA: Singular Publishing Group, Inc.

Robey, R. (2004). A five-phase model for clinical outcome research. *Journal of Communication Disorders, 37,* 401–411.

Robey, R., & Schultz, M. (1998). A model for conducting clinical/outcome research: An adaptation of the standard protocol for use in aphasiology. *Aphasiology, 12,* 787–810.

Rosner, J., & Rosner, J. (1986). The clinical management of perceptual skills disorders in a primary care practice. *Journal of the American Optometry Association, 57*(1), 56–59.

Russo, N. M., Nicol, T. G., Zecker, S. G., Hayes, E. A., & Kraus, N. (2005). Auditory training improves neural timing in the human brainstem. *Behavioral Brain Research, 156*(1), 95–103.

Sackett, D. L., Richardson, W. S., & Rosenberg, W. M. C. (1997). *Evidence based medicine.* London: Churchill Livingstone.

Sackett, D. L., Straus, S. E., Richardson, W. S., Rosenberg, W., & Haynes, R. B. (2000). *Evidence-based medicine: How to practice and teach EBM* (2nd ed.). Edinburgh: Churchill Livingston.

Schiavetti, N., & Metz, D. E. (2002). *Evaluating research in communicative disorders* (4th ed.). Boston: Allyn and Bacon.

Schlosser, R. W., & Raghavendra, P. (2004). Evidence-based practice in augmentative and alternative communication. *Augmentative and Alternative Communication, 20*(1), 1–21.

Seminars in Hearing. (2002). Management of auditory processing disorders. *Seminars in Hearing, 23.* New York: Thieme.

Sweetow, R., & Palmer, C.V. (2005). Efficacy of individual auditory training in adults: A systematic review of the evidence. *Journal of the American Academy of Audiology, 16,* 494–504.

Tallal, P., Miller, S. L., Bedi, G., Byma, G., Wang, X., Nagarajan, S. S., Schreiner, C., Jenkins, W., & Mezenich, N. M. (1996). Language comprehension in language-learning impaired children improved with acousti-cally modified speech. *Science, 271,* 81–84.

Tomatis, A. A. (1991). *The conscious ear.* New York: Station Hill Press.

Tremblay, K., & Kraus, N. (2002). Auditory training induces asymmetrical changes in cortical neural activity. *Journal of Speech, Language, and Hearing Research, 45,* 564–572.

U.S. Bureau of the Census. (2000). *Statistical abstract of the United States* (120th ed.). Washington DC: Author.

Wallace, G., Inglebret, E., & Friedlander, R. (1997). American Indians: Culture, com-munication, and clinical considerations. In G. L. Wallace (Ed.), *Multicultural neuro-genics: A resource for speech-language*

pathologists (pp. 193–225). Tucson, AZ: Communication Skill Builders.

Wertz, R. T., & Irwin, W. H. (2001). Darley and the efficacy of language rehabilitation in aphasia. *Aphasiology, 15,* 231–247.

Wertz, R. T., & Katz, R. C. (2004). Outcomes of computer-provided treatment for aphasia. *Aphasiology, 18,* 229–244.

World Health Organization. (2001). *ICF: Inter-national classification of functioning, disability, and health.* Geneva: Author.

Worrall, L. E., & Bennett, S. (2001). Evidence-based practice: Barriers and facilitators for speech language pathologists. *Journal of Medical Speech-Language Pathology, 9*(2), xi–xvi.

Zipoli, R. P., & Kennedy, M. (2005). Evidence-based practice among speech-language pa-thologists: Attitudes, utilization, and barriers. *American Journal of Speech-Language Pathology, 14,* 208–220.

CHAPTER 3

ACOUSTIC FOUNDATIONS OF SIGNAL ENHANCEMENT AND ROOM ACOUSTICS

JACEK SMURZYNSKI

Sound Wave Phenomena

Air molecules while being in constant random motion create static air pressure that is proportional to the density of the molecules. Under particular conditions, changes in existing air pressure may be perceived as sounds. Those pressure variations may be local or spread out, minuscule or massive, slow or fast. The task of the auditory system is to detect and to process them in such a way that a meaningful message may be sent to the brain.

Sound originates from the vibration of an object. When the object moves outward away from its resting position, the molecules next to it are jammed into the adjacent molecules and create an area of increased density (condensation), that is, an area of pressure higher than the static

one. Through multiple collisions, extra energy given to the molecules is transferred to other molecules and the region of condensation moves away from the vibrating object. When the object moves back toward its original position, an area of a partial vacuum (rarefaction) is created before molecules fill the space vacated by the vibrating object. Now the density of air molecules has decreased locally. Thus, the movement of an object to and fro around its resting position creates a disturbance or a local variation of air pressure and that disturbance initiates a wave that may travel through a medium, for example, air. The object represents a source that delivers energy to the medium and a wave carries this energy away from the source. It is important to recognize the fact that even though the air through which the wave

51

travels may experience some local oscillations as the wave passes, the air particles do not travel with the wave. A sound wave in air is an example of a longitudinal wave: the displacement of the medium (air particles) occurs along an axis that is aligned with the direction of sound propagation.

The disturbance that initiates the wave may have a variety of shapes, from a short pulse to a long-lasting oscillation. An impulsive wave may be generated by a single short stimulation of a vibrating object. Common examples of impulsive sounds are those produced from plucked or struck musical instruments (e.g., the guitar, the piano, and most percussion instruments). It is important to point out that a wave that travels on a guitar string when it is plucked is a transverse wave; the particles of the string move perpendicular to the direction in which the wave travels (along the string). However, the energy of a vibrating string creates a longitudinal wave propagated in the air and traveling away from the instrument. An impulsive wave may be also created by an abrupt change of air pressure (e.g., by clapping hands or resulting from an explosion). Oscillatory waves have a pattern that is repeated over and over. A sine wave, the simplest type of sound, is created when displacement of a vibrating object to and fro around its resting position over time can be described mathematically by a sine function. A vibrating tuning fork produces a sine wave, also called a simple tone or a "pure tone." Musical instruments generate oscillatory waves that are complex but can be represented by a sum of sine waves by doing Fourier analysis.

Three parameters must be specified to describe an oscillatory wave: amplitude, wavelength, and the period (or the frequency which is the reciprocal of the period). The amplitude of the wave represents the greatest amount by which the instantaneous pressure is changing above and below the existing static air pressure. The distance between each successive condensation (or rarefaction) is the wavelength of sound, symbolized by the Greek letter λ. The time interval that separates the arrival of the two condensations at any fixed location is called the period of the wave (often written as T). The wave's period (in seconds) or its frequency and the wavelength (in meters) are related as follows:

$$\lambda = cT \text{ or } \lambda = c/f \qquad \text{(Eq. 3.1)}$$

where c is the velocity of sound (in meters per second) and f is the frequency (in Hz) or the number of times per second the waveform repeats itself. The speed of sound in dry air at 20 degrees Celsius is approximately 343 meters per second; however, it varies as a function of the temperature, density, and humidity of air (Cramer, 1993).

The simplest three-dimensional source of sound waves may be described by a uniformly pulsating sphere whose radius alternately expands and contracts according to a sine function. If the size of such a sphere is much smaller than the wavelength of sound it emits (λ), it can be represented by a "monopole" or a "point source." This source radiates sound equally well in all directions under a free-field condition. The point source model is a good approximation for the sound field created by a boxed loudspeaker at low frequencies. The concept of a free field assumes that the space has no boundaries and the medium (air) is homogeneous and motionless; thus, there are no reflections. Under free-field conditions, the sound intensity is described by the inverse square law, which states that the intensity varies inversely with the square of the distance from the source. Therefore, sound intensity I (in W/m^2) measured at distance r (in m) from the source producing the power P (in W) is described as:

$$I = P/(4\pi r^2). \qquad \text{(Eq. 3.2)}$$

Thus, if distance is doubled, sound intensity decreases by a factor of four. When expressed in decibels, level decreases by 6 dB for each doubling of the distance from the source to the point of measurement.

During the process of wave generation, some of the energy delivered by a source is dissipated in the form of heat and therefore some degree of damping must be anticipated. With resistance added to the system, the amplitude of oscillation will not have a constant value but rather will decay over time. The amount of resistance is associated with how rapidly damping occurs. The greater the amount of resistance in the system, the more the oscillation is damped. As resistance is increased, a condition known as critical damping will be reached when the system no longer oscillates but simply relaxes to the equilibrium position. Thus, damping provides a force that acts to stop objects vibrating. The effect of damping may be used beneficially to control acoustical properties of a room, as discussed later in this chapter.

Sound Reflection, Absorption, Diffusion, and Transmission

Major departures from the inverse square law occur in most listening conditions (including in the classroom) whenever there is an obstacle in the sound path. These obstacles may alter the sound wave in a number of ways, including reflection, absorption, diffusion, and transmission. These alterations occur any time there is a change in the physical properties of the medium through which a wave travels (e.g., when a wave propagating in air strikes a brick wall). Then, part of the acoustic energy carried by the wave is reflected from the barrier, part absorbed by it, and part transmitted through into the space beyond it. Also, a sound/surface interaction may create a scatter of the wave in many directions (i.e., diffusion).

The characteristic impedance, Z, represents the opposition of a medium to the passage of sound waves; a medium with high impedance obstructs the movement of acoustic energy more than a medium with low impedance. Impedance is proportional to both the density of the medium (ρ; mass per unit volume) and the speed of sound propagation (c) or $Z = \rho c$. How much energy is reflected or transmitted depends on the impedance of the medium in which the wave is initially traveling, Z_1, (e.g., air), the impedance of the material in which the wave travels when it crosses the boundary, Z_2, and on the size of the boundary in relation to the wavelength of the sound. Reflection is quantified by the reflection coefficient, R (i.e., the ratio of pressure amplitude in reflected and incident wave) and it depends on the acoustic impedances of the two media, Z_1 and Z_2. If the wave is normally incident to the boundary between the two media, the pressure reflection coefficient is expressed by:

$$R = (Z_2 - Z_1) / (Z_2 + Z_1). \qquad \text{(Eq. 3.3)}$$

The ratio of intensities in reflected and incident waves is called intensity reflection coefficient, R_{int}. It shows what fraction of the energy reaching the boundary is reflected from it:

$$R_{int} = |R|^2 \qquad \text{(Eq. 3.4)}$$
$$= |(Z_2 - Z_1) / (Z_2 + Z_1)|^2$$

Absorption coefficient, α, is defined as

$$\alpha = 1 - R_{int} \qquad \text{(Eq. 3.5)}$$

and it represents energy of the incident wave minus that of the reflected sound. For example, if $\alpha = 0.9$, 90% of acoustic energy is transported into the second medium and 10% is reflected from the boundary. It needs to be kept in mind that some energy absorbed by a barrier may be transmitted into the space beyond it, that is, sound may penetrate the barrier. This is an important aspect of room acoustics because a part of acoustic energy created by a source in a room will be transmitted outside through walls or ceiling, between spaces within a building, through ventilation systems and other structures of a building.

Acoustic isolation is a measure of the decrease in sound level (attenuation) when sound passes from one room to another. It depends on the sound reduction through building elements, on their size, on sound leakage around their periphery, and on the frequency of the sound.

Transmission loss (TL) describes the amount of sound pressure level reduction that a partition imparts to the transmitted acoustic wave. Typically, TL decreases with a decrease of frequency and it increases with an increase in the mass of a partition. Attenuation properties of partitions are described quantitatively by a single number rating called sound transmission class (STC). The STC value is determined in an acoustical testing laboratory by measuring the transmission loss of partitions in 1/3-octave bands (e.g., The American National Standards Institute [ANSI], 2002). A higher STC rating provides more sound attenuation through a partition. Similarly, noise isolation class (NIC) is a single-number rating of the noise isolation between two enclosed spaces that are connected acoustically by one or more paths. The procedure used for calculating NIC is the same as that used for calculating STC except that noise reduction between the two spaces in 1/3-octave bands is used instead of transmission loss.

Reflection and diffraction provide the possibility of hearing sound around barriers. Diffraction involves a change in direction of a wave as it passes through a small opening or around a barrier in its path. The effects of diffraction are more pronounced for low rather than for high frequencies; in other words, the effects increase with decreasing the frequency (see Equation 3.1). When the wavelength of a wave is smaller than the obstacle no noticeable diffraction occurs; small objects present no barrier to sound waves that have a wavelength longer than the object's size. Larger objects create shadows for sound with wavelengths shorter than the object's size; longer wavelengths bend (diffract) in behind the object. This principle is also important for binaural hearing if the interaural level difference is considered as one of several cues available for sound source localization. Low-frequency sounds have a wavelength which is long compared with the size of the head. Therefore, the sound bends around the head and, due to diffraction, no shadow is cast by the head. At high frequencies, the wavelength is short compared with the size of the head, little diffraction occurs, and a shadow is cast by the head creating an interaural level difference which is a useful cue for pure tones with frequencies above 2 kHz.

Another aspect of diffraction is exhibited when waves spread out past small openings. A small (relative to the wavelength) gap between acoustic spaces causes the sound waves to be reradiated; the small opening is a source of a sound wave itself. Larger gaps between barriers are no obstacle to the waves; lower frequencies bend around the edges of the gap and higher frequencies are shadowed.

Standing Waves

When two waves pass though a medium simultaneously, the resulting acoustic pressure is the sum of the acoustic pressure of each individual wave at that particular location and at that moment. An interesting wave interference pattern, called a standing wave, is produced by two sine waves of equal amplitude and frequency traveling in opposite directions. Standing waves are characterized by the absence of propagation and by alternating nodal and antinodal regions, where the pressure is zero and maximum, respectively.

When a wave is incident on a boundary, an acoustic field is created with wave interference resulting from an interaction between the incident and reflected waves. In the case of total reflection, that is, for $R = R_{int} = 1$, the amplitude of reflected pressure is the same as that of the incident pressure. A standing wave may be created if a sound is perfectly reflected back and forth between two parallel surfaces located at a distance L from each other. In such a simple one-

dimensional room model, resonance frequencies at which standing waves occur (f_n) are given by:

$$f_n = nc/2L \qquad (Eq.\ 3.6)$$

where n is an integer ($n = 1, 2, 3, \ldots$) and c is the speed of sound in the room. In other words, a standing wave exists when a frequency is such that the distance L is equal to an integer multiple of one half of a wavelength λ, or:

$$L = n\lambda/2 \qquad (Eq.\ 3.7)$$

For example, if the room has a length of $L = 10$ m, then the longest wavelength of the standing wave (for $n = 1$) is 20 m. Therefore, assuming that $c = 343$ m/s, the lowest resonance frequency is approximately 17 Hz (c/λ; 343/20). Consecutive resonance frequencies are 34, 51, 68 Hz, and so forth.

The pressure is always at a maximum at the wall when the room is driven at any of its resonance frequencies. When the sound source is located at an antinode for a given resonance frequency, the maximum pressure is twice the source amplitude because the incident and reflected waves are in phase at the wall. With the source located at a node, the room response drops to zero; the amplitude of the pressure wave as a function of position in the room will be zero regardless of the pressure amplitude at a source.

A standing wave pattern will only occur when the room is driven at a resonance frequency. At any other frequency, the wave radiated from the source reflects from the walls, but it does not combine to create a standing wave. Thus, there are no antinodes and nodes, and the pressure may reach zero at a wall.

Typically, an incident wave is not completely but rather partially reflected, that is, $R < 1$. Standing waves may be still formed by an interaction of incident and partially reflected waves; however, the maximum pressure will be smaller than twice the source amplitude and will be greater than zero at a node.

In a three-dimensional enclosed space, a complicated pattern of three-dimensional standing waves, or room modes, exists. There are three basic types of room modes. Axial modes take place between two opposing parallel surfaces as described above for a one-dimensional model. Axial modes are a function of the linear dimensions of a room. Tangential modes occur between four surfaces and oblique modes between all six surfaces of the room. Therefore, tangential and oblique modes are a function of two or all three of the dimensions of the room, respectively.

Modes are described by mode numbers $n1$, $n2$, $n3$ which are integers (0, 1, 2, etc.). For a rectangular room of dimensions L (length), W (width), and H (height), the frequencies of the room modes are given by the equation:

(Eq. 3.8)
$$f_{n1n2n3} = c/2 \, [(n1/L)^2 + (n2/W)^2 + (n3/H)^2]^{1/2}$$

If two mode numbers are zero, then Equation 3.8 represents axial modes (e.g., $f_{1,0,0}$). When one of three mode numbers is zero, the equation provides values of frequencies of tangential modes. If all three numbers are different from zero, oblique modes may be described. The combination of these three mode types forms a set of possible standing wave frequencies in a room.

A distribution of room modes is important because it directly affects the frequency response of a room when stimulated by a sound source, especially at low frequencies, because of the relatively low modal density in small rooms. It is desirable to space room modes as evenly as possible to avoid the situation of multiple modal frequencies falling within a small bandwidth or bandwidths with absence of modes. If a room is a perfect cube, there will be a large resonance at a low frequency corresponding to the lowest axial mode which is the same for all three dimensions ($f_{1,0,0}$, $f_{0,1,0}$, and $f_{0,0,1}$). Therefore, it is better to design a room where all three dimensions are different. Equation 3.8 also shows that if any of the dimensions are integer multiples of each other, then some of the frequencies of the room modes will be the same. Therefore, it is better to choose noncommensurate (i.e., not harmonically related) ratios for the room dimensions to obtain the modes that are spread out as much as possible.

Many methods and optimum room ratios have been suggested over the last 60 years to minimize the absence or boosting of certain frequencies in the room response. Often the most favorable dimensions are given in terms of the ratios to the smallest room dimension. Bolt (1946) provided a chart to determine good room ratios under the assumption that evenly spaced modal frequencies would create fewer problems with peaks and dips in the modal response. He suggested the ratio of 1:1.26:1.59, but also noted that there was a broad area over which the average modal spacing criterion would be acceptable. Louden (1971) used the standard deviation of the inter-mode spacing and recommended a room ratio of 1:1.4:1.9.

In general, the number of resonances within a given frequency bandwidth increases with frequency. The top panel of Figure 3-1 displays frequencies of modes up to 275 Hz for a rectangular room with a height of 3.5 m and the ratio of dimensions of 1:1.26:1.59, as suggested by Bolt. Modal frequencies are relatively equally spaced with no coincident modes as indicated by the same mode strength for all components depicted. However, some of the frequencies are very close to each other (e.g., a tangential mode and an axial mode around 63 Hz).

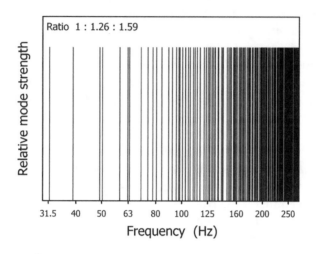

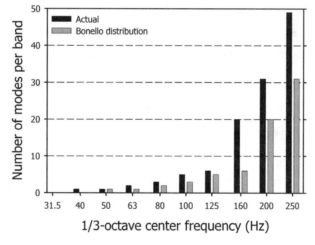

Figure 3-1. *Top:* Distribution of room modes for a rectangular room with a height of 3.5 m and the ratio of dimensions as indicated. Relative mode strength is shown in arbitrary units. There are no coincident modes as indicated by the same mode strength of all components. *Bottom:* Distribution of modes in 1/3-octave bands for the room with modal frequencies depicted in the top (*black bars*) and for Bonello's criteria (*gray bars*). See text for more information.

Bonello (1981) developed criteria for assessing the modal behavior in a room based on perceptual terms. The number of modes is counted in 1/3-octave bands, which represent an approximation of critical bands. If the number of modes per band increases monotonically, then it is assumed that the room will be perceived as having a smooth frequency response. In addition, modes with coincidental frequencies are not expected to create perceptually noticeable response peaks in a band when there are at least three additional noncoincident resonances to balance the two that are coincident. The bottom panel of Figure 3–1 represents the distribution of modes per 1/3-octave bands for the room with modal frequencies depicted in the top panel. It is assumed that if the bar calculated according to Bonello's criteria (gray) in any 1/3-octave exceeds the actual bar (black) in the same 1/3-octave, the room is "nonideal." If this is the case, an alternate ratio of room dimensions should be considered, or if altering the room dimensions may not be feasible, adaptation of the room acoustics should be planned. The frequency range below approximately 200 Hz is acoustically the most challenging because of the spatially and frequency-wise distribution of room modes. Computer programs are available that provide the calculations of the resonant modes of a given room and suggestions for optimum sound source (e.g., a loudspeaker) and listener placements.

Reverberation

Below approximately 200 Hz the acoustics of different locations in the room are dominated by a particular distribution of discrete room resonances. For frequencies above 200 Hz, these modes become tightly packed in frequency (see Figure 3–1), the room behaves more uniformly, and is better described by its reverberation properties. When a sound source, such as a loudspeaker or a talker, is located inside a room, the waves from the source travel in diverging directions. Part of a sound that arrives directly to the listener's ears is called direct sound. The rest strikes surrounding boundaries. At each encounter with the boundaries of the room, the waves are partly absorbed (representing the loss of energy) and partly reflected. Reflected waves, after a single or multiple reflections, reach the listener's ears with a delay of some milliseconds after the direct sound. Thus, the direct sound is followed by the reverberant sound arriving at the ears with a variety of delays and intensities. In a room with a sound source emitting a constant acoustic power, the reverberant sound builds up to a constant level. The equilibrium level occurs when the total loss of energy related to sound absorption by the boundaries of the room equals the rate at which the energy is being injected into the enclosure by the source. To predict reverberation characteristics of a room with given acoustic properties, one needs to know the total sound absorption, which depends on the areas and absorptive properties of the materials covering room boundaries.

The room absorption (also known as absorptivity or room constant), A, is described by the sum of absorption coefficients, α, weighted by their areal contribution to the room:

$$A = \alpha_1 S_1 + \alpha_2 S_2 + \alpha_3 S_3 + \ldots \quad \text{(Eq. 3.9)}$$

where α_n is an absorption coefficient of a material covering a boundary surface segment with the area of S_n. Note that A

has a unit of square meters. It is called metric sabin (named after W. C. Sabine) and it is equivalent to one square meter having an absorption coefficient α, of 1, as would be the case for an open window (no energy reflected back to the room). It is important to point out that α depends on frequency and it is usually measured at 125, 250, 500, 1000, 2000, and 4000 Hz. Also, the sum expressed in Equation 3.9 includes dissipation of energy in the medium within the room and absorptions due to objects (including people) placed in a room. Statistical approach assumes that, except close to the source or to the absorbing surfaces, the energy distribution in the room is uniform and has random local directions of flow. In such conditions, the intensity of the reverberant sound created by the source producing the power P is given by:

$$I = 4P/A. \qquad \text{(Eq. 3.10)}$$

Note that all the information on the room is expressed by the room absorption A. Let us assume that in a busy classroom with the initial value of $A = 40$ sabins, all internal sources (e.g., air conditioning and conversation) generate a sound level of 60 dB. After installing wall and ceiling acoustic treatments, A increased to 400 sabins. Then, the reverberant sound level would be reduced by 10 dB, from 60 to 50 dB.

Most rooms have a mixture of reverberant and direct sound. At a point that is close to the sound source, more energy comes directly from the source than from the reverberant field. Then, the directivity factor of the source needs to be taken into account. That aspect of energy propagation may be related to the source per se or to a location of a source relative to room boundaries. As described above, a monopole radiates sound equally well in all directions under a free-field condition. However, if the monopole is placed on a floor that is a perfectly reflecting surface ($\alpha = 0$), then it radiates only into the upper half of the space. Therefore, the intensity at a distance r from it would be twice that given by Equation 3.2; the extra power would come from the floor reflection. Similarly, if the source is located in a three-surface corner of a room (e.g., , where two walls and the ceiling meet), then the intensity would be eight times higher than that of a free-field condition.

Most sound sources, for example the human mouth, do not radiate energy equally well in all directions, that is, they are not omnidirectional. They are characterized by their directionality. The directivity factor, Q, is defined as the ratio of the intensity of a source in some specified direction (usually along the acoustic axis of the source) to the intensity at the same point in space due to an omnidirectional point source with the same acoustic power. Thus, Q indicates how much more effectively a directional source concentrates its available acoustic power into a preferred direction. Typically, the value of Q increases with an increase of frequency and therefore it must be expressed as a function of f or $Q(f)$. For a source that is different from a monopole (then $Q = 1$), Equation 3.2 should be modified:

$$I = Q(f) \, P/(4\pi r^2). \qquad \text{(Eq. 3.11)}$$

The total intensity obtained by combining the direct and reverberant sound is given by:

$$I = Q(f) \, P/(4\pi r^2) + 4P/A. \qquad \text{(Eq. 3.12)}$$

Converting the above equation into a logarithmic scale would allow calculating contributions of the direct and reverberant sound in terms of sound intensity level:

$$L = L_p + 10\log[Q(f)/ (4\pi r^2) + 4/A] \quad \text{(Eq. 3.13)}$$

where L_p is the power level from the source referenced to one picowatt or 10^{-12} watts.

At any point in a room, a listener receives both direct sound, which follows the inverse square law (or the 6-dB rule), and reverberant sound, the level of which is independent of distance from the source. Equation 3.13 is presented graphically in Figure 3–2 assuming that a sound source is a talker with a directivity factor $Q = 3.5$ placed in a small room

$(9 \times 6 \times 2.75$ m$)$ with the room constant $A = 50$ sabins. When the listener (e.g., a child in a classroom) is close to the source, the level of the direct sound exceeds that of the reverberant sound. When the listener is far from the source, the reverberant sound dominates. The so-called critical distance, D, is defined as the distance from a sound source at which direct sound and reverberant sound are at the same level. For the example depicted in Figure 3–2, D = 1.9 m. At distances less than approximately one third of the critical distance, the direct sound level is at least 10 dB stronger than the reverberant sound and the contribution of reverberation can generally be ignored. The sound level depends on the directionality of the source and, therefore,

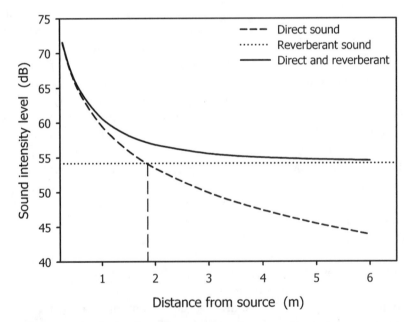

Figure 3–2. Sound intensity level in a room, with parameters described in the text, as a function of a distance from a source. Dashed line corresponds to direct sound, dotted line to reverberant sound, and solid line to total sound energy. Dashed vertical line corresponds to the critical distance from the source at which the levels of direct and reverberant sounds are equal.

may vary with a change in the position of a listener or of a microphone measuring sound pressure distribution across different locations. At distances greater than approximately three times the critical distance, the direct sound is at least 10 dB weaker than the reverberant sound and the contribution of the direct signal is negligible.

Reverberation Time

Equations 3.12 and 3.13 represent an equilibrium situation of a uniformly diffuse acoustic field reached when a sound source emits a constant acoustic power and the reverberant sound builds up to a constant level. When the sound source is turned off, the reverberant sound level begins to decrease because the waves emitted by the source have repeated collisions with the room boundaries losing energy with each collision as determined by the absorption coefficients. The energy will gradually decay until all sound energy gets absorbed by the boundaries. The time taken for the energy density to decrease to one-millionth of its initial value, that is, for the sound level to drop by 60 dB, is defined as the reverberation time, T_r. Sabine (1927) developed an equation for calculating the reverberation time, which remains a fundamental parameter in studies of room acoustics:

$$T_r = (0.161V)/A \qquad \text{(Eq. 3.14)}$$

where V is the cubic volume of a room in m^3.

Following the pioneering work of Sabine, reverberation time was measured by exciting a room into a steady state by a noise signal and recording graphically the decay curves (sound pressure level plotted against time) after the sound source was turned off. The shortcoming of that procedure was a substantial test/retest variability of decay curves, especially in the initial portion of the curves, due to the randomness of the amplitudes and phases of the normal room modes at the moment when the excitation signal was turned off. To minimize the effect of the fluctuations in decay curves, multiple measurements were performed and the results were averaged to determine the reverberation time. Schroeder (1965) proposed a new method based on applying tone bursts to excite the enclosure and then calculating the backward integration of room response. In that method, the last energy is integrated first and the initial arrival is integrated last, similar to the integration of a backward-played tape recording of the decaying signal. The data obtained from a single measurement result in a decay curve which theoretically equates to the ensemble average of infinitely many decay curves measured using interrupted noise. The work of Schroeder started a new area of research and practical applications based on the impulse response of a room.

Early and Late Reflections

The impulse response describes the propagation of a brief pressure impulse that is generated at some point inside a room and recorded by a microphone placed in another location. An example of the impulse response of a room is presented in Figure 3–3. The direct sound arrives first at the point of the microphone with a short latency, t_0, relative to

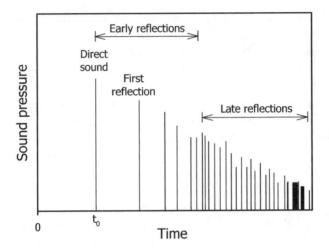

Figure 3–3. An example of the impulse response of a room. A brief pressure impulse is generated at time equals zero. Direct sound arrives first at the point of the measurement, followed by single and multiple early reflections, and a series of late reflections coming closer and closer in time.

the time of the initial pulse generation. The second impulse is smaller than the direct sound and it corresponds to the first reflection from the surface closest to the microphone. Then, other pulses corresponding to single reflections from the walls, the ceiling, and the floor are recorded followed by a series of multiple reflections coming closer and closer in time. The reflected sounds become smaller and smaller because they have more encounters with the boundaries and thus are increasingly absorbed by the surface. Sounds that strike multiple surfaces represent the reverberant energy that persists for some extended period of time (expressed quantitatively by the reverberation time).

The impulse response can be used to evaluate acoustic properties of an existing room and to suggest modifications that can be made to improve communication in the room. In addition, the analy-

sis of a predicted impulse response is useful during the process of designing a room. Many computer programs have the capability of creating models of acoustical properties of a room by simulating propagation of signals generated by virtual sound sources placed in various locations within the room of a particular shape, dimensions, and materials used to cover the boundaries (e.g., Siebein, 2004).

When analyzing the impulse room response, it is important to distinguish between early and late components (see Figure 3–3). Hass (1972) described the beneficial effect of sound reflections arriving at a listener's ears within short time periods after the direct sound. Two brief sounds are heard as a single sound if the interval between them is short. The limit is about 5 ms for clicks, but may be 40 ms for complex signals such as speech. The lagging sound is suppressed. If two successive sounds are heard as fused, the location of the total sound is determined largely by the location of the first sound; a listener makes his or her localization judgments instantly based on the earliest arriving waves in the onset of a sound. This phenomenon is called the precedence effect (or Haas effect) because the earliest arriving sound wave, the direct sound with accurate localization information, is given precedence over the reverberation that conveys inaccurate information.

The precedence effect influences speech perception in rooms designed for the purpose of speech communication, such as small meeting rooms, classrooms, and auditoria. Early reflections (occurring within a 50–80-ms time window after the direct sound) can be integrated with the direct sound. They are considered a useful portion of the energy because they generally increase the audibility of a speech source without degrading intelligibility (e.g., Bradley, Sato, & Picard, 2003). A study of Nábělek and Robinette (1978) performed for normal and hearing-impaired listeners indicated that reflections arriving shortly after the direct sound may enhance word identification in both groups of subjects if the direct sound level was not sufficient. Later reflections (greater than 50–80 ms) are perceived as a prolongation of the sound and "smear out" the temporal information. For speech signals, those later reflections cause a decrease in intelligibility. Therefore, in a room where speech communication is the deciding factor for evaluating its acoustical quality, reverberation is often considered in negative terms, together with background noise that can originate from outside or inside a room. Some of the most common sources of noise include air and road traffic, heating, ventilating and air

conditioning systems, human activity in adjacent rooms, and internal human activity (including speech). The effect of noise can be considered negligible if its level is at least 10 dB below that of the late reverberation. Similarly, the effect of late reverberation is insignificant if its level is at least 10 dB below that of the noise.

By recognizing different contributions of early versus late reflections to speech intelligibility, Lochner and Burger (1961) introduced the useful-to-detrimental energy ratios. These measures relate the useful portion of energy in a signal (for example in speech), consisting of the direct sound and early reflections, to the detrimental energy, which consists of reverberant energy and background noise. Bradley (1986) evaluated different acoustical measures as predictors of speech intelligibility in rooms of varied size and acoustical conditions. He showed high predictive accuracy of the U_{80} parameter, that is, a useful-to-detrimental energy ratio calculated with the value of 80 ms selected as the dividing point between the early energy that is useful and contributes to the loudness of the direct sound and the detrimental energy. Similarly, there are other early/late ratio measures, U_{35}, U_{50}, U_{90}, when the value of 35, 50, or 95 ms is defined as the dividing point between the early and late energy, respectively. These latter parameters are related to the effective signal-to-noise (S/N) ratio; the effective signal is a combination of the direct signal and early reverberation, whereas the effective noise is a combination of actual noise (from external and internal sources) and late reverberation. It is generally agreed that if the listener is to have access to all the useful information in the speech signal, the effective S/N needs to be at least 15 dB across a broad frequency region (e.g., Boothroyd, 2004). One possibility for reaching this requirement would be to minimize T_r.

Maximizing Room Acoustics

The recent ANSI standard (ANSI, 2002) specifies maximum reverberation times in unoccupied, furnished learning spaces measured in octave bands with center frequencies of 500, 1000, and 2000 Hz. The recommended value of T_r is 0.6 seconds or lower in small to medium classrooms (with enclosed volume <10,000 ft³) and 0.7 seconds or lower in large classrooms (with enclosed volume >10,000 ft³ and <20,000 ft³). The presence of 20 to 25 students in a room is expected to lower T_r by approximately 0.05 seconds. A position statement of the American Speech-Language-Hearing Association (ASHA, 2005) recommends acoustical criteria that are essentially identical to the ANSI standard. The ANSI and ASHA recommendations suggest a need for minimizing reverberation times. Very short values of T_r may be obtained by increasing absorption of room surfaces. However, that solution is likely to lead to reduced early reflection energy and therefore to reduced speech intelligibility (see above). Bradley et al. (2003) reported data on speech intelligibility tests in simulated sound fields for normal-hearing and hearing-impaired listeners. The results showed that increased early reflection energy (arriving within the first 50 ms after the direct sound) had the same effect in increasing speech intelligibility scores as increased direct sound level; therefore, adding early reflections increases the effective S/N. More-over, both groups of subjects benefitted similarly from added early reflections. The results also confirmed that listeners with hearing impairment required approximately 5 dB higher S/N values to have similar intelligibility scores as normal-hearing listeners (Bradley et al., 2003).

The directionality of the human voice may also influence the amount of the direct energy available to a listener. For example, when the talker's head is turned away from the listener, the listener will experience reduced direct speech sound, especially for the high frequencies, which are critical for speech recognition. By modifying the spectrum of the direct speech sound, Bradley et al. (2003) simulated changes in the talker's head angle relative to the listener. When early reflections were added, there was only a small reduction in intelligibility scores for the situation of the talker's head turned 180 degrees (i.e., facing away from the listener) compared to the zero-degree position (i.e., the talker situated straight ahead). Those results clearly indicated that in many situations, where the direct sound is reduced due to the talker who is not facing the listener, speech understanding is possible only because of the benefits of early reflections.

Analyses of impulse response measurements in typical rooms used for speech communication included in the study of Bradley et al. (2003) indicated that the effect of early reflections in rooms is equivalent to an increase in the direct speech level of up to 9 dB. Moreover, the benefit of the early reflection energy tended to increase with an increase of a distance between a source (talker) and a receiver (listener). That finding emphasizes that a correct design which enhances early reflections provides the greatest increase in intelligibility where it is most needed, that is, the farthest from the source.

In recent years, many computer programs have been developed to assist architects, acousticians, and engineers in designing new rooms and modifying existing rooms (e.g., Bradley, et al., 2003; Siebein, 2004). Software resources may be used to construct computer models for evaluating and maximizing room acoustics at different stages of such projects. As described above, the major goal in the acoustical design of rooms for speech communication should be to maximize the energy of the direct sound and early reflections (i.e., the speech signal).

Computer models allow evaluation of different options for placement of sound-reflecting surfaces to enhance the signal. Optimal location of acoustic reflectors on a ceiling depends on teaching strategy and may be different for a typical lecture-type classroom than for a room designated for small group instruction with general movement throughout the classroom by the teacher. Different options for spatial distribution of absorbing materials also may be tested using computer models to ensure that there is no excessive later-arriving reflection energy and to optimize frequency characteristics of the reverberation time.

Clearly, model studies are helpful in evaluating the geometry of a room in terms of a distribution of room modes that should be spaced as evenly at low frequencies as possible. Strong specular (mirrorlike) reflections should be limited in small rooms where standing waves modes are well separated at low frequencies. One method of reducing specular reflections involves placing diffusing surfaces. Diffusing surfaces, such as a roughened or textured surface, create random scattering of incident waves. Such an option is relatively easy to implement; however, the response of a diffusing surface is difficult to predict due to random characteristics of the reflections. Specially designed diffusers provide a uniform diffraction pattern over a specified frequency range, defined as the operating bandwidth.

Very often the term "damping" rather than "absorption" is used to describe properties of absorbers that are designed to maximize the conversion of acoustic energy to heat and thus result in minimizing late reflections and detrimental resonances. In physics, damping describes an effect that tends to reduce the amplitude of oscillations. It seems more appropriate, therefore, to relate damping to the characteristics of a sound source and absorption to a decrease of acoustic energy that has been generated by the source and decays, while propagating in a room, due to the characteristics of the boundaries. During the process of designing acoustical properties of a room, placement of absorbing materials should be carefully arranged to enhance speech communication in the room. There are four general categories of sound absorbers.

The first type includes porous absorbers. Materials such as mineral wool, fiberboard, or plastic foams dissipate acoustic energy by friction that air molecules encounter while moving through pores. When such absorbers are applied directly to a reflecting surface (e.g., to a hard wall of a room), their effectiveness depends on the thickness of the matter. For a sound wave which is incident on a rigid wall, the maximum particle velocity occurs at $\lambda/4$. If the thickness of the absorber is less than one quarter of the wavelength, the damping effect is small. Therefore, even relatively thick porous sheets placed on a solid wall are effective primarily for high frequencies with short wavelengths (see Equation 3.1).

The second type of absorber, panel absorbers, is often used when low-frequency absorption is required. Thin wood panels are mounted away from the wall, creating an air cavity. Incident sound at a particular frequency causes the panel to vibrate. Due to inherent resistance of the panel to rapid flexing and to the resistance of the enclosed air to compression, some of the sound energy is converted into heat by the internal damping. Panel absorbers are most effective at their resonant frequency (typically around 100 Hz) which depends upon density of the surface material and the width of the enclosed space. Filling the cavity with a porous material results not only in broadening the frequency range over which some absorption occurs, but also in decreasing the peak value of the absorption coefficient (i.e., the "tuning" characteristic of the absorber becomes shallow).

Cavity absorbers, also known as resonators or Helmholtz resonators, represent a large cavity with a port on its front to couple the enclosed volume of the airspace to the air in the room. These absorbers give a high absorption coefficient in a narrow frequency band around the resonant frequency which is defined by the cross-sectional area and the length of the port and by the volume of air trapped in the cavity. At resonant and neighboring frequencies, the air moves in and out of the cavity, causing the acoustic energy to be converted into heat. Cavity absorbers are often used in noise control applications when energy of noise generated by machines occurs in a narrow range of frequencies. An absorber "tuned" to a targeted frequency provides high absorption efficiency.

All three of the mechanisms described above may be combined in slot and perforated panel absorbers. The panel itself may be plywood, hardboard, or metal and, therefore, it may act as a membrane absorber. The panel is spaced away from one of the walls and may have perforations, holes, or slots that create multiple cavity resonators. Absorption properties are improved by placement of porous materials between the wall and the panel. The frequency characteristic of the absorption coefficient depends on the width and depth of slots, pattern of perforations (hole size and spacing), the thickness of the panel and its distance from the wall, and the thickness and the placement of the porous material. There are various commercially available products that may provide required absorption properties and those are often used to reduce low-frequency reverberation time without affecting it in the high-frequency range.

Measuring Sound

The pascal (or N/m^2) is a unit of the amplitude of the pressure fluctuations created by sound propagation. Due to the wide dynamic range of the human auditory system the decibel (dB) scale, which is a logarithmic measure, is more useful for measuring sound affecting human listeners. A signal with a root-mean-square (RMS) pressure, p, has a sound pressure level, L (in dB SPL), of:

$$L = 20\log(p/p_0) \qquad \text{(Eq. 3.15)}$$

where p_0 is the reference value of 20 µPa. The RMS value of a time-varying signal is defined as the numerical value of a constant which would have the same average power as the signal. For a sine wave, the RMS value is 0.707 times the amplitude of the sine.

Sound pressure levels are measured by a sound level meter (SLM) that consists of a pressure-sensitive microphone, amplifier, weighting filter, temporal averaging circuit, and a display providing the result in dB SPL re: 20 μPa. Typically, condenser microphones are used in SLMs because of high precision and stability. The electrical signal produced by the microphone is relatively small and needs to be amplified before being further processed.

The weighting filters are designed to simulate the equal loudness contours by attenuating low- and high-frequency signals. There are three internationally standardized characteristics termed A, B, and C weightings (ANSI, 2001); however, the B-weighting filter is not widely used. The A-weighting filter resembles the response of the human auditory system to sine signals of low to intermediate levels (e.g., Moore, 2003). It attenuates low frequencies substantially, for example, by 19 dB at 100 Hz relative to 1 kHz. The A-weighted measures are most often used in evaluating sound annoyance. The C-weighting filter approximates equal loudness contour at high SPLs. Its response is almost flat with a small attenuation for frequencies below 200 Hz (e.g., 2 dB at 40 Hz) and above 1250 Hz (e.g., 3 dB at 8 kHz).

Most sounds that need to be measured fluctuate in level over time. Different settings of the temporal averaging circuit of an SLM allow a selection of response characteristics most appropriate to obtain an RMS value of a signal depending on its rate of fluctuation. A time constant of 125 ms (a "fast" setting) enables one to measure and follow sig-nals fluctuating slowly. A time constant of one second (a "slow" option) gives a response that averages out fast fluctuations. For measurements of very short (impulse) signals, SLMs have impulse characteristics with a time constant of 35 ms which is short enough to enable detection of a transient sound. In addition, some SLMs include a circuit for measuring the peak and the maximum RMS values of the sound level, regardless of its duration and fluctuations. Modern SLMs have digital displays that depict results and information of settings (e.g., A-weighting, F-time constant).

Annoyance of noise depends not only on its level, but also on its duration. For constant sound levels, the measurement is straightforward. If the signal varies over time, the level must be sampled repeatedly over a specified time period. Most commonly, level-fluctuating sounds are described in terms of an average level that has the same acoustic energy as the summation of all the time-varying events. This energy-equivalent sound descriptor is called the equivalent continuous sound level, L_{eq}. The most common averaging period is hourly. For example, a one-hour-average A-weighted sound level is a single-value measure corresponding to the time-mean-square A-weighted sound pressure averaged over a one-hour period.

Noise Sources in a Classroom

In addition to specifying maximum reverberation times, the recent ANSI standard (ANSI, 2002) provides criteria for background noise in classrooms. According to ANSI (2002), the one-hour-average

A-weighted steady background noise in a classroom shall not exceed 35 dB. For large spaces with volumes >20,000 ft^3, the limit is 40 dBA SPL. These limits apply to the noisiest continuous one-hour period during times when learning activities take place and while exterior and interior noise sources are operating simultaneously.

According to Siebein (2004), poorly designed heating, ventilation, and air conditioning (HVAC) systems are the primary sources of noise in classrooms. Siebein provided recommendations for designing air handling units to achieve background noise criteria of ANSI. Noise from students within the classroom, in adjoining rooms, and in outdoor areas add significant amounts of energy to the unwanted background. Absorbers placed in a classroom reduce noise from students' activities within the room, in addition to optimizing reverberation. Installing carpet on the floor may decrease impact sounds propagating within multistory school buildings. Walls, windows and doors with high transmission loss also lower the noise level of exterior sources. This is especially important if a site for a school is located near a major road, airport, railway line, or industrial noise source. One needs to keep in mind that acoustic isolation of a classroom is limited by the weakest element in the entire acoustic system. For example, a gap between a window frame and a wall can negate high transmission loss of the wall.

In some situations, a sufficient S/N ratio cannot be achieved by modifying room acoustics or by lowering the influence of noise sources. In such cases, amplification provided by FM systems should be considered. These systems consist of a wireless microphone used by a teacher, an amplifier, and loudspeakers carefully located in the classroom to increase the level of speech signals (see Chapter 7).

High-Fidelity Transducers

High-fidelity or *hi-fi* reproduction is defined as the reproduction of sounds that is as close as possible to the original. A hi-fi system contains several different devices and any device within that system may distort signals in various ways or add some amount of noise. The performance of the entire system is determined by the performance of its weakest element. A set of measurements is performed to assess the sound quality of each element.

One specification which is commonly evaluated is frequency response. A sine wave of constant amplitude and varying frequency is used as an input signal to the device and the output signal is expected not to vary as a function of frequency. Typically, there are some irregularities in the response and the frequency range that is reproduced is limited. For example, the frequency response of a loudspeaker may be stated as 60 to 18,000 Hz ± 3 dB, meaning that the sound level would not vary over more than a 6-dB range for any frequency from 60 Hz to 18 kHz. From a perceptual standpoint, it is not necessary to extend the response of a hi-fi device below 30 Hz, as there is little audible energy in musical signals below that frequency, except for synthesized sounds and some organ sounds of a very low pitch. Because the frequency limits of hearing are generally stated to lie between 20 Hz and 20 kHz for normal young human ears, it also is assumed that, in the absence of distortions, energy in the range above 16 kHz would not make a significant contribution to the perceived sound quality. Thus, a frequency response extending from 30 Hz to 16 kHz is perfectly sufficient for hi-fi reproduction.

Significant irregularities in the frequency response may affect the timbre of the reproduced sound. A series of studies reported by Green (1988) on a so-called profile analysis suggested that listeners cannot detect changes in spectral shape when the level in a given frequency region is changed by less than 2 dB relative to the level in other frequency bands. A response that is flat within ±1 dB, therefore, would not be perceptually different from a completely flat one. A frequency response specified as 30 to 16,000 Hz ±1 dB would be ideal in term of perceptual relevance.

In general, all elements of a hi-fi system exhibit some degree of nonlinearity or, in other words, they generate distortion (i.e., the presence of some frequency components in the output signal that are not present in the input signal). One method of evaluating the degree of nonlinearity is to measure harmonic distortions. A pure tone of a particular frequency is used as an input signal. Due to nonlinearities, the output signal would contain a fundamental component with the same frequency as that of the input signal and a series of harmonics, that is, components with frequencies corresponding to integer multiplications of the fundamental frequency. The total amplitude of the second and higher-order harmonics, expressed as a percentage of the amplitude of the fundamental, is called the total harmonic distortion, *THD*. The

audibility of harmonic distortion depends on the spectrum of the input signal and on the distribution of energy among harmonics. If the second and third harmonics dominate, THD of 2 to 3% would not be noticed if the signal is a piece of music; however, if the distortion produces significant energy at high-order harmonics, TDH above approximately 0.1% may be audible (Moore, 2003).

Another method of measuring distortion is to apply simultaneously two pure tones (primary tones) with frequencies f_1 and f_2 at the input and to measure combination products in the output signal with frequencies such as $f_1 - f_2$, $2f_1 - f_2$, or $f_1 + f_2$ (intermodulation distortions). The total amplitude of the intermodulation signals is expressed as a percentage of the amplitudes of the primary tones. The audibility of intermodulation distortion may be difficult to predict; however, in general a value smaller than 0.5% is not expected to be detected (Moore, 2003).

Some amount of undesired noise, in the form of a low-frequency hum due to the frequency of the alternating current (AC) power supply and/or in the form of a high-frequency hiss, may be expected to be added to the signal by many devices. The S/N ratio, expressed in decibels, is specified as the ratio of the output power for a relatively high-level signal to the output power due to hum and noise alone. A ratio greater than 70 dB is adequate for listening to music at moderate sound levels (Moore, 2003).

A basic sound reinforcement (i.e., amplification) system consists of an input device (e.g., a microphone, a cassette deck, and a CD player), an amplifier, and an output device (one loudspeaker or a set of loudspeakers). The primary goal of the sound system in a room designed for speech communication is to deliver clear, intelligible speech to each listener. The performance of modern hi-fi amplifiers and CD players is likely to be more than adequate for limits required by the ear (Moore, 2003). The sound quality of the entire system, therefore, typically is determined by the performance of the microphone and loudspeakers. The microphone is the first link in the audio system and thus a poor quality microphone may result in preventing the rest of the system from functioning to its full potential.

There are two basic microphone transducer types: dynamic and condenser. In a dynamic microphone, a coil of wire is mounted on a diaphragm surrounded by a magnetic field. When the diaphragm is moved by a change of air pressure (sound), the resulting fluctuations in the magnetic field create the electric signal corresponding to the sound picked up by a microphone. Dynamic microphones are economical, but still provide excellent sound quality; therefore, they are the most widely used in general sound reinforcement systems (Shure, 2006). A condenser microphone is based on an electrically charged diaphragm/backplate assembly which forms a sound-sensitive capacitor. When a sound wave vibrates the diaphragm, a variation of the spacing between the diaphragm and the backplate is created that produces the electric signal corresponding to the sound picked up by the microphone. The construction of a condenser microphone must include a source of electric charge, either an internal battery or a phantom power. Condenser microphones are more complex than dynamic ones and tend to be more expensive; however, a condenser microphone can provide a flat frequency response, especially in the extended frequency range and can be made small

physically without significant loss of high performance (Shure, 2006). In an environment like a boardroom, auditorium, or a courthouse, when the highest sound quality is desired, a condenser microphone rather than a dynamic microphone might be preferred.

The sensitivity of a microphone is defined as the level of its electrical output for a sound of a particular level at its input. For weak sounds, a microphone of high sensitivity is desirable. The directional characteristic of a microphone is defined as the variation of its output when it is oriented at different angles relative to the direction of the sound source. An omnidirectional microphone is equally sensitive to sound coming from all directions and its characteristics will show on a polar graph as a smooth circle. A unidirectional microphone is most sensitive to sound coming from a particular direction. A cardioid microphone, with a heart-shaped polar pattern, is the most common type of unidirectional microphones. The cardioid microphone is most sensitive to sound coming from the front of the microphone and least sensitive to sound from the rear; therefore, it may be directed toward the desired sound source and away from the undesired source. In addition, a cardioid microphone picks up less ambient noise than an omnidirectional microphone (Shure, 2006). Directional characteristics may vary as a function of frequency, but high-quality microphones maintain their polar pattern over a wide frequency range.

Microphones used for speech communication include several designs: handheld, user-worn (clip-on, lavalier styles worn on a lanyard around the neck, or head-worn types), free-standing mounted, or surface mounted. For optimum operation of a microphone, it should be placed much closer from a talker than the critical distance (*D*) to get an acceptable ratio of direct-to-reverberant sound. In general, an omnidirectional microphone should be placed no farther from the talker than 30% of *D* (see earlier comments related to Figure 3–2) and a unidirectional microphone should be positioned closer than 50% of *D*.

Any type of microphone (except phantom-powered condensers) may be used as part of a wireless system, which needs to include a radio transmitter and a radio receiver to replace the microphone cable with a radio link. The transmitter uses the audio signal from the microphone to vary frequency of a radio signal based on frequency modulation (FM) and broadcasts the microphone signal to the receiver.

Loudspeakers are transducers that convert electrical energy of a signal delivered by an amplifier into sound energy. The frequency response of a loudspeaker is typically measured in an anechoic chamber where there are no reflections from walls, ceiling, or floor. A loudspeaker's efficiency is expressed in dB/W by measuring the sound pressure level at a distance of one meter from the loudspeaker for an input of one watt. The efficiency determines the power of an amplifier needed to produce a particular sound level. Loudspeakers often generate significant amounts of harmonic and intermodulation distortion, with a common THD value of approximately 1 to 2%; therefore, a loudspeaker is most likely to be the weakest element of a hi-fi system (Moore, 2003).

It is desirable to reproduce the full range of audio frequencies (from 30 to 16,000 Hz) uniformly for the playback frequency band of the speaker system, but it is difficult for one loudspeaker unit to reproduce such a wide range of frequencies. Therefore, it is common practice to adopt a system of dividing the bandwidth and using individual speakers for high, middle, and low ranges. The dividing network divides and applies electric input to each speaker. The frequency at the boundary for dividing the electric input is called the crossover frequency. Using more than one transducer also helps to partially solve the problems related to the directional characteristics of a loudspeaker. (See earlier discussion on the directivity factor Q for sound sources.) The frequency response of a loudspeaker is typically measured with a microphone placed directly in front of the loudspeaker. If the microphone is placed at some angle to the loudspeaker but at the same distance from it, the measured sound pressure level may decrease due to directional characteristics. In conventional loudspeakers, the beam of energy radiated by a loudspeaker grows narrower as the frequency increases. Using multiple transducers, each of which produces a reasonable wide beam over the range of frequencies it reproduces, may create a directional characteristics that is more independent of frequency than that of a single-transducer speaker (Moore, 2003).

Room acoustics also influence the perceived sound quality reproduced by a loudspeaker because: (1) reflections are always present, (2) high frequencies are usually absorbed more than low frequencies, and (3) at low frequencies room resonances may be excited by acoustic energy radiated by the loudspeaker. Peaks and dips of the frequency response measured in an anechoic chamber may be combined with peaks and dips produced by room acoustics to produce a substantially irregular response of the loudspeaker in a particular room. To minimize this effect, the frequency response recorded in the anechoic chamber should be as smooth as possible. If loudspeakers are part of a sound system in a room, their parameters and location should be carefully designed to provide the most even distribution of sound throughout the space and to minimize acoustic feedback which arises when the sound from the loudspeakers recirculates and is picked up by a microphone.

Summary

Sound waves carry acoustic energy generated by a source (e.g., loudspeaker, musical instruments, or a speaker) away from that source. In a free-field condition (i.e., in a space with no boundaries), the sound intensity decreases inversely with the square of the distance from the source. Major departures from the inverse square law occur in most listening conditions (including the classroom) due to obstacles in the sound path resulting in reflection, absorption, diffusion, and altered transmission of sound waves. Interference of waves reflected within a three-dimensional enclosed space may create a complicated pattern of standing waves. Computer programs are available to optimize room geometry and the placement of sound sources (e.g., loudspeakers) and listeners to maximize the uniform distribution of acoustic energy within the room. Some of the sound generated by a source located inside a room arrives directly at the listener's ears. Other waves reflected by the boundaries of the room reach the listener's ears with a delay subsequent to the direct sound. The listener's ability to integrate early reflections (occurring within 50 ms) with the direct sound can increase speech intelligibility. Excessive reverberation (i.e., extended persistence of sound in a room due to multiple reflections) may reduce intelligibility; therefore, a room design that enhances early reflections and controls reverberation (but not necessarily decreasing it too much) benefits room acoustics. It is important to recognize that acoustic conditions of a room that are tolerable for normally hearing adults in informal conversation can be difficult for children in learning situations, especially for individuals with deficits of hearing, language, attention, or processing. A carefully designed amplification system may be helpful to deliver clear speech signals to each listener within the room.

References

American National Standards Institute. (2001). *American National Standard specification for sound level meters.* ANSI S1.4. New York: Author.

American National Standards Institute. (2002). *Acoustical performance criteria, design requirements, and guidelines for schools.* ANSI S12.60. New York: Author.

American Speech-Language-Hearing Association. (2005). *Acoustics in educational settings* [Position statement]. Available at http://www.asha.org/members/deskref-journals/deskref/default.

Bolt, R. H. (1946). Note on normal frequency statistics for rectangular rooms. *Journal of the Acoustical Society of America, 18,* 130–133.

Bonello, O. J. (1981). A new criterion for the distribution of normal room modes. *Journal of the Audio Engineering Society, 29,* 597–605.

Boothroyd, A. (2004). Room acoustics and speech perception. *Seminars in Hearing, 25*, 155-166.

Bradley, J. S. (1986). Predictors of speech intelligibility in rooms. *Journal of the Acoustical Society of America, 80*, 837-845.

Bradley, J. S., Sato, H., & Picard, M. (2003). On the importance of early reflections for speech in rooms. *Journal of the Acoustical Society of America, 113*, 3233-3244.

Cramer, O. (1993). The variation of the specific heat ratio and the speed of sound in air with temperature, pressure, humidity and CO_2 concentration. *Journal of the Acoustical Society of America, 93*, 2510-2516.

Green, D. M. (1988). *Profile analysis.* Oxford: Oxford University Press.

Haas, H. (1972). The influence of a single echo on the audibility of speech. *Journal of the Audio Engineering Society 20*, 146-159.

Lochner, J. P. A., & Burger, J. F. (1961). The intelligibility of speech under reverberant conditions. *Acustica, 11*, 195-200.

Louden, M. M. (1971). Dimension-ratios of rectangular rooms with good distribution of eigentones. *Acustica, 24*, 101-104.

Moore, B. C. J. (2003). *Psychology of hearing.* San Diego: Academic Press.

Nábělek, A. K., & Robinette, L. (1978). Influence of the precedence effect on word identification by normally hearing and hearing-impaired subjects. *Journal of the Acoustical Society of America, 63*, 187-194.

Sabine, W. C. (1927). *Collected papers on acoustics.* Cambridge, MA: Harvard University Press.

Schroeder, M. R. (1965). New method of measuring reverberation time. *Journal of the Acoustical Society of America, 37*, 409-412.

Shure Inc. Web site. http://www.shure.com/shurenotes/feb2003/mic.asp. Retrieved January 7, 2006.

Siebein, G. W. (2004) Understanding classroom acoustic solutions. *Seminars in Hearing, 25*, 141-154.

SECTION II

Intervention

CHAPTER 4

AUDITORY TRAINING

**FRANK E. MUSIEK, GAIL D. CHERMAK, AND
JEFFREY WEIHING**

Auditory Training Defined

The perspective and approach to auditory training (AT) discussed in this chapter differ somewhat from classic views and definitions of AT. Traditional AT focused on utilizing residual hearing. For example, Goldstein (1939) stated that AT "involved the development and or improvement in the ability to discriminate various properties of speech and non-speech signals" (Schow & Nerbonne, 1996, p. 95). Carhart (1960) described AT as "the process of teaching the child or adult with hearing impairment to take full advantage of available auditory cues" (Schow & Nerbonne, 1996, p. 95). Erber (1982) viewed AT as "the creation of special communication conditions in which teachers and audiologists help hearing impaired children acquire many of the auditory perception abilities that normally hearing children acquire naturally without their intervention" (p. 1). Although these traditional definitions of AT are appropriate in the context of peripheral hearing impairment, they do not emphasize the intimate linkage of AT to auditory plasticity and other brain functions and, therefore, are not particularly relevant to AT for central auditory dysfunction.

In viewing AT in the context of (central) auditory processing disorder ([C]APD), it is imperative to understand that plasticity takes place in the brain, it is a central phenomenon, and it is key to changing auditory performance. In order to expand the definition of AT to include peripheral and central auditory performance, and also to recognize the association between AT and brain function, the following definition is offered. Auditory training is *a set of (acoustic) conditions and/or tasks that are designed to activate auditory and related systems in such a manner that their neural base and associated auditory behavior are altered in a positive way.*

In some cases, simple (i.e., passive) acoustic stimulation can improve auditory performance. This is often seen in experiments with animals that have been acoustically deprived or experienced damage to their auditory systems. In an all-encompassing sense, stimulation alone could be considered a form of AT; however, improving auditory performance is more likely to occur when the subject is actively involved (see Bao, Chang, Woods, & Merzenich, 2004; Musiek & Berge, 1998). Although passive listening (i.e., stimulation that is not contingent on performing a task) in an acoustically rich environment can enhance auditory skills, active listening (i.e., performing auditory tasks) is much more likely to make a difference (Greenough & Bailey, 1988; Hassmannova, Myslivecek, & Novakova, 1981; Recanzone, Schreiner, & Merzenich, 1993). In reviewing AT methods, the theme that constantly emerges is that the patient, student, or subject needs to be engaged and motivated to do the task. This principle and many other important principles in AT are not new; in fact, they have been part of AT's long history.

Significant Events in the History of AT

The concept of AT as sound stimulation has been known for centuries. In Wedenburg's (1951) wonderful review of AT,
it was related that in the sixth century doctors used large ringing bells in an attempt to stimulate a hearing response in people who were considered deaf. Although this primitive method was traced back centuries, it really was the initial work of Itard in the 1800s at the Paris School for the Deaf that is often considered the beginning of systematic AT. Itard had his students identify and discriminate vowels and consonants, as well as tonal stimuli of different pitches (Hudgins, 1954). It was reported that this training yielded improvements in hearing. In England in the mid to late 1800s, Toynbee and Urbantschitch, two therapists who followed the work of Itard, conducted AT with individuals with hearing impairment. They ad-vanced Itard's work and did much to establish the concept of AT in England (Wedenburg, 1951). Max Goldstein, a student of Urbantschitch, founded the Central Institute for the Deaf (CID) in the United States. Goldstein brought many ideas about AT to the CID and conducted some of the early efficacy studies on AT. Interestingly, over the past 50 years, AT has continued to employ exercises involving identification and discrimination of various sounds, similar to Itard's early approach.

After World War II, audiology was founded in the United States, and because so many soldiers suffered from hearing loss, AT became quite popular. DiCarlo, Carhart, Huizing, Doehring, and Ling were major names associated with rehabilitation and AT. In general, these clinicians focused on identification and discrimination of rhythmic patterns, isolated phonemes, letters, digits, and minimally different words. They also trained intensity and frequency discrimination tasks using pure tone stimuli (Carhart, 1960;

DiCarlo, 1948). (See Musiek & Berge, 1998, for a review.)

In the 1950s and 1960s, AT was tied to helping patients fitted with hearing aids accommodate to amplification. During the late 1960s and 1970s, interest in AT began to wane. It was difficult to obtain reimbursement by third-party payers, there was little efficacy data, and audiologists and patients felt the procedures were tiring (Musiek & Berge, 1998).

In addition, there seemed to be little concern as to the underlying mechanisms that might enhance one's auditory skills and perception. Focus was primarily on peripheral hearing loss and there seemed to be little interest in the role that the central auditory nervous system (CANS) and neural plasticity played in AT.

As interest in AT waned, some important events were emerging that would eventually reinvigorate interest in AT—although in a different direction. Webster (1977) showed that auditory deprivation reduced auditory cell volumes in the brainstem. Hassmannova et al. (1981) demonstrated that AT with young mice (which involved passive daily exposure to a wide variety of sounds) enhanced auditory cortex activity as recorded by near-field evoked potentials. These studies showed the effects of peripheral hearing loss (i.e., auditory deprivation) on the CANS and the potential of the CANS to enhance auditory function.

Timing could not have been better because at about the same time clinicians were directing greater attention to children with learning problems who appeared to have (C)APD (Pinheiro, 1977; Willeford, 1977). Because (C)APD arises from dysfunction in the auditory substrate of the brain, it was logical to consider AT, which seemed to be based on brain plasticity, as a possible tool for remediation of (C)APD. In the ensuing years, breakthroughs in auditory neuroscience, particularly with regard to plasticity, garnered increasing interest in AT and (C)APD, interest that continues to gain momentum today (as discussed later in the section, The Role of Auditory Neuroplasticity). A major finding that emerged from the many animal studies of AT, as well as from other types of behavioral training, is that brain plasticity is critical for successful AT. Also, it became clear that the CANS is plastic and that the peripheral auditory system is not (Lund, 1978).

Following the early breakthroughs in auditory neuroscience, AT techniques began to emerge for use with children with language impairments, learning problems, and presumed (C)APD. One of the early programs, developed by Katz and Harmon (1982), introduced phonemic synthesis training for (C)APD. This program centered on blending sounds into words. At about the same time, Alexander and Frost (1982) introduced an AT program that focused on temporal facets of speech. It was designed to decelerate the speech signal and enhance the perception of transitions by increasing the intensity of these speech segments. In fact, this program was quite similar to the Fast ForWord© program introduced many years later. The Alexander and Frost program demonstrated improvements in auditory discrimination in children with language delays—perhaps one of the first extensive efficacy studies on AT. Other AT programs emerged, some commercial and others not. These more modern AT approaches are discussed below (see Clinical Training of Temporal Processing below.).

Diagnostic Information: Deficit-Specific Intervention

A full (C)APD diagnostic evaluation must be completed prior to undertaking AT with older children (i.e., ages 7–8 years and older) and adults. The diagnostic test battery should provide information about the patient's particular auditory strengths and weaknesses. Unfortunately, most clinics that perform central auditory processing evaluations today do not have the full range of capabilities, or otherwise choose to assess only a subset of the known auditory processes, thereby often generating an incomplete profile of the patient's auditory strengths and weaknesses. Most clinics do assess temporal and dichotic processes; therefore, these processes will serve as examples of how diagnostic information can lead to specific interventions. For younger children suspected of (C)APD for whom current behavioral tests may be inappropriate and lead to invalid results, it may be reasonable to introduce listening games similar to those described in the final section of this chapter.

The central auditory test results depicted in Figure 4–1 reveal deficits for frequency pattern recognition, dichotic digits, and competing sentences. AT

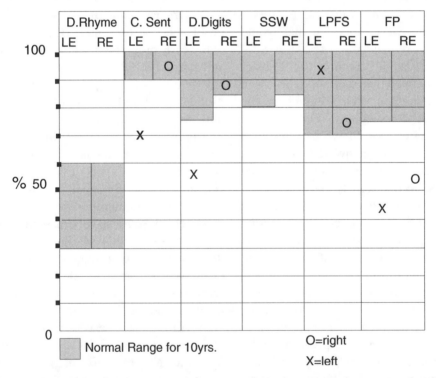

Figure 4–1. Central auditory test battery results with deficits for dichotic listening and frequency pattern perception. Please see discussion in the text. Key: tests from left to right are: dichotic rhyme, competing sentences, dichotic digits, staggered spondaic words, low-pass filtered speech, and frequency patterns.

designed to strengthen temporal processing (following from the poor scores on the frequency pattern test) might range from work on the *Simon Game*™ to enrolling the child in the Fast ForWord program. AT exercises directed to improve deficient dichotic listening range from dichotic interaural intensity difference (DIID) training to drilling speech recognition in competition. All of these training procedures, as well as other examples of AT procedures appropriate to specific deficits identified through diagnostic evaluation, are elaborated later in this chapter. (See also Chermak & Musiek [2002] for additional examples.)

Formal and Informal Approaches to Auditory Training

The concept of formal and informal approaches to AT grew out of an obvious need that was recognized at the Dartmouth Hitchcock Medical Center which is located in a rural area. It was realized that many patients in need of AT could not travel to the clinic as often as needed to effectively conduct treatment. An attempt was made, therefore, to modify some of the procedures performed in the lab or clinic in a way that they could be used in everyday training environments, such as at school or home (Musiek, 1999). Informal procedures are conducted by school personnel (e.g., speech pathologist, educational audiologist) or in some cases parents.

Formal AT procedures are conducted by audiologically trained personnel in a clinic or lab setting that permits control over stimulus generation and presentation. For example, for formal frequency

discrimination AT, tones of slightly different frequency are generated on a computer and the patient is required to decide if the tones are the same or different. Adaptive approaches also can be employed whereby the stimulus parameters vary on the basis of the patient's performance on preceding trials. The frequency, duration, interstimulus interval, and overall intensity are all controlled in formal AT.

Informal AT is used to complement formal AT. Training the patient to discriminate similar sounding notes on a keyboard provides informal AT for temporal processing that complements formal frequency discrimination training. Coupling informal with formal AT offers a more powerful approach, as it provides for more intensive and extensive practice, including real-world, everyday settings that are functionally significant to the patient. This should maximize generalization and treatment efficacy.

Auditory Training Principles

Regardless of the type of AT approach, several principles have emerged that should guide AT. Most of these principles are logical, but often overlooked in AT programs. See Chapter 6 for additional illustration of the application of the principles discussed below to computerized AT.

Age- and Language-Appropriate Training

One of the primary considerations is to be sure that the materials and the tasks used are age- and language-appropriate for the patient. If materials and tasks exceed the patient's cognitive, language, or communication skills, interest and progress will be stymied. Conversely, for older children and adults materials should not be childlike. This latter situation is perhaps more common than the former —primarily because most AT materials are developed for children. AT materials that are age and communication level appropriate will engage the patient and help the clinician maintain the patient's motivation.

Developing and Maintaining Motivation

Motivation is perhaps the pivotal factor in AT, as it is for most other behavioral, rehabilitation, and learning in general (Reagan, 1973). Patients who are not motivated, for whatever reason, are not likely to be successful in an AT program. To maintain motivation, the patient must understand the rationale underlying the AT. Even children need to understand that they are enrolled in AT to improve their listening abilities, which in turn may impact their social and academic success. Teachers, parents and clinicians should explain to children, using real-world and functional examples (e.g., ability to follow a coach's directions or segment words into syllables) why they are in therapy and how it will help them.

Also heightening motivation is the use of subject matter of interest to the patient. Although it is advantageous to design AT to reinforce the academic curriculum, it is also worthwhile to include other topics of high interest to the child that might not pertain directly to the classroom but rather to the child's hobbies and social and recreational activities.

Encouragement also is crucial to maintaining motivation. Parents and teachers should encourage the child to do his or her best in therapy and in the classroom. Because AT must be intensive and can be quite repetitive, children can lose interest in AT and become bored with the tasks. Tasks must be varied; there is no substitute for variety and innovative approaches to therapy.

When a child has lost motivation or is poorly motivated at the outset, it is necessary to determine why. Is the child bored with the AT tasks? Are classmates making fun of the fact that the child attends therapy (i.e., peer pressure or ridicule)? Perhaps the child has detected parental discomfort with the therapy program, or perhaps the child has become aware of parental disagreements about the treatment program. These are just a few examples of underlying reasons why motivation toward therapy may be low. Unless these underlying issues are addressed, the effectiveness of AT will be compromised.

Motivation is so important, yet can be so fragile, that at times it may be better, especially when working with adolescents and teenagers, not to enroll the youngster in therapy rather than compromise their self-sense or overall outlook. The adolescent and teenage years are times when most students do not wish to be seen as different—they want to fit in. AT conducted using a pull-out model, which requires students to leave class, often makes this age group feel uncomfortable, especially because they fear they appear *different* to peers. Sometimes the use of the computer promotes interest and acceptance in AT, as the computer is a tool that typically engages this generation of school-aged youngsters. Despite the use of technology, for some students motivation and acceptance of AT is difficult to obtain. In these cases, offering informal approaches using AT software or other exercises that can be done at home may be the best approach. Formal AT can be postponed temporarily until circumstances permit heightened motivation and acceptance. Clearly, there are many complex issues surrounding motivation, a pivotal issue in successful AT.

Varying AT Tasks

As briefly mentioned in regard to motivation, varying AT tasks helps to maintain motivation and prevent boredom. Varying tasks also leads to greater performance gains. For example, greater gains in animals' motor skills are seen when motor training tasks vary as opposed to repetitions of the same task or set of tasks (Greenough & Bailey, 1988). An AT program targeting improved temporal resolution should include a variety of tasks, such as click discrimination, gap detection, and backward and forward masking. Each of these training tasks exercises temporal processing, providing more intensive practice while reducing the potential loss of motivation and *burnout.*

Progression of AT Tasks

In addition to varying AT tasks, it has also been shown that the tasks should be graduated in difficulty over time, as a function of the patient's performance (Greenough & Bailey, 1988). The clinician can chart patient progress manually or rely on computer software adaptive programming to determine when and by what increment

to increase task difficulty. (Adaptive algorithms automatically adjust the progression in task difficulty: as the patient reaches a certain performance criterion level, the program advances to a more demanding level of task difficulty.) The amount or degree of progression is sometimes difficult to determine; most software programs have sufficient flexibility to adjust incremental levels. The issue is the step size of the progression. If the step size is too large, performance will not improve, signaling that a smaller increment in difficulty level should be introduced (see Erber [1982], pp. 82–102). Appropriate increments in task difficulty have been shown in animal studies to be critical to improvement seen from training (Linkenhoker & Knudsen, 2002).

A Balanced Success-Failure Rate

Another important principle underlying AT is the success/failure criterion ratio to be targeted. This criterion is related to progression (i.e., incremental difficulty level) in that the level of difficulty influences an individual's ability to successfully perform a task. Therapy programs should be designed so that the client experiences success sufficient to maintain motivation at high levels. Success rates approaching 100%, however, usually indicate that the task is too easy and that the patient's auditory system is not sufficiently challenged to elicit optimal change.

One of the few studies that speaks to this issue is the work of Edeline and Weinberger (1993) who measured behavioral and electrophysiologic changes in animals that received two types of AT for frequency discrimination, one considered to be easy and the other highly difficult (i.e., requiring discriminations beyond the capability of the animals). Interestingly, the *easy* AT yielded definite improvements in frequency discrimination measured behaviorally, while the *difficult* AT yielded essentially no improvement. Direct measurements at the auditory cortex, however, showed improved receptive field response for both easy and difficult tasks. Based on their findings, training tasks should be designed to maintain motivation; however, difficulty level should not be excessive such that performance plummets and behavioral change is jeopardized.

Also related to training and performance is degree of arousal. As Wingfield (1979) noted, as arousal level progresses along the continuum from sleepiness to boredom, to mild alertness to optimal alertness, performance improves with each successive level until one reaches optimal alertness, which is equated with the highest level of performance. On the other hand, high arousal levels that are associated with stress, anxiety, and panic lead to decreased performance; therefore, one must balance task difficulty and arousal level to optimize the benefits of AT. AT tasks must be presented systematically and appropriately graduated in difficulty to ensure persistence on task and challenge, but should not be overwhelming to the patient.

Sufficient Time Must Be Allotted for Therapy

Sufficient time must be devoted to any therapeutic program, including AT, to induce change. Intensive therapy requires considerable time, which can be distributed in regard to the length of the training session, the number of training sessions, the time intervals between sessions, and the period of time over which training is conducted (Tallal et al., 1996). Duration of the training session can be limited by intrinsic factors such as attention level and performance. Unfortunately, extrinsic factors such as caseload, therapy environment, cost, schedule conflicts, and so forth are probably more common issues that frequently reduce therapy time.

Obviously, once the client makes marked improvement to the point where little or no residual problem exists, therapy can be terminated. It is more difficult to decide how long to continue training when little, slow, or no progress is being made. It is important to consider that sometimes progress is not made because insufficient time has been devoted to the training: therapy sessions are too few, and they have not spanned the necessary time frame. Although much is not known about how much therapy is needed for improvement, and certainly there are many factors that influence this calculation, it does seem based on both experimental and clinical findings and experience that considerable time is needed to evoke change in the nervous system (Delhommeau, Micheyl, Jouvent, & Collet, 2002; Greenough & Bailey, 1988; Recanzone et al., 1993; Tallal, et. al., 1996). Although the specific parameters remain to be delineated, it is fair to say that therapy sessions that last half an hour and meet only once a week are not sufficient to change the function of the auditory system. Of course, this determination will fluctuate across patients. Finally, realistic goals must be set. Unrealistic goals are not likely to be attained no matter the frequency of sessions or the duration of therapy.

Monitoring and Feedback

Careful monitoring of patient progress is important as it allows the clinician to gauge the appropriateness of the AT program and provides the basis for feedback to the client. Feedback and reinforcement must be included in the design of tasks regardless of the delivery system (i.e., manual vs. computer-assisted) (Erber, 1982). In computer-based AT, feedback is automatic: the adaptive algorithm provides positive feedback as it advances the patient through the program based on successful performance (Tallal et al., 1996). This feedback is also reflected in reward and progress animations.

Monitoring also means using appropriate testing methods to determine if progress is being made (Erber, 1982; Sanders, 1971). Ideally three types of measures should be considered in monitoring auditory changes: (1) psychophysical, (2) electrophysiologic, and (3) questionnaires and scales. These measures should be completed pre- and post-therapy, as well as during the course of treatment. Questionnaires should be completed by the patient where appropriate as well as by individuals who interact with the client in a variety of settings (e.g., other professionals, parents, teachers). (See Chapter 1 for discussion of outcome measures.)

Acoustical Control

In many cases, it is important to be able to control precisely the acoustic stimulus to achieve the desired type of training, especially when conducting formal AT. Generally, comfortable loudness levels are necessary for most effective training, although for some patients and in some situations, levels slightly above or below comfortable loudness levels are needed to achieve best results. For example, specific level differences between ears are required in the DIID training procedure (as discussed below under Recent Human Studies in Auditory Discrimination Training [Intensity-Frequency]). In all cases, however, acoustical control is an important principle guiding effective and safe delivery of AT.

The Role of Auditory Neuroplasticity

Brief Orientation to Neuroplasticity

Auditory plasticity is discussed in Chapters 1 and 3 of this volume; however, a brief orientation is provided here, with a focus on several particularly relevant aspects of neuroplasticity for AT. Auditory plasticity underlies the alteration of the brain evoked by appropriate AT. Neural plasticity can be defined as the alteration of nerve cells to better conform to immediate environmental influences, with this alteration often associated with behavioral change (Musiek & Berge, 1998). Scheich (1991) described three types of neural plasticity. *Developmental plasticity* results from the maturation of the nervous system as more connections are made between neurons and myelination of neurons progresses. Neural maturation is dependent on stimulation: enriched stimulation increases maturational rate (Kalil, 1989). *Compensatory plasticity* occurs after damage to the nervous system as other areas of the brain assume functions of the damaged areas.

The third type of plasticity is *learning-related*. Although all three types can play a role in AT, learning-related plasticity is the primary plasticity underlying the success of AT and other behavioral rehabilitation efforts. Plasticity permits changes in the neural substrate that supports performance on a particular task or related tasks. Most importantly, it must be recognized that plasticity is a function of the CANS; plasticity is not a feature of the peripheral auditory system.

Long-Term Potentiation

Long-term potentiation (LTP) is thought to be the mechanism underlying learning and memory (Hebb, 1949). Specifically, LTP refers to an increase in strength of synaptic transmission related to repetitive use of the neurons involved (Bliss & Lomo, 1973). In a general sense, LTP can be considered a form of plasticity. Exposing an animal (or human) repeatedly to acoustic stimuli should enhance the LTP and also the perception of that repeated stimulus. AT and other behavioral interventions may increase synaptic activity and thereby facilitate behavioral change. Interestingly, LTP has been measured months after repetitive exposure has ended (Greenough & Bailey, 1988). This finding bodes well for long-term maintenance of changes observed immediately following treatment.

What Has Been Learned from the Vestibular System?

Perhaps not well known have been the insights suggesting the potential of AT derived from studies and observation of the vestibular system. It is now well known that the human brain accommo-

dates after surgical ablation of the vestibular labyrinth. Immediately following a labyrinthectomy, patients will experience dizziness and feel imbalanced; however, over the course of the next few days, their balance will return due to compensation by central mechanisms, provided the patient is somewhat active during this postsurgical period (Ludman, 2003; Bamiou & Luxon, 2003 for review). Another example of the accommodative capability of central mechanisms can be seen in benign positional vertigo, a condition associated with particular positions or movements. One of the most successful treatments for this condition is repeated movements that actually induce the dizziness. This "vestibular training" forces the central system to accommodate, and in time the dizziness ceases to be a problem (Bamiou & Luxon, 2003). These findings in the vestibular system reflecting compensation by the central nervous system provide insight as to how training and plasticity work together to improve patients' function. Given the close association between the vestibular system and the auditory system, one would expect that training and plasticity work similarly in the auditory system as observed in the vestibular system.

Results of CANS Stimulation/Training— Selected Animal Models

It has been well established using animal models that auditory stimulation induces changes in the underlying neural substrate of the CANS (Hassmannova et al., 1981; Knudsen, 1988; Linkenhoker, von der Ohe, & Knudsen, 2004; Recanzone et al., 1993). CANS plasticity is the basis of these physiologic changes (Salvi &

Henderson, 1996). The inference drawn from these animal studies is that if these stimulation paradigms can induce CANS changes in animals, then stimulation delivered through AT of the human auditory system should induce similar neurophysiologic changes. Considered briefly below are some results from selective animal studies that may apply to human AT. (See Chapter 3 in Volume I of this Handbook for additional discussion of neurophysiologic changes induced by training.)

Perhaps most directly relevant to AT are the findings of Recanzone and colleagues (1993). In their studies, owl monkeys were trained on an auditory task which required the monkeys to complete a series of frequency discrimination trials using a specific reference frequency. When cortical responses were obtained following training, results indicated that the sharpness of tuning and latency of the evoked response for the trained frequency was greater when compared to untrained controls. Perhaps most importantly, however, was that the amount of cortical tissue that was associated with the trained frequency was greater than that of untrained controls. This indicates substantial cortical reorganization (e.g., plasticity) for stimuli used in the AT paradigm.

Stimulation of the CANS also has been noted as a direct precursor to cell growth. Hassmannova et al. (1981) observed functional and biochemical changes in the juvenile rat cortex following acoustic stimulation with tone pips. Among changes seen was a significant increase in total RNA content in cortical neurons following training relative to the no-stimulation control group. This difference persisted and was maintained up to 4 weeks after the end of training. Their results suggest that stimulation initiated processes by which new cell division could occur.

Interestingly, the CANS can be modified regardless of whether stimulation increases *or* decreases (Hassmannova et al., 1981; Webster & Webster, 1977). These modifications occur so that the CANS can process acoustic cues optimally when performing a specific function, as seen in the localization research of Knudson and colleagues (Knudsen, 1988; Linkenhoker & Knudsen, 2002; Linkenhoker et al., 2004).

Knudsen (1988) modified the localization cues presented to barn owls by decreasing the amount of stimulation in one ear (i.e., inserting an ear plug unilaterally). This temporary unilateral loss was created to interfere with the normal binaural localization cues utilized by the owls in hunting. Although localization ability was initially impaired after the loss, performance gradually returned to normal as the CANS adjusted to this new pattern of stimulation. When the ear plug was removed and the unilateral loss corrected, localization performance was again impaired. However, as the CANS again adjusted, this time to increased stimulation, performance returned to normal.

Although training-induced localization changes are generally greater in juvenile owls, there is evidence to suggest that adult owls also demonstrate the plasticity necessary for effective AT (Linkenhoker & Knudsen, 2002; Linkenhoker et al., 2004). For instance, adult barn owls, which learned to localize using incongruent visual-auditory cues as juveniles, showed abnormal anatomic projections in the auditory cortex that were attributed to this early experience. This persistence of the projections may benefit any readaptation which may occur later in life (Linkenhoker et al., 2004). Additionally, adult barn owls that undergo incremental change, rather than a single large change in visual-auditory cues, learn to adapt better to subsequent large changes in these cues (Linkenhoker & Knudsen, 2002). This finding speaks to the advantage of incremental training in adult subjects (as alluded to earlier under Progression of AT Tasks).

The additional benefits of using training to reorganize the CANS rather than using stimulation alone has been demonstrated by Bao and colleagues (Bao et al., 2004). In this study, rats had to find food in a maze while noise pulses were presented. The rate of noise pulse presentation indicated distance to the food source. As the rats approached the food, the rate of noise pulse presentation increased. The response of auditory cortical neurons to fast-rate noise pulses was compared among this group of rats, a second group which received auditory stimulation (i.e., white noise pulses) but were given food freely, and a third control group which did not experience auditory stimulation. Results indicated that greater neural responses were obtained in the trained group. The responses obtained from the second and third groups did not differ significantly. These findings speak to the importance of using structured AT rather than relying on passive stimulation when attempting to induce lasting cortical changes.

Recent Human Studies in Auditory Discrimination Training (Intensity-Frequency)

One of the most fundamental abilities of the auditory system is discrimination of frequency, intensity, and timing differences within the acoustic signal. The abil-ity to discriminate auditory information is essential for many obvious reasons, including basic orientation and survival. Perhaps the most important use of auditory discrimination for our purposes is its role in the detection and processing of the rapid acoustic changes in speech that underlie language processing and in particular phonologic awareness (Tallal et al., 1996). Children with learning disabilities and associated disorders often demonstrate deficits in phonologic awareness and abnormal neurophysiologic representation of auditory stimuli in the CANS despite having a normal peripheral auditory system (Hayes et al., 2003, King et al., 2002; Kraus, 1999). Auditory discrimination training can benefit these children, as well as other children and adults demonstrating listening difficulties.

Much of the evidence for the efficacy of auditory discrimination training comes from the work of Kraus, Tremblay, and colleagues (Kraus et al., 1995; Kraus, 1999; Tremblay, Kraus, Carrell, & McGee, 1997; Tremblay, Kraus, & McGee, 1998; Tremblay, Kraus, McGee, Ponton, & Otis, 2001; Tremblay & Kraus, 2002). Kraus et al. (1995) exposed participants with normal peripheral and central hearing to an auditory discrimination protocol and obtained pre- and post-training behavioral and electrophysiologic measures. The training protocol consisted of discrimination of two synthesized /da/ tokens that differed in the onset frequencies of the second and third formant (F2 and F3) transitions. Training was divided into six, one-hour sessions over the course of one week, during which participants determined whether two successive tokens were the same or different. The mismatched negativity response (MMN), an auditory cortical response that occurs as a result of acoustic change in a repetitive sequence of stimuli, served as the electrophysiologic outcome measure.

Efficacy of training was documented in both the behavioral and the electrophysiologic measures. For half the participants, discrimination of /da/ tokens increased from 56% pre-training to 67% post-training. This behavioral increase persisted one month following the termination of training. Following discrimination training, the duration and amplitude of the MMN was larger for the vast majority of the participants. Interestingly, some of the electrophysiologic changes were not reflected in behavioral change. Whereas only half the sample could behaviorally identify the changes between the two /da/ tokens post-training, electrophysiologic changes were observed in the large majority of participants following training. Taken together, these findings suggest that training-related changes may be below the threshold of conscious detection in this subset of participants. Additionally, although training requires the attention of the participants, the measurement of training-induced physiologic changes can occur in the absence of attention, as indicated by the MMN results.

Tremblay and colleagues (1997) also investigated the efficacy of discrimination training in a manner similar to Kraus et al. (1995) using normal hearing participants. In addition to determining training efficacy, Tremblay et al (1997) sought to determine to what extent discrimination training with one set of tokens would transfer (i.e., generalize) to another set of tokens not used in training. The training stimuli were two consonant-vowel (CV) continua with voice onset times (VOTs) of different, but similar, durations. The training continuum was comprised of labial consonants, whereas the post-training measures utilized both labial and alveolar continua. In addition to discriminating stimulus pairs, participants were asked to identify, from a closed set, which CV (differing by VOT duration) had been presented. Training extended over a five-day period for the experimental group; a second control group did not receive any training. Behavioral outcome measures included measures similar to those used during training. As in the Kraus et al. (1995) study, Tremblay and colleagues recorded the MMN as the electrophysiologic outcome measure. Post-training results revealed that the trained group, but not the control group, showed increases in behavioral discrimination for both the labial (trained) and alveolar (untrained) CVs. The effect was smaller, however, for the alveolar tokens. For the behavioral identification measure, post-training improvements were seen for the trained group on the labial (trained) VOTs only; however, MMN responses showed an increase in area and duration for both the labial (trained) and alveolar (untrained) VOTs, although the effect was smaller for the alveolar tokens. An increase in MMN duration was greater over the left frontal lobe.

Similar to the findings of Kraus et al. (1995), the results of Tremblay et al. (1997) speak to the efficacy of AT in improving auditory discrimination ability. In addition, the results demonstrate how the effects of training can generalize beyond the stimuli used during the training session. Although the effects were smaller, improvements in the ability to detect differences in alveolar tokens were noted even though these tokens were not used during training. The increased MMN duration in the left hemisphere reflects the greater benefit of training to this hemisphere probably due to the greater activity in the left frontal lobe because of the linguistic nature of the stimuli.

Although the MMN response has shown some promise as a research tool, it has yet to show high clinical utility (Tremblay et al., 2001; Tremblay & Kraus, 2002). For this reason, Tremblay and colleagues (2001, 2002) conducted additional AT studies that were similar in nature to those described above, with the exception that the N1-P2 was used as the electrophysiologic outcome measure. It has been suggested that the N1-P2 may be more clinically feasible than the MMN (Tremblay et al., 2001).

Participants were again normal hearing individuals who underwent right ear discrimination and identification training with labial CV tokens (differing by VOT duration) over a period of one week. A similar task was used to obtain post-training behavioral outcomes. The N1-P2 response was recorded from several locations on the scalp and separate recordings were made for the two VOT stimuli (e.g., the CV at either end of the continuum). Post-training, behavioral discrimination performance increased almost 30% (Tremblay et al., 2001). Similarly, post-training improvements were seen in the amplitude of the N1-P2 complex at Cz when the stimuli were presented at a slow rate (Tremblay et al., 2001). When the amplitudes of P1, N1, and P2 were measured relative to baseline, it was noted that the P1 and the N1 increased over the right frontal lobe only, whereas P2 increases were noted bilaterally (Tremblay & Kraus, 2002). These differences in the late potentials were the same regardless of which CV stimulus was used.

These post-training improvements are consistent with the MMN trends reported earlier by Kraus et al. (1995) and Trem-

blay et al. (1997). The N1-P2 potential likely reflects early cortical processes relevant to stimulus encoding and the detection of speech. The MMN likely reflects later processes involving the discrimination of changes in the speech signal (Tremblay et al. 2001; Tremblay & Kraus, 2002). The series of Kraus and Tremblay studies using MMN and N1-P2 suggest that training-induced changes using a discrimination paradigm may not only impact auditory processes involved in discrimination, but also the earlier encoding of auditory stimuli as well. The laterality effect noted for P1 and N1 was interpreted by Tremblay & Kraus (2002) to mean that small voicing distinctions are processed as nonlinguistic acoustic cues. This interpretation was suggested as right, not left, hemisphere changes were primarily observed for these potentials. The bilateral P2 changes, on the other hand, may represent a cognitive increase in attention that is necessary for learning to occur.

The effects of auditory discrimination training also have been examined using functional magnetic resonance imaging (fMRI). Jancke, Gaab, Wustenberg, Scheich, and Heinze (2001) trained normal hearing participants for a total of nine hours using an oddball paradigm, similar to that used to evoke the MMN. A frequent 950-Hz tone was presented along with a less frequent 952-, 954-, or 958-Hz tone. Participants were asked to press a button whenever they heard one of the infrequent tones. fMRI imaging was conducted pre-, post-, and during training. A control (C) group also was recruited which did not participate in the training, but did participate in imaging for the pre- and postsession. Subsequent analysis revealed that the experimental group could be further divided into one that demonstrated (T+) post-training improvement and one group that did not show improvements (T−). Compared to the T− and the C groups, following training the T+ group showed a decrease in response from the superior temporal gyrus (bilaterally) and from the planum polare (right hemisphere) for the 954- and 958-Hz tones. fMRI images for the T+ group are presented in Figure 4–2. Consistent with Kraus et al. (1995), this research demonstrates that auditory discrimination training can improve behavioral auditory discrimination ability. In addition, Jancke et al. (2001) demonstrated increased discrimination ability paired with a reduction in activation from certain auditory areas within the cortex. Jancke and colleagues suggested that this decrease in activation is consistent with "fast learning theories." These theories suggest that as optimal sensory units are selected for a task, processing becomes more efficient and automatic. As a result, less activation corresponds to a streamlining of auditory processing for optimal performance.

Similar to the work of Tremblay et al. (1997) on generalization of training effects reported in this section, Delhommeau and colleagues (Delhommeau et al., 2002; Delhommeau, Micheyl, & Jouvent, 2005) examined to what extent training generalizes to untrained stimuli. Delhommeau et al. (2002) asked normal hearing participants to determine which of two 1000-Hz tones of variable duration was most similar to a 200-ms, 1000-Hz reference tone, thereby establishing a duration discrimination threshold re: 200 ms. This training was conducted using the right ear for eight sessions over a period of four weeks. Baseline and post-training outcomes were measured using three different durations as a reference (i.e., 40, 100, and 200 ms) to examine transfer of training across different stimulus durations. Following training, participants improved their ability to correctly identify the most similar tone for each of three 1000-Hz duration reference tones, demonstrating that training generalized beyond the trained reference stimulus (i.e., 200 ms). The performance improvement was larger

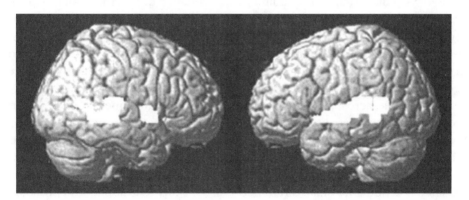

Figure 4–2. White areas reflect significant decreases in activation for the T+ group following frequency discrimination training. Decreases in activation may be consistent with "fast learning theories." (Adapted from Jancke, Gaab, Wustenberg, Scheich, & Heinze [2001]).

for the 100- and 200-ms duration stimuli than for the 40-ms duration stimulus, perhaps a consequence of reduced temporal integration, although other possibilities were considered by the researchers (Delhommeau et al., 2002). These results suggest that discrimination training using temporal information is relatively non-duration-dependent and generalizes reasonably well.

Delhommeau et al. (2005) also investigated the degree to which frequency discrimination training generalizes to other frequencies. Participants were trained for six sessions in a manner similar to Delhommeau et al. (2002), with the exception that participants were trained on only a single reference frequency. The reference frequency varied, however, across participants and included: 750, 1500, 3000, or 6000 Hz. Baseline and post-training measures included all four frequencies as a reference. Post-training measures were recorded at three separate times. Organized in this way, the study was able to examine the generalizability of frequency discrimination training to untrained frequencies over a period of time following the termination of training.

Several important findings emerged. Discrimination thresholds improved following training. There was no interaction between session and training frequency, suggesting that the benefit from training was comparable across all frequencies, whether or not they were used in training. However, additional analysis challenged this second finding. When measures from the three post-training sessions were examined individually, a small difference between the trained and untrained frequencies was observed for the first post-training session, but not for the later two. The difference between the trained and untrained frequencies disappeared

in the later two sessions because performance for untrained frequencies became better, not because performance for the trained frequency deteriorated over time. This finding suggests that a difference in discrimination ability for trained and untrained frequencies may exist immediately following training, even if the difference is very small; however, performance for untrained frequencies quickly improves following exposure to the untrained stimulus.

Delhommeau et al. (2005) explained their findings as evidence of metalearning, or learning about the basic nature of the discrimination task, which leads to improved performance for untrained frequencies. This notion of metalearning may also explain the post-training bilateral P2 increases reported by Tremblay & Kraus (2002). Although both findings might be somewhat incongruous with the findings of Recanzone and colleagues (1993) reported earlier in this chapter (i.e., that the amount of cortical tissue associated with trained frequencies exceeded that for untrained frequencies), utilization of general cognitive resources to enhance task performance is not necessarily mutually exclusive of neurophysiologic changes that are specific to the central auditory system. (See Chapter 5 for discussion of metacognitive processes and their role in intervention.)

Moore, Rosenberg, and Coleman (2005) looked at the generalization of AT in a broader sense. They used a phoneme continuum discrimination task to examine the affects of AT on receptive language skills, skills that are auditory-based, but only indirectly related to the phoneme discrimination task employed. To this end, they recruited normal-hearing children and exposed them to four weeks of training (i.e., three days a week for

30 minutes a day) using a computerized discrimination task in which participants were required to determine which of two alternatives was identical to a reference. Each participant was exposed to several different phoneme continua. The procedure was adaptive, becoming more difficult as participants improved. Assessment measures, administered pre- and post-training, included a phonologic assessment battery and a word discrimination test. A second group was recruited that did not participate in the training and was used as a control.

Results provided some evidence for the efficacy of the AT program. Phonologic awareness and word discrimination scores were significantly higher post-training for the experimental group only and these scores remained high when reassessed some time after the initial post-training measure. There was no correlation, however, between performance on the training game and improvement in word discrimination and phonologic awareness, suggesting that, although mean differences were found, it was difficult to tease out these effects at the individual level. Moore et al. (2005) mentioned that nonauditory factors (e.g., attention) may have benefitted from training and this may complicate interpretation of some analyses. Additionally, because many phoneme continua were used, the amount of training received on any one set may have been too small to produce measurable auditory changes at the individual level. That being said, the mean differences noted for the experimental group on the outcome measures, especially for phonologic awareness, speak to some aggregated effect of the training protocol on the auditory discrimination performance of the participants.

Recent Studies in Temporal Processing Training

Like auditory discrimination, temporal processing, or the sequencing, ordering, discrimination, and integration of acoustic events over a period of time, also is integral to auditory processing. Temporal response patterns in the brain have been attributed a very important role as organizing structures that aid in the development and maintenance of unique neural representations, such as speech sounds (Tallal, Merzenich, Miller, & Jenkins, 1998). Temporal processing also has been shown to be important in the normal development of reading. For instance, Kujala et al. (2000) found that children with dyslexia often show a fundamental deficit in temporal processing skills. Training temporal processing, therefore, could potentially have many far-reaching, secondary effects, beyond the direct remediation of auditory processes.

To investigate the role of temporal processing in the dyslexic population, Kujala et al. (2001) provided nonverbal AT to a pediatric dyslexic population. Central to this investigation was an attempt to determine the role of an auditory deficit in dyslexia as comorbid or causal. To this end, AT involved stimuli with no linguistic features. Kujala and colleagues reasoned that if training was not speech related and still successfully treated the disorder to some degree, then auditory processing must play a causal role in dyslexia at some level.

Training was conducted for 10 minutes twice a week for a total of seven weeks. The training stimuli consisted of sound elements which varied in frequency, intensity, or duration. Participants were asked to match a sound sequence to visual analogs of the sequence on the computer screen (e.g., duration was conveyed by the length of the bar, intensity by the height, etc.). As participants were asked to choose a correct response among several options, this was technically both a temporal processing and a discrimination task. By removing all linguistic elements from the stimuli and the response, the task isolated the fundamental elements of reading that are dependent on temporal processing. The MMN and four measures of reading-related skills, including spelling and phonologic awareness measures, were obtained before and after training. A dyslexic group that did not undergo training was used as a control.

Although both the experimental and the control groups showed numerical improvement on the reading skills outcome measures, only the experimental group showed a statistically significant increase in the number of words read correctly and the rate at which words were read. Additionally, the experimental group showed greater amplitude of the MMN following training. Interestingly, the MMN also showed a moderate correlation with some of the behavioral reading measures: as reading scores improved, the amplitude of the MMN tended to increase.

Kujala and colleagues (2001) interpreted this pattern of results to suggest that reading difficulties in dyslexia originate from bottom-up deficits in auditory processing. Their conclusion follows from finding improvements in the MMN, an auditory measure, correlated with reading improvements, in the context of an experimental manipulation that was auditory but nonlinguistic. Their findings suggest the utility of temporal processing training as a treatment for both audi-

tory processing and other processes mediated by auditory processing (e.g., reading). Kujala et al. (2001) emphasized, however, that training also was successful because it was conducted early (children were approximately 7 years of age) and the semantic component was removed from the training paradigm. Training paradigms that do not take such steps may not be as successful.

Foxton, Brown, Chambers, and Griffiths (2004) administered temporal processing training to a normal hearing population using a paradigm very similar to Kujala et al. (2001). Training was conducted over seven sessions for 25 minutes a session with no more than three days separating a session. Participants were included in one of four groups. The visual-auditory contour comparison task (VAC) group was trained using reference stimuli represented both visually and auditorily (e.g., frequency of the reference stimulus was represented aurally, as well as visually by representing the spatial location of bars: the higher the bar, the higher the frequency). Following the reference, participants were required to determine if auditory sequences in a subsequent trial were the same as or different from the reference trial. Participants were instructed to attend only to the relative contour of the sequence and not to the actual frequency value. The absolute frequency of tones in a sequence could diverge from the reference; however, if the relative frequency differences between each tone in a sequence were identical to the reference, then the contour was deemed to be identical.

Training for the pitch contour discrimination (PCD) group was identical to that of the VAC group, with the exception that their training included no visual information during the reference trial.

Training of the actual pitch discrimination (AD) group was identical to the PCD group with the exception that participants were trained to attend to actual frequency changes in the sequence and not just the contour. The AD group was asked to identify which sequence sounded identical in pitch *and* contour to the reference trial. Finally, a control (C) group that did not undergo training was utilized. Despite different training regimens, each group completed all three tasks pre- and post-training (e.g., the PCD group completed the AD and VAC tasks in addition to the PCD task before and after training).

Significant differences among groups were seen in the amount of improvement on the PCD measure. Specifically, both the PCD and AD groups showed improvement on this measure, with the effect being much bigger for the former group. The VAC and C groups did not show any improvement on this measure. No group showed any improvement on the AD and VAC measures following training. Foxton et al. (2004) explained the finding that frequency discrimination alone (e.g., AD group) aided in contour discrimination by suggesting that proper frequency discrimination also requires proper contour discrimination. The AD group may not have shown a benefit on AD measures because the attended-to tones may have been masked by surrounding tones (i.e., informational masking).

Foxton et al. (2004) interpreted their results as evidence of the importance of contour training. Contour perception is important for frequency and duration pattern tasks, for speech perception and auditory-language processing (conveying many properties such as stress and intonation), for music perception, and for reading (Musiek, Kibbe, & Baran, 1984).

Foxton et al. (2004) suggested that AT using contour discrimination tasks and training on a musical instrument may aid in both the improvement of pitch contour perception skills and literacy.

Clinical Training of Temporal Processing

A popular computerized AT program currently used clinically to train temporal processing and phonologic awareness is Fast ForWord (FFW) (Merzenich et al., 1996; Tallal et al., 1996). This program presents training within the context of language (in some ways similar to the approach incorporated in Earobics discussed below under Auditory-Language Training Approaches); however, the scientific foundation of FFW and the acoustic manipulations introduced lead us to categorize FFW as a temporal processing training program. (See Chapter 6 for discussion of computerized auditory training.)

Several studies have demonstrated the efficacy of FFW. Temple et al. (2003) trained dyslexics on FFW for 100 minutes a day, five days a week, for almost a month. Pre- and post-training measures included fMRI. During the fMRI sessions, participants were asked to perform a rhyming task (i.e., push a button if the sounds associated with two letters rhyme, for instance "T" and "D"). A normal non-dyslexic control group also completed the rhyming task but did not participate in the training. Increased activation in the left temporoparietal cortex and inferior frontal gyrus were observed following training and these increases were positively correlated with improvements on some nonreading, language tasks.

Increased activation also was seen in the right inferior and superior frontal gyri and middle temporal gyrus, and these increases were positively correlated with a measure of phonologic processing.

Temple and colleagues (2003) observed changes in activation of cortical areas known to support phonologic processing; however, the primary benefits of increased activation in these areas would be expected to be seen for auditory processing. Moreover, cortical activation changes in these areas suggest that treatment exerted both normalizing and compensatory effects. Normalizing effects were seen in the temporoparietal and frontal gyrus regions, where previously depressed activity relative to normal controls increased. Compensatory effects were seen in the remaining cortical areas displaying increased activation, as these are areas that are not typically activated in normal hearing individuals but which nonetheless showed benefit from training. It should be noted that these increases in activation are somewhat inconsistent with the "fast learning theories" described previously in this chapter for discrimination training (Jancke et al., 2001), whereby activation decreases as processing becomes more efficient and automatic. Differences in the direction of activation changes following training may be attributed to the type of training used (frequency discrimination vs. temporal processing training) and/or the clinical status of the participants (normal hearing vs. dyslexic) across the two studies.

FFW also has been investigated in a population with specific language impairment (Agnew, Dorn, & Eden, 2004). This group was trained for 100 minutes a day, five days a week, for four to six weeks. Outcome measures included an auditory duration discrimination task and a visual duration discrimination task. For the auditory duration discrimination task, participants were required to judge whether the duration of a second tone was shorter or longer relative to a preceding 800-ms reference tone. Although technically a discrimination measure, duration discrimination also is an important element in temporal processing and was, therefore, a relevant outcome measure for a study of FFW. The visual task was identical in design to the auditory task, with the exception that pictures were used as stimuli instead of sounds. This visual task was included to determine to what extent AT benefits generalized to other modalities. Two phonologic awareness measures were administered to assess reading benefits.

Pre- and post treatment comparisons revealed significantly improved auditory duration discrimination by almost 15%. No significant improvements were seen on the visual duration discrimination task or the two measures of phonologic awareness; hence, AT did not generalize to the visual modality, suggesting the specificity of this type of training to the auditory domain. AT, as administered through FFW, does not appear to benefit nonauditory skills related to learning, such as attention. That is, if attention were influenced, then multimodality effects would have been expected. This contrasts somewhat with the generalizability of auditory discrimination training discussed earlier (Delhommeau et al., 2002; Delhommeau et al., 2005; Tremblay et al., 1997). However, in the auditory discrimination paradigms, generalization was examined within the auditory modality. The Agnew et al. (2004) study suggests that auditory discrimination training may not generalize across modalities.

Despite the findings of improved performance described above, the overall efficacy of FFW has been challenged for several reasons (Friel-Patti, Loeb, & Gilliam, 2001; Gilliam, Loeb, & Friel-Patti, 2001). For instance, Gilliam et al. (2001) argued that FFW does not truly train temporal processing, noting that no clear relationship has been established between several indirect measures of temporal processing (e.g., perception of backward masked speech) and treatment using FFW. These researchers do not deny, however, that FFW may benefit some aspects of language comprehension and production.

A new training strategy being developed at the University of Connecticut (UCONN) Neuroaudiology Lab utilizes the game SIMON™ to treat temporal processing deficits (Musiek, 2005). The training is incremental in difficulty, starting with simple sequencing tasks and progressing to more complicated temporal ordering based on the patient's success. Because the SIMON game provides visual cues, the patient is instructed to perform pertinent tasks without looking at the table-top electronic device. The simplest task requires the patient to label tones. Tones can be labeled in any fashion; for instance, "one" may correspond to the lowest pitch tone and "four" may be assigned to the highest pitch tone. Following success on this simple labeling task, the patient can then be asked to indicate any time a target tone occurs. Similarly, this is followed by the more difficult task of identifying a sequence of target tones (e.g., tone "one" followed by tone "three"). Once proficiency is gained on all of the above relatively simple tasks, the patient is ready to tackle more complex tasks. In the next phase of training, again without visual cues, the patient plays a tone, to which the device generates a second tone. The patient is required to label the new tone played back by SIMON as higher or lower in frequency than the last tone in the sequence.

Although no efficacy data have yet been collected for this training technique, positive results have been found by Pisoni and colleagues (Cleary, Pisoni, & Geers, 2001; Karpicke & Pisoni, 2004; Pisoni & Cleary, 2004) using a similar paradigm to examine memory. Developed concurrently and independently from the approach used at UCONN, this treatment approach uses a SIMON-like instrument to play verbal stimuli connected to each of four buttons (i.e., labeled either by color or digits) and includes an option to present visual patterns alone without any audio input. Participants are asked to repeat sequences presented by the device. The device has been used successfully to quantify implicit memory differences between a cochlear implant population and normal hearing controls (Cleary et al., 2001). Additionally, and perhaps more relevant to the present chapter, their approach has been shown to induce learning.

Karpicke and Pisoni (2004) found that when normal hearing participants were trained on sequences which, unbeknownst to the participants, followed grammatical rules, they performed better on novel post-training sequences that followed those grammatical rules than for novel sequences that followed a grammar, but not the one used during training. That is to say, participants' memory was better for sequences that followed ordering rules that they had previously learned during training. Although Karpicke's and Pisoni's training objectives and stimuli differ from that of the UCONN SIMON protocol, the use of similar procedures and the reliance on brain plasticity suggest that the SIMON training protocol may also prove to be efficacious.

Other AT paradigms, which also focus on temporal processing tasks, are being developed at UCONN. One such paradigm utilizes a keyboard or piano to train temporal sequencing abilities. Initially, two different notes are played for the patient in the absence of visual cues. The patient must label them each as high or low pitch in the order that they were played. As the patient improves, task complexity can be increased in at least three ways. First, progressively more notes can be added to the series and labeled by the patient accordingly. Second, the pitch of the notes can be made more similar by selecting keys which are closer together. Third, the interval between each note can be decreased, requiring faster processing of the series in order to provide a correct response. A paradigm which is similar to the piano protocol uses note cadences. The patient is asked to replicate a particular finger tapping cadence, which can be increased in complexity as the task is mastered. Both of the above paradigms train the patient's ability to order a sequence of rapid auditory events.

Dichotic Training

Children with (C)APD often demonstrate a left ear deficit on dichotic speech tasks (Musiek, Gollegly, & Baran, 1984). A published case study in 1998 reported significant improvement in binaural listening tasks and academic performance when dichotic training tasks were incorporated in the AT program (Musiek & Schochat 1998). The dichotic interaural intensity difference training (DIID) procedure was used in that case study.

The DIID is derived from research conducted on *split-brain* patients in the late 1970s and throughout the 1980s. These studies demonstrated that split-brain patients are not able to transfer information from the right to left hemisphere due to sectioning of the corpus callosum (Musiek, Kibbe, & Baran, 1984b). Kimura (1961) demonstrated suppression of the ipsilateral pathways during dichotic listening, rendering the auditory system a crossed system. This means that during dichotic listening right ear information is routed to the left cortex and left ear information is routed to the right cortex. Because most people are left hemisphere language dominant, words, numbers, or sentences presented to the right ear are conducted to the speech hemisphere and are easily repeated. Speech stimuli presented to the left ear must cross the corpus callosum to access the language dominant hemisphere in order for the patient to verbally respond. Because the corpus callosum is severed in split-brain patients, this crossover cannot occur and a severe left ear deficit on dichotic listening occurs. Interestingly, Musiek, Kibbe & Baran, (1984) reported that major left ear deficits also occur in children—especially those with learning disabilities, probably due to delayed myelination of the corpus callosum.

Musiek and Schochat (1998) found that if dichotic stimuli with greater intensity were presented to the left ear relative to the right ear, scores for the left ear increased and scores for the right ear decreased for both split-brain patients and children with left ear deficits. By training children with various dichotic stimuli using greater intensity to the poorer ear (typically the left ear) to maintain good performance in that ear, the intensity level of the stronger ear could be gradually raised over a period of time and the poorer ear would maintain its high performance. Some children required more training than others; however, a high percentage did improve their left ear performance. Often after training, both ears performed well on subsequent dichotic listening tests. Though the mechanisms underlying this "dichotic improvement" remain under investigation, it appears that greater intensity to the left ear releases the left auditory pathway from right auditory pathway suppression.

Ongoing research has revealed the DIID to be a highly promising tool for improving left ear deficits in children with (C)APD (Figure 4–3). A recent report on a patient with mild head trauma who demonstrated a left ear deficit on dich-otic digits and showed marked improvement on dichotic listening after DIID training, demonstrated the potential of the DIID to improve dichotic listening across a range of patients, not only children with learning difficulties (Musiek et al., 2004). A number of clinical trials are underway to test the clinical feasibility of DIID training.

Administering the DIID is straightforward. A variety of dichotic test materials (e.g., digits, words, sentences, CVs) and a two-channel audiometer are essentially all that is required. The DIID should be applied as both a binaural integration and

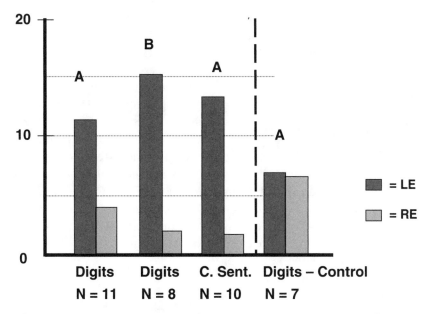

Mean % Dichotic Improvement from DIID Training

Figure 4–3. Mean dichotic listening performance from training on the DIID from two preliminary studies indicated by *A* (Musiek, unpublished data) and *B* (Wertz & Moncrieff, unpublished data). Note the improvement primarily for the left ear. Training for study *A* was approximately three months and two to three 20-minute sessions per week. Training for study *B* was for 30 minutes, three times a week for four weeks. The tests administered were the dichotic digits (Digits) and competing sentences (C. Sent.).

a separation task. The integration task requires the patient to respond to the stimuli in both ears; the separation task requires the patient to ignore one ear and respond to stimuli presented in the other ear. If the patient shows a greater problem with binaural integration than separation, DIID training should emphasize this aspect of dichotic listening and vice versa. The amount and length of training that is needed is determined by the patient's own progress; however, we generally suggest training three to four times per week for 20 to 30 minute sessions. Further research, however, may provide more direction in regard to the optimal intensiveness and frequency of DIID training. The DIID training procedure can be adapted for application in school and at home using modifications of a stereo system and interchangeable earphones. This informal approach is still considered experimental (Musiek et al., 2004).

Auditory-Language Training Approaches

Several AT approaches do not fit easily into the categories previously discussed in this chapter. These approaches usually include a variety of AT procedures that are included in one training session or possibly over several sessions. Two such training programs serve as good examples of this general category of AT. One is a workbook-based approach developed by Christine Sloan (Sloan, 1986) and the other is Earobics®, a well-known computerized program. These two general AT programs focus on basic phonemic awareness, and acoustic discrimination and identification using speech-language

tasks. Because these programs cover auditory-language training in broad terms they can be used to treat some of the associated phonologic awareness deficits often presented by individuals diagnosed with (C)APD.

The Sloan workbook and the Earobics program incorporated some of the same stimuli and approaches to AT first introduced by Carhart and DiCarlo, mentioned earlier in this chapter. Earobics includes some exercises with time- and intensity-altered stimuli, which certainly supports temporal training. The focus of this program, however, is directed to phonological awareness training. Several versions of Earobics are available for different age levels (4–7, 7–10, adolescent and adult), as well as a version for home use. The home version is a valuable tool that allows the clinician to extend training into the home.

Some evidence suggests the efficacy of the Earobics program in improving language processing in children with learning problems. Increases in the amplitude of evoked responses to speech stimuli related to brainstem and cortical substrate indicated possible improvements in electrophysiologic representation in the CANS following training with Earobics (Russo, Nicole, Zecker, Hayes, & Kraus, 2005; Warrier, Johnson, Hayes, Nicol, & Kraus, 2004).

AT with Preschool Children

Unfortunately, it is not easy to definitively diagnose (C)APD in children under 7 years of age due to the difficulty posed by central auditory tests designed to challenge a redundant CANS. This does not mean however, that one should not begin AT with younger children deemed at-risk for auditory/listening problems (Musiek & Chermak, 1995). Indeed, listening activities typically are part of the preschool curriculum, as they should be given that listening activities occupy approximately 75% of a school day (Hubble-Dahlquist, 1998). It is appropriate to involve all young children in listening activities and games, not just those who may be at risk for (C)APD. These games can be conducted at home or at school, by parents or teachers. There are a variety of commercial listening games on the market that can be used with preschoolers including Earobics, which has a version for young children (4–7 years) that can be used by parents. With some ingenuity, a number of listening games can be formulated easily. Following are several examples of listening activities for children 4 year of age and older. The reader is referred to Chermak and Musiek (2002) and Musiek and Chermak (1995) for more expansive discussions of AT for young children, as well as activities for school-aged children.

Finding the Target Sound or Word

An adult reads a story to a child or group of children. Before reading, the children are asked to listen for a certain word or sound that occurs in the story. The children are required to raise their hands each time a target word or sound is heard or to keep track of the number of times the target is heard and report at the story's end. The latter variation trains memory as well as selective attention. The former variation might interfere with comprehension; therefore, it is

important to encourage the listener to attend to the story and not only to the individual target.

Localization

The child is blindfolded and asked to point to the location of the person who is speaking while roaming across the room. Task difficulty can be increased by reducing the length or intensity of the speech segment produced at any given location.

Walking and Listening

While accompanying a child on an outdoor field trip, the child is encouraged to listen for sounds and to label these environmental sounds when heard (e.g., a dog barking). This activity can be combined with localization requiring the child to point to the location of the sound after labeling the sound.

Following Directives

The child is asked to follow one-, two-, or three-step motor tasks verbally conveyed by a parent or teacher (e.g., go to the kitchen and turn on the light). The child should be able to easily perform the required motor activity.

Interhemispheric Processing

Practice at transferring information from one hemisphere to another can be a valuable training task—especially with the long maturational course of the corpus callosum (Musiek, Kibbe, & Baran,

1984). Playing "name that tune" likely requires activity between cortices. Also, having children close their eyes and name objects felt with their left hand also is an enjoyable game that likely requires information exchange between hemispheres.

Listening to Rhymes

Exposing young children to nursery rhymes, as well as singing songs, helps develop temporal processes that underlie prosody. These activities are enjoyable, employ accessible and varied material, and can be done repetitively without the child tiring or becoming bored.

Musical Chairs

Musical chairs is a game that requires a number of auditory, motor, and cognitive processes. Sustained attention is pivotal to the multiple processes and skills trained through this game. Children walk around chairs (equal to the number of children at the outset of the game) set in a circle while music plays in the background. When the music stops, the children must sit in a chair. After each music segment, a chair is removed resulting in one child left standing and eliminated from the game. The game continues until only one chair remains to accommodate one child. The game can be modified to increase the challenge by having the children listen for specific targets within the music (e.g., when the music becomes louder or softer sit down). Also, the time between musical segments can be varied greatly introducing unpredictability and challenge that should exercise the child's ability to maintain attention to the task.

Summary

Auditory training (AT) is no longer a rehabilitative approach directed primarily to those with peripheral hearing loss. Recent studies in both animals and humans have demonstrated that AT improves basic central auditory processes and skills. This improvement in auditory capability is linked to plastic changes in the brain. In fact, auditory plasticity underlies the success of AT. To ensure success, however, the principles derived from neuroscience and learning theory reviewed in this chapter must be followed to ensure maximal improvement at an optimal pace. AT is an essential component of a comprehensive approach to treat (C)APD. The reader is referred to Chapters 5 and 7 for elaboration of the other elements (i.e., central resources training and signal enhancement, respectively) of the recommended comprehensive approach to intervention for (C)APD.

References

Agnew, J., Dorn, C., & Eden, G. (2004). Effect of intensive training on auditory processing and reading skills. *Brain and Language, 88,* 21-25.

Alexander, D., & Frost, B. (1982). Decelerated synthesized speech as a means of shaping speed of auditory processing of children with delayed language. *Perceptual and Motor Skills, 55,* 783-792.

Bamiou, D., & Luxon, L. (2003). Medical management of balance disorders and vestibular rehabilitation. In L. Luxon (Ed.), *Textbook of audiological medicine: Clinical aspects of hearing and balance* (pp. 839-916). London: Martin Dunitz.

Bao, S., Chang, E., Woods, J., & Merzenich, M. (2004). Temporal plasticity in the primary auditory cortex induced by operant perceptual learning. *Nature Neuroscience, 7,* 974–981.

Bliss, T., & Lomo, T. (1973). Long-lasting potentiation of synaptic transmission in the dentate area of the anaesthetized rabbit following stimulation of the perforant path. *Journal of Physiology, 232*(2), 331–356.

Carhart, R. (1960). Auditory training. In H. Davis (Ed.), *Hearing and deafness.* New York: Holt, Rinehart and Winston.

Chermak, G., & Musiek, F. (2002). Auditory training: Principles and approaches for remediating and managing auditory processing disorders. *Seminars in Hearing, 23,* 297–308.

Cleary, M., Pisoni, D., & Geers, A. (2001). Some measures of verbal and spatial working memory in eight and nine year old hearing impaired children with cochlear implants. *Ear and Hearing, 22,* 395–411.

Delhommeau, K., Micheyl, C., & Jouvent, R. (2005). Generalization of frequency discrimination learning across frequencies and ears: Implications for underlying neural mechanisms in humans. *Journal of the Association for Research in Otolaryngology, 6,* 171–179.

Delhommeau, K., Micheyl, C., Jouvent, R., & Collet, L. (2002). Transfer of learning across durations and ears in auditory frequency discrimination. *Perception and Psychophysics, 64,* 426–436.

DiCarlo, L. (1948). Auditory training for the adult. *Volta Review, 50,* 490.

Edeline, J., & Weinberger, N. (1993). Receptive field plasticity in the auditory cortex during frequency discrimination training: Selective retuning independent of task difficulty. *Behavioral Neuroscience, 107,* 82–103

Erber, N. (1982). *Auditory training.* Washington DC: Alexander Graham Bell Association for the Deaf.

Foxton, J., Brown, A., Chambers, S., & Griffiths, T. (2004). Training improves acoustic pattern perception. *Current Biology, 14,* 322–325.

Friel-Patti, S., Loeb, D., & Gilliam, R. (2001). Looking ahead: An introduction to five exploratory studies in Fast ForWord. *American Journal of Speech-Language Pathology, 10,* 195–202.

Gilliam, R., Loeb, D., & Friel-Patti, S. (2001). Looking back: a summary of five exploratory studies of Fast ForWord. *American Journal of Speech-Language Pathology, 10,* 269–273.

Goldstein, M. (1939). *The acoustic method.* St. Louis, MO: The Laryngoscope Press.

Greenough, W., & Bailey, C. (1988). Anatomy of a memory: Convergence of results across a diversity of tests. *Trends in Neuroscience, 11,* 142–146

Hassmannova, J., Myslivecek, J., & Novakova, V. (1981). Effects of early auditory stimulation on cortical centers. In J. Syka & L. Aitkin (Eds.), *Neuronal mechanisms of hearing* (pp. 355–359). New York: Plenum.

Hayes, E., Warrier, C., Nicol, T., Zecker, S., & Kraus, N. (2003). Neural plasticity following auditory training in children with learning problems. *Clinical Neurophysiology, 114,* 673–684.

Hebb, D. O. (1949). *The organization of behavior.* New York: John Wiley & Sons.

Hubble-Dahlquist, L. (1998). Classroom amplification: Not just for the hearing impaired anymore. CSUN '98 Papers [online]. Available at http://www.dimf.ne.jp/doc/english/Us_Eu/conf/csun_98/csun98_124.htm.

Hudgins, C. V. (1954). Auditory training: Its possibilities and limitations. *Volta Review, 56,* 339.

Jancke, L., Gaab, N., Wustenberg, H., Scheich, H., & Heinze, H. (2001). Short-term functional plasticity in the human auditory cortex: An fMRI study. *Cognitive Brain Research, 12,* 479–485.

Kalil, R. (1989). Synapse formation in the developing brain. *Scientific American, 261,* 76–87.

Karpicke, J., & Pisoni, D. (2004). Using immediate memory span to measure implicit learning. *Memory and Cognition, 32,* 956-964.

Katz, J. & Harmon, C. (1982). *Phonemic synthesis: Blending sounds into words.* Allan, TX: Developmental Learning Materials.

Kimura, D. (1961). Some effects of temporal lobe damage on auditory perception. *Canadian Journal of Psychology, 15,* 157-165.

King, C., Warrier, C., Hayes, E., & Kraus, N. (2002). Deficits in auditory brainstem pathway encoding of speech sounds in children with learning problems. *Neuroscience Letters, 319,* 111-115.

Knudsen, E. (1988). Experience shapes sound localization and auditory unit properties during development in the barn owl. In G. Edleman, W. Gall, & W. Cowan (Eds.), *Auditory function: Neurological bases of hearing.* New York: John Wiley & Sons.

Kraus, N. (1999). Speech sound perception, neurophysiology, and plasticity. *Pediatric Otorhinolaryngology, 47,* 123-129.

Kraus, N., McGee, T., Carrell, T., King, C., Tremblay, K., & Nicol, T. (1995). Central auditory system plasticity associated with speech discrimination training. *Journal of Cognitive Neuroscience, 7,* 25-32.

Kujala, T., Karma, K., Ceponiene, R., Belitz, S., Turkkila, P., Tervaniemi, M., & Naatanen, R. (2001). Plastic neural changes and reading improvement caused by audiovisual training in reading-impaired children. *Proceedings of the National Academy of Sciences of the United States of America, 98,* 10509-10514.

Kujala, T., Myllyviita, K., Tervaniemi, M., Alho, K., Kallio, J., & Naatanen, R. (2000). Basic auditory dysfunction in dyslexia as demonstrated by brain activity measurements. *Psychophysiology, 37,* 262-266.

Linkenhoker, B., & Knudsen, E. (2002). Incremental training increases the plasticity of the auditory space map in adult barn owls. *Nature, 419,* 293-296.

Linkenhoker, B., von der Ohe, C., & Knudsen E. (2004). Anatomical traces of juvenile learning in the auditory system of adult barn owls. *Nature Neuroscience, 8,* 93-98.

Ludman, H. (2003). The role of surgery in the management of the dizzy patient. In L. Luxon (Ed.), *Textbook of audiological medicine: Clinical aspects of hearing and balance* (pp. 917-928). London: Martin Dunitz.

Lund, R. (1978). *Development and plasticity of the brain: An introduction.* New York: Oxford University Press.

Merzenich, M., Jenkins, W., Johnston, P., Schreiner, C., Miller, S., & Tallal, P. (1996). Temporal processing deficits of language-learning impaired children ameliorated by training. *Science, 271,* 77-81.

Moore, D., Rosenberg, J., & Coleman, J. (2005). Discrimination training of phonemic contrasts enhances phonological processing in mainstream school children. *Brain and Language, 94,* 72-85.

Musiek F. E. (1999) Habilitation and management of auditory processing disorders: Overview of selected procedures. *Journal of the American Academy of Audiology, 10,* 329-342

Musiek, F. (2005). Temporal (auditory) training for (C)APD. *The Hearing Journal, 58,* 46.

Musiek, F., Baran, J., & Shinn, J. (2004). Assessment and remediation of an auditory processing disorder associated with head trauma. *Journal of the American Academy of Audiology, 15,* 133-151.

Musiek, F., & Berge, B. (1998). A neuroscience view of auditory training/stimulation and central auditory processing disorders. In M. Masters, N. Stecker, & J. Katz (Eds.). *Central auditory processing disorders: Mostly management* (pp. 15-32). Boston: Allyn & Bacon.

Musiek, F. E., & Chermak, G. D. (1995). Three commonly asked questions about central auditory processing disorders: Management. *American Journal of Audiology, 4*(1), 15-18.

Musiek, F., Gollegly, K., & Baran, J. (1984a). Myelination of the corpus callosum and auditory processing problems in children: Theoretical and clinical correlates. *Seminars in Hearing, 5,* 231-241.

Musiek, F., Kibbe, K., & Baran, J. (1984). Neuroaudiological results from split-brain patients. *Seminars in Hearing, 5*, 219-229.

Musiek, F., & Schochat, E. (1998). Auditory training and central auditory processing disorders. *Seminars in Hearing, 9*, 357-366.

Musiek, F., Shinn, J., & Hare, C. (2002). Plasticity, auditory training, and auditory processing disorders. *Seminars in Hearing, 23*, 263-275.

Pinheiro, M. (1977). Tests of central auditory function in children with learning disabilities. In R. Keith (Ed.), *Central auditory dysfunction* (pp. 223-256). New York: Grune & Stratton.

Pisoni, D., & Cleary, M. (2004). Learning, memory, and cognitive processes in deaf children following cochlear implantation. In F. Zeng, A. Popper, & R. Fay (Eds.), *Cochlear implants: Auditory prostheses and electric hearing* (pp. 407-418). New York: Springer.

Reagan, C., (1973). *Handbook of auditory perceptual training* (pp. 11, 30, 65-66). Springfield, IL: Charles C. Thomas.

Recanzone, G., Schreiner, C., & Merzenich, M. (1993). Plasticity in the frequency representation of primary auditory cortex following discrimination training in adult owl monkeys. *Journal of Neuroscience, 13*, 97-103.

Russo, N., Nicole, T., Zecker, S., Hayes, E., & Kraus, N. (2005). Auditory training improves neural timing in the human brainstem. *Behavioural Brain Research, 156*, 95-103.

Salvi, R., & Henderson, D. (1996). *Auditory system plasticity and regeneration*. New York: Thieme Medical Publishers, Inc.

Sanders, D. A. (1971). *Aural rehabilitation.* Englewood Cliffs, NJ: Prentice-Hall.

Scheich, H. (1991). Auditory cortex: Comparative aspects of maps and plasticity. *Current Opinion in Neurobiology, 1*, 236-247.

Schow R, & Nerbonne M. *Introduction to audiologic rehabilitation* (3rd ed). Boston: Allyn & Bacon.

Sloan, C. (1986). *Treating auditory processing difficulties in children.* San Diego: College-Hill Press.

Tallal, P., Merzenich, M., Miller, S., & Jenkins, W. (1998). Language learning impairments: integrating basic science, technology, and remediation. *Experimental Brain Research, 123*, 210-219.

Tallal, P., Miller, S.L., Bedi, G., Byma, G., Wang, X., Nagarajan, S., Schreiner, C., Jenkins, W., & Merzenich, M. (1996). Language comprehension in language-learning impaired children improved with acoustically modified speech. *Science, 271*, 81-84.

Temple, E., Deutsch, G., Poldrack, R., Miller, S., Tallal, P., Merzenich, M., & Gabrieli, J. (2003). Neural deficits in children with dyslexia ameliorated by behavioral remediation: evidence from functional MRI. *Proceedings of the National Academy of Sciences of the United States of America, 100*, 2860-2865.

Tremblay, K., & Kraus, N. (2002). Auditory training induces asymmetrical changes in cortical neural activity. *Journal of Speech Language and Hearing Research, 45*, 564-572.

Tremblay, K., Kraus, N., Carrell, T., & McGee, T. (1997). Central auditory system plasticity: generalization to novel stimuli following listening training. *Journal of Acoustical Society of America, 102*, 3762-3773.

Tremblay, K., Kraus, N., & McGee, T. (1998). The time course of auditory perceptual learning: neurophysiological changes during speech-sound training. *NeuroReport, 16*, 3557-3560.

Tremblay, K., Kraus, N., McGee, T., Ponton, C., & Otis, B. (2001). Central auditory plasticity: changes in the N1-P2 complex after speech-sound training. *Ear and Hearing, 22*, 79-90.

Warrier, C., Johnson, K., Hayes, E., Nicol, T., & Kraus, N., (2004). Learning impaired children exhibit timing deficits and training-related improvements in auditory cortical responses to speech and noise. *Experimental Brain Research, 157*, 431-441.

Webster, D., & Webster, M. (1977) Neonatal sound deprivation affects brainstem auditory nuclei. *Archives of Otolaryngology, 103*, 392-396.

Wedenburg, E. (1951). Auditory training of the deaf and hard of hearing children. *Acta Otolaryngologica, 94*(Suppl.), 1–29.

Wertz D., & Moncrieff, D. (Unpublished data). Dichotic Interaural Intensity Difference (DIID).

Willeford, J. (1977). Assessing central auditory behavior in children: A test battery approach. In R. Keith (Ed.), *Central auditory dysfunction* (pp. 43–72). New York: Grune & Stratton.

Wingfield, A. (1979). *Human learning and memory*. New York: Harper & Row.

CHAPTER 5

CENTRAL RESOURCES TRAINING

Cognitive, Metacognitive, and Metalinguistic Skills and Strategies

GAIL D. CHERMAK

Intervention for central auditory processing disorder ([C]APD) should commence as soon as possible following diagnosis to take advantage of the plasticity of the central nervous system and thereby maximize therapeutic effectiveness and minimize functional deficits (ASHA, 2005; Chermak & Musiek, 1997). Intervention should be comprehensive and multidisciplinary, given the potential impact of (C)APD on listening, communication, and learning, as well as the frequent comorbidity of (C)APD with language, learning, attention, and related disorders (Chermak, Hall, & Musiek, 1999; Chermak & Musiek, 1992, 1997; Musiek, Bellis, & Chermak, 2005). The influence of higher-order, non-modality-specific processes such as attention, executive control, memory, and decision making on all auditory tasks further underscores the need for

comprehensive intervention (Musiek et al., 2005; Salvi, Lockwood, Frisina, Coad, Wack, & Frisina, 2002). This undergirding of basic perceptual events by supramodal cognitive processes is demonstrated, for example, by the integral role of working memory in numerous auditory processes, including localization, temporal resolution, and pattern recognition (Marler, Champlin, & Gillam, 2002; Martinkauppi, Rama, Aronen, Korvenoja, & Carolson, 2002; Zattore, 2001). Notwithstanding the primacy of auditory processing deficits in (C)APD, comorbid supramodal cognitive, attention, language, and related deficits can compound auditory processing deficits and exacerbate the adverse impact of (C)APD for listening, communication, and learning (Chermak & Musiek, 1997). Indeed, links between inefficient auditory processing and language or learning problems have been documented both behaviorally and electrophysiologically (e.g., Bellis & Ferre, 1999; Kraus et al., 1996; Moncrieff & Musiek, 2002; Wible, Nicol, & Kraus, 2005). Similarly, even though (C)APD is not posited as a direct cause of all or even most cases of academic failure, learning disability, or reading disability, (C)APD certainly can exacerbate academic challenge (e.g., listening in noisy classroom environments) (Musiek, Bellis, & Chermak, 2005). Comorbid deficits can impede generalization of strategic listening behaviors across settings and may jeopardize treatment effectiveness and efficacy (Borkowski & Burke, 1996; Chermak & Musiek, 1997). Intervention to address the clinical and functional deficit profile that accompanies (C)APD must be comprehensive in scope. Nonetheless, the effectiveness and efficacy of (C)APD intervention should not be gauged primarily by academic outcomes or social skills, but rather by improvements in auditory function. These, in turn, will support improvements in those functions (e.g., listening and spoken language processing) that are dependent upon audition (Musiek et al., 2005).

Although the complex organization of the brain, involving interactive and interfacing sensory, cognitive, and linguistic networks may underlie comorbidity and compound the impact of (C)APD, that same complex organization presents opportunities to benefit intervention (Chermak & Musiek, 1997; Merzenich, Schreiner, Jenkins, & Wang, 1993; Poremba et al., 2003). Central resources, comprised of cognitive (i.e., processes involved in *knowing*), metacognitive (i.e., use of knowledge), and language resources, can be engaged to buttress central auditory processing and complement direct auditory skills training, thereby minimizing the functional consequences of (C)APD (Chermak & Musiek, 1997). This chapter focuses on the role of central resources training in comprehensive intervention to enhance central auditory processing, listening, and spoken language understanding.

Theoretical Framework for Central Resources Training

Brain Organization and Neuroplasticity

A comprehensive approach to intervention capitalizes on the complex organization of the brain and its neuroplasticity. The neural substrate of the auditory system is large, interfacing with other sensory, cognitive, motor control, and linguistic networks (Poremba et al., 2003). Conversely, widespread cortical networks spanning temporal, frontal, and parietal lobes sustain cognitive processes (e.g., attention and memory) that support auditory processing (Gaffan, 2005; Thiebaut de Schotten et al., 2005).

Consistent with a network model, emphasizing the distributed nature of information processing within the nervous system, perceptual responses to sensory stimuli are mediated across a large number of brain regions involving multiple serial, parallel, and dispersed neural networks (ASHA, 1996; Masterton, 1992; Ungerleider, 1995). Neuroplasticity is induced through experience and stimulation and leads to reorganization (i.e., remapping) of the cortex and cognitive and behavioral change (Elbert, Pantev, Wienbruch, Rockstroh, & Taub, 1995; Merzenich et al., 1993; Moore, 1993; Recanzone, Schreiner, & Merzenich, 1993; Robertson & Irvine, 1989; Weinberger & Diamond, 1987; Willott, Aitken, & McFadden, 1993). An array of plastic changes underlie cortical reorganization, including the potential for enlargement of a region's function (i.e., map expansion), compensatory allocation (i.e., novel allocation of particular process to another brain region), crossmodal reassignment (i.e., region of the brain accepting input from a new sensory modality), and homologous area adaptation (i.e., same area in opposite hemisphere assuming processing responsibility) (Grafman & Litvan, 1999). Because all auditory skills are affected by higher-order, non-modality-specific factors (e.g., attention, memory, motivation, and decision processes) and the underlying multimodal, crossmodal, and supramodal neural interfaces that support performance, the array of potential neuroplastic changes bodes well for successful outcomes when intervention is undertaken comprehensively and broadly.

The plasticity of the central auditory nervous system (CANS) provides tremendous opportunity to improve central auditory processes and skills through direct treatment (i.e., auditory training). This neuroplasticity also compels us to undertake central resources training to engage related systems that interface with the CANS and can, through those interactions, potentially reduce the functional impact of (C)APD and enhance listening, communication, social and learning outcomes. (See Chapter 1 of both Volume I and Volume II of this Handbook for additional discussion of neuroplasticity.)

Modeling (Central) Auditory Processing: Information Processing

Recent developments in cognitive neuroscience underscore the highly complex, multistage, interactive, and integrative nature of central auditory processing and the complementary interplay of both bottom-up and top-down information processing strategies (Chermak & Musiek, 1992, 1997; Massaro, 1987). Also becoming clear is the essential role of neurotransmitters and molecular mechanisms, triggered by sensory stimulation, in facilitating central auditory processing (Aoki & Siekevitz, 1988; Gopal et al., 2004a, 2004b; Kalil, 1989; Morley & Happe, 2000; Musiek & Hoffman, 1990; Sahley, Musiek, & Nodar, 1996; Sahley & Nodar, 1994; Syka, 2002).

The emerging conceptualization of central auditory processing views information processing as neither exclusively bottom-up nor top-down (Chermak & Musiek, 1997). Bottom-up processing encompasses data-driven strategies in which the listener is alerted to novel or incompatible information. Complementary top-down strategies emphasize context and assimilation of lower order information within the experience and expectations of the listener (Chermak & Musiek, 1992; Neisser, 1976; Rumelhart, 1984). According to information processing theory, an active listener selectively attends, processes data, and imposes higher level constraints to construct the signal or message (Borkowski & Burke, 1996; Flavell, 1981; Gibson, 1966; Watson & Foyle, 1985). Listeners assign meaning to audible discourse based on the extraction of information through various interactions among central auditory processing and cognitive, language, and metacognitive functions (Chermak & Musiek, 1997; Massaro, 1975a, 1975b, 1976). Skilled listeners are actively engaged in discovering the speaker's message. They orchestrate various bottom-up (e.g., segmenting, discriminating, and sequencing) and top-down strategies (e.g., question formulation, paraphrasing, mnemonics, note-taking, drawing, verbal rehearsal, mental imaging, and summarizing) to monitor listening and extract information from the spoken message (Chermak & Musiek, 1997).

The relative contribution of bottom-up and top-down processes is driven by the changing demands of the listening situation. The influence of top-down processes is more substantial when stimuli are presented in degraded form, including noisy environments and linguistically ambiguous contexts (Marslen-Wilson & Tyler, 1980; Neisser, 1976; Rumelhart, 1980, 1984; Warren & Warren, 1970). For persons with (C)APD who routinely confront internal distortions that degrade the signal, top-down processing exerts a more significant influence in all listening situations, especially in noisy and reverberant environments and when coupled with complex linguistic and cognitive demands (e.g., in classrooms).

Comprehensive intervention for (C)APD is structured consistent with information processing models that involve the complementary interplay of both bottom-up and top-down strategies (Chermak & Musiek, 1997). Skilled listeners, actively engaged in discovering what speakers are communicating, rely on central auditory processes to segment, discriminate, integrate, and organize the acoustic information inherent to the auditory signal, as well as various executive strategies to monitor their listening and extract meaningful information from the spoken message (Chermak & Musiek, 1997). They must organize and elaborate information and deploy executive strategies and self-regulatory processes to guide the flow of information processing and coordinate knowledge sources (Borkowski & Burke, 1996; Flavell, 1981; Gibson, 1966). Conceptualized within this framework in which

processes at various sensory and central levels influence information processing, (C)APD resulting from specific, sensory processing deficiencies may be exacerbated by higher order (i.e., top-down) deficiencies in regulating or coordinating central auditory and cognitive and linguistic processes (ASHA, 1996; Chermak & Musiek, 1992, 1997; Swanson, 1987). In addition to deficits in specific central auditory processes (e.g., auditory discrimination, temporal processing, performance with competing or degraded acoustic signals), individuals with (C)APD may lack listening strategies or employ inappropriate strategies and fail to engage in self-monitoring behavior (Chermak & Musiek, 1997).

Consistent with information processing theory, bottom-up and top-down approaches form two complementary components of a comprehensive intervention program for (C)APD (see Table 5-1). Bottom-up approaches for (C)APD focus on auditory training and enhancement of the acoustic signal and the listening environment. Top-down approaches focus on central resources, including cognitive skills (e.g., attention, working memory); metacognitive knowledge and skills (e.g., monitoring, coordinating, and deploying strategies); language (e.g., metalinguistic) skills and strategies; classroom, instructional, and learning strategies; and workplace, recreational, and home accommodations (ASHA, 2005; Chermak, 2002; Chermak & Musiek, 1997, 2002).

Systems Theory

The tenets of systems theory support a collaborative and ecologic or context-based approach to intervention (Chermak

Table 5–1. Components of Comprehensive Intervention for (Central) Auditory Processing Disorder

Bottom-Up Treatment
Auditory Training
Signal Enhancement (e.g., assistive listening systems, clear speech)
Environmental (Listening Environment) Modifications (e.g., reduce noise and reverberation)
Top-Down Approaches
Language Strategies
Cognitive Strategies
Metacognitive Strategies
Classroom, Instructional, and Learning Strategies
Workplace, Recreational, and Home Accommodations

& Musiek, 1997). The study of systems as entities rather than a conglomeration of parts has received broad application across disciplines, including the social sciences, education, and health and rehabilitation sciences (Bartoli & Botel, 1988; Damico, Augustine, & Hayes, 1996; Duranti & Goodwin, 1990; Weaver, 1993). A systems perspective considers an individual as a system of interacting cognitive, affective, and physiologic subsystems and as a part of larger social systems, including the family, school, workplace, and community. Environmental events are seen as directly impacting the individual's function. In contrast to a medical model in which behavioral problems are attributed solely to the neurobiologic problems of the individual, a systems approach encompasses a broad perspective whereby factors external to the individual are seen as interacting with internal neurobiologic predispositions, thereby contributing to behavioral deficits (Chermak & Musiek, 1997). In effect, an individual's behavior is the culmination of numerous transactional interactions between the individual and his or her context (i.e., environment, culture, society) (Chermak & Musiek, 1997). Notwithstanding the neurobiologic basis of (C)APD, environmental expectations and demands (e.g., listening to sophisticated language in a noisy classroom) exacerbate the mismatch between internal capacity and external structure and lead to communication dysfunction and academic underachievement (Chermak & Musiek, 1997).

The assumptions of systems theory reinforce the importance of collaboration and empowerment for successful intervention. These assumptions translate into interventions that include attention to interacting internal and external factors, interventions directed toward the individual, including central resources training, as well as environmental interventions, in the classroom, workplace, and recreational settings (Bartoli & Botel, 1988; Chermak & Musiek, 1997; Gibson, 1966; Maag & Reid, 1996; Poplin, 1988a, 1988b; Weaver, 1985, 1993).

Central Resources Utilization Strategy

A central resources utilization strategy is derived from a processing model in which resources are finite and must be efficiently allocated across sensory and central systems (Pichora-Fuller, Schneider, & Daneman, 1995). Emerging from that *finite pie* model, a comprehensive intervention approach develops auditory perceptual skills and fortifies central systems to efficiently and effectively allocate resources across sensory and central systems proportionate to the demands of a particular listening task. In so doing, resources are available *downstream* (i.e., peripheral) or *upstream* (i.e., central) to most efficiently and accurately execute the task.

Strengthening central resources does not target central auditory processes directly; however, augmenting central resources complements and supplements direct treatment provided through auditory training (described in Chapter 4) and signal enhancement (discussed in Chapter 7), providing a more thorough and encompassing approach to remediating and minimizing (C)APD and related functional deficits. Although a growing number of published reports document improved psychophysical performance, neurophysiologic representation of acoustic stimuli, and listening and related function in children and adults following

auditory training (e.g., Hayes, Warrier, Nicol, Zecker, & Kraus, 2003; Jirsa, 1992; Kraus & Disterhoft, 1982; Kraus et al., 1995; Merzenich, Grajski, Jenkins, Recanzone, & Peterson, 1991; Merzenich et al., 1996; Miller & Knudsen, 2003; Musiek, Baran, & Pinheiro, 1992; Musiek, Baran, & Shinn, 2004; Russo, Nicol, Zecker, Hayes, & Kraus, 2005; Tallal et al., 1996; Tremblay & Kraus, 2002; Tremblay, Kraus, Carrell, & McGee, 1997; Tremblay, Kraus, & McGee, 1998; Tremblay, Kraus, McGee, Ponton, & Otis, 2001; Warrier, Johnson, Hayes, Nicol, & Kraus, 2004), central resources training complements these remedial efforts, providing buttressing and compensatory techniques (e.g., bolstered metacognitive knowledge and strategies to strengthen self-regulation of spoken language processing) to more effectively address functional deficits. These techniques will also mitigate auditory processing deficits more resistant to treatment. Components of central resources training are listed in Table 5–2.

Fortified central resources (i.e., cognitive, metacognitive, and language and metalinguistic skills and knowledge) promote improved listening and spoken language comprehension (Chermak & Musiek, 1997). To the extent central resource augmentation improves listening and reading comprehension, such augmentation also may reduce learning problems. For example, training in deducing word meaning from context should benefit both listening and reading comprehension, given the robust correlations among vocabulary, reading comprehension, and listening comprehension (Perfetti, 1985; Samuels, 1987; Stanovich, 1993; Sticht & James, 1984; Wiig, Semel, & Crouse, 1973). Similarly, therapy to increase phonologic awareness and segmentation skills should aid both reading

Table 5–2. Components of Central Resources Training for (Central) Auditory Processing Disorder ([C]APD)

Metacognitive Resources: Skills and Strategies	Cognitive Resources: Skills and Strategies
Attribution Retraining	Sustained Auditory Attention (Auditory Vigilance)
Self-Instruction	Memory
Cognitive Problem Solving	Mnemonics
Self-Control (Self-Regulation)	Auditory Memory Enhancement (AME)
Cognitive Strategy Training	Mind Mapping
Cognitive Style and Reasoning	Working Memory
Reciprocal Teaching	
Assertiveness Training	

Metalinguistic Resources: Skills and Strategies

Schema Induction and Discourse Cohesion Devices

Auditory Closure

Vocabulary Building

Phonologic Awareness (Phonemic Analysis and Synthesis)

Prosody (Temporal Processing)

and listening comprehension (Agnew, Dorn, & Eden, 2003; Ehri et al., 2001; Gillon, 2005; Liberman, Cooper, Shankweiler, & Studdert-Kennedy, 1967; Mann, 1991; Mattingly, 1972; Perfetti & McCutchen, 1982; Swanson, Hodson, & Schommer-Aikins, 2005).

Pivotal Role of Metacognition and Executive Function in Central Resources Training

Metacognition refers to the active monitoring and consequent regulation and orchestration of attention, memory, learning, and language processes in the service of some goal (Flavell, 1976). Executive function, a component of metacognition, refers to the self-directed actions of an individual that are used to self-regulate to accomplish self-control, goal-directed behavior, and maximize future outcomes (Barkley, 1997a, 1997b). These general control processes coordinate knowledge (i.e., cognition) and metacognitive knowledge, transforming such knowledge into behavioral strategies, which ensure that an individual's behavior is adaptive, consistent with some goal, and beneficial to the individual (Chermak & Musiek, 1997). Because listening takes place within the multiple contexts of the acoustic, phonetic, linguistic, and social domains, simultaneous and integrated orchestration of multiple knowledge bases and skills is required for spoken language comprehension (Chermak & Musiek, 1997). Metacognition drives this coordi-nated effort and is, therefore, pivotal to central resources training.

Metacognition directs the allocation of central resources for self-regulation of skills and strategies (Chermak & Musiek, 1997). Moreover, by directing the allocation of central resources, metacognition indirectly influences bottom-up perceptual events (Ahissar & Hochstein, 1993). The observation that listeners require a larger interval of silence (i.e., gap) to perform a *between channel* versus a *within channel* gap detection task demonstrates how central resource allocation influences auditory perception (Phillips, Taylor, Hall, Carr, & Mossop, 1997; Phillips, Hall, Harrington, & Taylor, 1998). By engaging metacognitive processes, we promote a client-centered approach to therapy that should maximize intervention efficiency as a self-regulating client generalizes skills and strategies to everyday settings, including the classroom, workplace, and home. Extending skills and strategies across settings provides considerable practice opportunities, which optimizes plasticity (Hassaman-nova, Myslivecek, & Novakova, 1981; Rumbaugh & Washburn, 1996). Metacognition is key to central resources training and ultimately to successful rehabilitation outcomes.

Metacognition and (C)APD

Although (C)APD, by definition, is not a metacognitive disorder, the experiential deficit suffered by individuals with (C)APD in processing the auditory signal can lead to metacognitive deficits, as metacognition develops through experience in a skill-based context, such as spoken language processing (Harris, Reid, & Graham, 2004; Wong, 1991). Whereas much of the evidence documenting metacognitive strategy deficits has been collected from subjects who were described as learning disabled, subject selection criteria and histories indicate the likelihood that these subjects also presented central auditory processing deficits (Bos & Filip, 1982; Gerber, 1993b; Hallahan & Kneedler, 1979; Kotsonis & Patterson, 1980; Paris & Myers, 1981; Pressley & Levin, 1987; Suiter & Potter, 1978; Swanson, 1989, 1993; Torgesen, 1979; Torgesen & Houck, 1980; Wiens, 1983; Wong, 1987; Wong & Jones, 1982). The evidence reveals that these individuals present a passive and inefficient approach to problem solving (Swanson, 1989; Torgesen, 1979), a lack of metacognitive awareness (Brown, Bransford, Ferrara, & Campione, 1983; Hallahan & Kneedler, 1979; Paris & Myers, 1981; Swanson, 1993; Wiens, 1983), and difficulty monitoring comprehension (Bos & Filip, 1982; Kotsonis & Patterson, 1980; Wong & Jones, 1982). They tend not to deploy strategies spontaneously, often requiring external prompting to mobilize a strategy, and have difficulty choosing appropriate problem-solving devices (Chermak & Musiek, 1997). Less likely to activate schematic knowledge, they do not elaborate and construct information that guides comprehension (Gerber, 1993b).

This evidence coupled with clinical experience suggests that individuals with (C)APD may not always exert executive control in deploying strategies to aid in organizing, monitoring, and understanding the acoustic signal, strategies that might facilitate information processing and enable them to compensate to some

extent for the deficient central auditory processes that characterize the disorder (Chermak & Musiek, 1992, 1997; Gerber, 1993b; Harris, Reid, & Graham, 2004; Pressley & Levin, 1987; Suiter & Potter, 1978; Torgesen & Houck, 1980; Wong, 1987). As passive or inactive listeners, they may fail to attend selectively, organize input, deploy listening comprehension strategies, maintain on-task behavior, or employ task-approach skills, including the ability to focus on relevant task information (Chermak & Musiek, 1997).

Metacognitive deficits in individuals with (C)APD are secondary deficits resulting from repeated failure and lack of task persistence, limited use of executive function, inadequate experience with successful listening strategies, and low motivation (Chermak & Musiek, 1997). Fortunately, metacognitive deficits are responsive to intervention directed toward informed strategy use (Borkowski, Weyhing, & Carr, 1988; Brown et al., 1983; Fabricus & Hagen, 1984; Kendall & Braswell, 1982; Moynahan, 1978; Paris, Newman, & McVey, 1982; Reid & Borkowski, 1987). If left untreated, metacognitive deficits can exacerbate the impact of (C)APD for spoken language understanding; with treatment, individuals with (C)APD can become skilled listeners who actively engage in discovering what speakers are communicating. To achieve this goal they must be trained to use their metacognitive knowledge and strategies (i.e., executive function) to regulate and guide their listening and extraction of information from the spoken message (Chermak & Musiek, 1992). Comprehensive treatment of (C)APD demands attention to both first-order problems of deficient central auditory processes and second-order metacognitive deficits.

Metacognition Promotes Generalization

Generalization of newly learned skills and strategies to contexts not employed during treatment is requisite to documenting change in function and treatment efficacy (Olswang & Bain, 1994). Failure to generalize may reflect metacognitive deficits and/or limitations of the treatment program (Borkowski, Johnston, & Reid, 1987; McReynolds, 1989). As argued by Borkowski, Estrada, Milstead, and Hale (1989), generalization of even ingrained strategy-specific knowledge to new stimuli and novel situations requires intact executive processing to guide selection and monitoring of strategies. Furthermore, to achieve generalization, specific strategy knowledge and executive processes must be coupled with appropriate attributional beliefs of the likelihood of success (Borkowski et al., 1989). The metacognitive fulcrum of central resources training reinforces a number of generalization strategies.

Generalization Strategies

Consistent with the neuroscience-based training principles discussed above, extensive training, increased practice, and rehearsal promote mastery of skills and automaticity of function (Chermak & Musiek, 1997). Role-playing and simulation provide opportunities to practice skills in contexts that are meaningful and relevant to the individual. Such activities also serve to reduce the differences between the treatment and natural environments, a strategy that has been identified as important to generalization (Stokes & Baer, 1977). Training that allows the client to explore the use of the target skill in multiple and diverse contexts expands the client's focus and is among the practices most often suggested to promote generalization of skills (Griffiths & Craighead, 1972; McReynolds, 1989; Murdock, Garcia, & Hardman, 1977; Rumbaugh & Washburn, 1996). Training in diverse contexts, with focus on multiple treatment settings and naturalistic settings including the home, school, and workplace, also underscores the importance of collaboration among professionals and families (Chermak & Musiek, 1997). Active client involvement in the therapy process through self-monitoring and ultimately self-regulation motivates the client to consider the use of a particular skill or strategy and is of great value in promoting generalization of behaviors (Guevremont, 1990; Koegel, Koegel, & Ingham, 1986). (See Chapter 1 for additional discussion of collaboration, and Chermak and Musiek [1997] for other suggestions to promote generalization.)

Using Feedback to Promote Executive Control and Generalization

Strong feedback is both positive and corrective (Chermak & Musiek, 1997). Effective feedback statements recognize effort and convey specific suggestions for improvement (Brophy, 1981). Moreover, feedback regarding the value of a strategy yields positive effects on strategy use and generalization (Ellis, Lenz, & Sabornie, 1987; Kennedy & Miller, 1976; Lenz, 1984; Ringel & Springer, 1980). Feedback need not avoid mention of errors. In fact, specific suggestions concerning how one might avoid particular errors further strengthens feedback (Ellis & Friend, 1991). Engaging clients in self-monitoring and recording their performance using charts, logs, or other devices is probably more reinforcing than providing extrinsic rewards (e.g., tokens, points, or prizes) (Ellis & Friend, 1991). Self-monitoring renders feedback more effective and develops executive control (Chermak & Musiek, 1997). Similarly, giving clients an opportunity to elaborate on the clinician's feedback, explaining the shortcomings of their strategies and steps that might be taken to improve their performance, also strengthens feedback, motivates clients, and promotes self-regulation (Adelman & Taylor, 1983; Ellis & Friend, 1991; Pressley, Johnson, & Symons, 1987). Hence, feedback serves an important function in promoting executive control.

As the client demonstrates greater skill level, the clinician should shift more responsibility for monitoring and adjusting behavior to the client, moving away from directive feedback statements and toward feedback that is more mediative (Ellis & Friend, 1991). Such mediative feedback provides cues to help clients discover and elaborate their own strategies and solutions rather than providing them directly to the client (Ellis & Friend, 1991; Ellis, Lenz, & Sabornie, 1987; Stone & Wertsch, 1984). Encouraging clients to monitor and track their progress through maintenance of a diary or log of reflections on strategy successes and failures increases the effectiveness of mediative feedback and promotes executive control (Chermak & Musiek, 1997). Moreover, encouraging clients to re-establish goals on the basis of feedback strengthens motivation. The reader is referred to Chermak and Musiek (1997) for additional discussion of feedback and goal structuring.

Central Resources: Knowledge, Strategies, and Skills

Metacognitive Knowledge and Strategies

Improved spoken language comprehension may be achieved through the development of listening strategies (Aarnoutse, Van Den Bos, Kees, & Brand-Gruwel, 1998; Brand-Gruwel, Aarnoutse, & Van Den Bos, 1998; Graham & Harris, 2003; Harris, Reid, & Graham, 2004; Harris & Sipay, 1990; McKenzie, Neilson & Braun, 1981; Palincsar & Klenk, 1992; Pearson & Fielding, 1982; Pratt & Bates, 1982; Reid, 1992; Wong, 1993). Similar to the gains in memory seen with increasing age that are attributed to the development of mnemonic strategies (discussed below) rather than capacity (Pressley, 1982), improved spoken language comprehension may be achieved through self-regulation of listening strategies (Chermak & Musiek, 1997; Harris, Reid, & Graham, 2004; Reid, 1992). Interventions combining performance strategies (e.g., metalinguistic strategies that make use of context to derive meaning or invoke schemata to guide interpretation) with self-regulation training are more successful than either approach in isolation (Brown, Campione, & Day, 1981; Graham & Harris, 2003). Moreover, the prospects for transfer or generalization of strategy use to other appropriate situations are excellent as metacognitive strategies (i.e., planning, checking, and monitoring) are not task specific, but rather constitute a general approach to problem solving (Brown, Campione, & Barclay, 1979; Lodico, Ghatala, Levin, Pressley, & Bell, 1983). Implementing executive or metacognitive strategies training in conjunction with other top-down and bottom-up approaches, particularly auditory training (e.g., auditory discrimination, temporal processing), provides a powerful intervention approach.

Metacognitive Knowledge

Regulation and deployment of metacognitive strategies require a motivated individual in control of certain executive knowledge and functions (Chermak & Musiek, 1997). In particular, three types of knowledge (i.e., declarative, procedural, and conditional) are needed to effectively implement metacognitive strategies.

Declarative knowledge refers to knowledge that is known in a propositional manner. For example, prior knowledge of the topic and pertinent vocabulary facilitate message comprehension. Procedural knowledge refers to awareness of the processes underlying effective listening and spoken language comprehension. An effective listener, for instance, knows how to scan the message for main ideas, how to paraphrase the message, and how to incorporate context to facilitate message comprehension (Chermak & Musiek, 1997).

Declarative and procedural knowledge are necessary but not sufficient for effective listening unless employed in conjunction with conditional knowledge (Chermak & Musiek, 1997). Being aware of conditions that affect listening is integral to conditional knowledge, as well as knowing why particular strategies work and when to use them. Conditional knowledge would enable an effective listener to parse a message for facts when precise detail is required in response, rather than to paraphrase it. Conversely, deficient conditional knowledge would

be evident in giving undue attention to a political theme of a message about voting irregularities at the expense of honing in on percentages and demographics detailed in the message. Informal assessment of metacognitive strategies, prior to and during the therapy process, can reveal a client's metacognitive knowledge and processes and better prepare the clinician to train metacognitive strategy use. Items of a metacognitive knowledge and strategies assessment developed for reading (*Index of Reading Awareness*) by Jacob and Paris (1987) can be adapted relatively easily to evaluate clients' awareness of the listening process (Chermak & Musiek, 1997).

Self-regulation is key to converting knowledge into practice. A skilled listener selectively deploys and coordinates resources and strategies using the executive processes of planning, evaluation, and regulation to achieve spoken language comprehension (Chermak & Musiek, 1997). Failed comprehension can be recognized through ongoing self-monitoring, after which the listener can modify strategies to meet the changing demands of the listening task, and ultimately enjoy successful message comprehension.

Metacognitive Strategies

Metacognitive strategies used for listening comprehension rely on the following skills and processes: (1) understanding task demands, (2) appropriately allocating attention, (3) identifying important parts of the message, (4) self-monitoring, (5) self-questioning, and (6) deployment of debugging strategies (Chermak & Musiek, 1997). Whereas skilled listeners use many of these processes automatically and tacitly, individuals with (C)APD may require direct instruction and opportunities for application and reinforcement. These practice opportunities will encourage individuals with (C)APD to take deliberate actions to enhance listening through conscious, metacognition (Chermak & Musiek, 1997).

(C)APD intervention programs may incorporate several metacognitive approaches, all of which promote active, self-regulation and share several distinguishing features (Chermak & Musiek, 1997). Notwithstanding their differences, these approaches typically provide explicit and detailed instruction regarding the goals of strategies and their application to tasks, as well as training self-regulation and self-monitoring of strategy deployment and outcomes of that deployment (Palinscar & Brown, 1987). They encourage self-identification of strategies employed and the rationale for their use, as well as feedback about the efficacy of strategies for particular tasks (Palinscar & Brown, 1987; Pressley, Borkowski, & O'Sullivan, 1984).

Elements of one metacognitive approach often reinforce aspects of another, a good reason to combine several metacognitive approaches in an intervention program (Chermak & Musiek, 1997). For instance, motivation underlies assertiveness training, and attribution training strengthens motivation. Similarly, self-instruction can be used to model cognitive problem solving. Also demonstrating the reinforcing linkages among metacognitive approaches, reciprocal teaching instills self-esteem and self-regulation and is highly motivating. Eight metacognitive approaches useful in managing (C)APD are discussed below.

Attribution Training

Chronic listening problems and the often associated academic or workplace failures, as well as the social frustrations inherent in the inability to integrate fully within the family or peer group, places individuals with (C)APD at risk for developing motivational problems (Chermak & Musiek, 1997). Some individuals with (C)APD become reconciled to the belief that their listening abilities (and perhaps intellectual abilities as well) are poor and cannot be improved and that their efforts to succeed are futile (Chermak & Musiek, 1997). These beliefs lead to poor motivation and deterioration in task persistence, and paradoxically, these beliefs often infiltrate their perception of their successes as well as their failures (Torgesen, 1980). Attribution problems occur, then, when these individuals attribute successes to luck, an easy task, or the benevolence of a teacher, coworker, or employer (Bryan, 1991; Butkowsky & Willows, 1980; Pearl, 1982; Torgesen, 1980).

Dysfunctional attributional patterns in which success is attributed to external factors (e.g., luck, a *nice* teacher) develop concurrent with an eroded motivation to learn, with failure being attributed to internal factors such as inability (Pearl, 1982). Academic failure underscores the futility of effortful learning, and results in low self-concept. These faulty beliefs and attributions engender low self-esteem and self-efficacy. Not unexpectedly, these individuals may avoid the challenging task of listening, particularly in competing backgrounds or when the message is otherwise degraded or difficult to sort. Moreover, they will fatigue and give up prematurely under these circumstances, failing to invoke listening strategies to meet task demands and achieve success. Because deployment of self-regulatory behavior depends on motivation, this sequence of events leads to deficits in executive functions and a passive approach to listening

(Chermak & Musiek, 1997). Passivity and inactivity, therefore, can be traced to a compromised self-system, a system that comprises self-efficacy, self-esteem, and attributions.

Rather than slide into passivity and low motivation, some maintain confidence by erroneously attributing their failings to teachers, parents, employers, or other external agents or circumstances. Others attribute difficulties to insufficient effort, an attribution tending to increase motivation (Licht, Kistner, Ozkaragoz, Shapiro, & Clausen, 1985; Speece, McKinney, & Applebaum, 1985). Attributions of failure to insufficient effort have, in fact, been shown to correlate with academic success (Kistner, Osborne, & LeVerrier, 1988).

Attribution retraining provides a direct approach to develop persistence and re-establish self-confidence in individuals who demonstrate a maladaptive motivational pattern (Licht & Kistner, 1986). Instilling causal attributions for failure to factors that are under the individual's control (e.g., insufficient effort) rather than to sensory or intellectual incapacity is a goal of attribution retraining, which should increase both self-esteem and persistence when individuals confront challenging listening tasks and conditions (Chermak & Musiek, 1997; Medway & Venino, 1982; Thomas & Pashley, 1982). Incorporating attribution training in therapy programs for young children with (C)APD offers a preventive approach to motivational problems (Chermak & Musiek, 1997).

Components of Attribution Training.
Attribution (re)training is a two-step procedure. As outlined by Chermak and Musiek (1997), the client is confronted with some failure (e.g., an incorrect response to a question posed following an oral-aural story presentation). The key component involves teaching the client to attribute the failure to insufficient effort. The clinician might tell the client that his or her answer was not correct, that he or she is working hard but should listen even more carefully. In a parallel manner, the clinician should attribute successes to effort, providing feedback that communicates that the response was correct and acknowledging that the client was listening carefully and trying hard.

Clients tend to be motivated to improve their performance and experience success when the wording of attributional statements (i.e., feedback) acknowledges hard work while urging even greater effort (Miller, Brickman, & Bolen, 1975; Schunk, 1982). Feedback that fails to recognize efforts already expended, indicating that the clinician perceived no effort or that the client was not indeed already working hard, are less likely to be effective (Miller et al., 1975; Schunk, 1982).

In addition to the specific wording of the attributional statements, the effectiveness of attribution retraining also depends on the proportion of successes and failures and scheduling of failures (Chermak & Musiek, 1997). Although confronting failure is integral to attribution retraining, some success is necessary to cultivate the self-efficacy needed to trust the method's premise that increased effort will lead to increased success (Clifford, 1978; Dweck, 1975). Tasks must be structured to allow that degree of success. Moreover, persistence is fostered by varying the number of difficult items, which demand increased effort, within an activity (Chapin & Dyck, 1976).

Payoff—improved performance resulting from increased effort—establishes the validity of attribution retraining.

Treatment effects will not persist or generalize without this validation or payoff (Dweck, 1977; Licht & Kistner, 1986). The client must be able to deploy appropriate metacognitive, cognitive, and metalinguistic strategies to maximize the chances that additional effort will lead to improved performance (Reid & Borkowski, 1987). Improved auditory skills developed through direct auditory training also are crucial to improved listening and hence the validation of attribution training. Knowing how to work harder, through sustained effort coupled with listening strategies, is more likely to lead to permanent improvements in performance and spontaneous deployment of these strategies (Borkowski, Weyhing, & Carr, 1988; Fabricus & Hagen, 1984; Kendall & Braswell, 1982; Moynahan, 1978; Paris et al., 1982). As stated by Reid & Borkowski (1987), "self-attributions about the importance of effort in producing success serve an energizing function in the deployment of available strategies and sustain the cognitive search for alternative strategies in the face of learning obstacles" (p. 306).

Cognitive Behavior Modification

Cognitive behavior modification depends on a client's use of strategies, notably executive and task-specific strategies (Lloyd, 1980). With the goal of self-control through a reflexive processing and response style, a client instructed in cognitive behavior modification employs, monitors, checks and evaluates behavioral strategies (Brown et al., 1981). Critical to this approach is the informed and active client.

Cognitive behavior modification is classified into four categories: self-instruction, problem solving, cognitive strategy train-

ing, and self-regulation (Whitman, Burgio, & Johnson, 1984). Although cognitive behavior modification methods fall into categories with distinct emphases and procedures, the commonality across methods is fundamental (Meichenbaum, 1986; Whitman et al., 1984). All cognitive behavior modification procedures include: (1) client involvement as active collaborators; (2) target strategies modeled during training; (3) a reflective processing and response style; and (4) analysis of the relationship between the client's actions and the task outcome (Lloyd, 1980; Meichenbaum, 1986). Also shared across the procedures is the use of daily logs or diaries. Encouraging the client to maintain a daily log exploring difficult listening situations and the relative value of strategies deployed to enhance listening promotes self-monitoring of the effectiveness of listening comprehension strategies (Chermak & Musiek, 1997). The use of diaries and logs as homework also benefits generalization of executive and task-specific strategies and skills (Guevremont, 1990).

Self-instruction, problem solving, self-regulation, and cognitive strategy training denote separate, but often interdependent, approaches in cognitive behavior modification. Demonstrating this overlap, self-instruction uses directive self-statements to train task-specific strategies and self-control, which are the foci of cognitive strategy training and self-regulation, respectively (Chermak & Musiek, 1997). Cognitive problem solving, while using self-instruction and self-regulation techniques, taps into a different aspect of the cognitive domain: reducing uncertainty and resolving problems (Chermak & Musiek, 1997). Clearly, combining procedures from more than one approach can increase training effectiveness (Whitman et al., 1984).

Self-Instruction. Self-instruction methods train clients to formulate adaptive and self-directing verbal cues before and during a task or situation (Chermak & Musiek, 1997). In addition to listening training, self-instruction is particularly useful in addressing academic difficulties, including reading comprehension problems, and impulsive and hyperactive behaviors (Hart & Morgan, 1993; Wong, 1993). Five sequential steps of self-instruction, outlined by Meichenbaum and Goodman (1971), promote the inculcation and generalization of the self-instructional routine: (1) the clinician performs the task while self-verbalizing aloud; (2) the client performs the task while the clinician verbalizes; (3) the client performs while self-instructing aloud; (4) the client performs while whispering; and (5) the client performs while self-instructing covertly (i.e., silently).

Several problem-solving skills are incorporated in self-instruction (Chermak & Musiek, 1997). The client must approach the listening situation with a plan and a reflective attitude, self-monitoring for any signs of inattention or distraction and assessing the purpose of the message. Next, the listener must focus on key words, examine context, and make predictions and draws inferences. The clinician may encourage general or more specific problem-solving instructions depending on the nature of the task. Drawing on the classification system of the cognitive domain developed by Bloom (1956) (i.e., knowledge, comprehension, application, analysis, synthesis, and evaluation), clients should be encouraged to pose more critical questions demanding higher level thinking commensurate with the message content and task requirements (Wilson, Lanza, & Barton, 1988). The clinician may find it helpful to move

problem-solving instructions from the specific to more general as the client's skills increase (Chermak & Musiek, 1997). Self-monitoring continues throughout the task, culminating in self-evaluation and feedback. Self-reinforcement, the final step in the self-instruction procedure, establishes a sense of pride and accomplishment and should increase the client's motivation to transfer the self-instructional technique to novel situations (Chermak & Musiek, 1997). If the client is not successful, the clinician should offer some guidance for coping with failure. As discussed in the preceding section, coping with failure may be best handled by self-attributions of failure to something under the client's control (e.g., improper strategy selection, insufficient effort).

Cognitive Problem Solving. Cognitive problem solving offers clients opportunities to resolve problems through systematic analysis and self-regulation. Basically a five-stage process, the clinician serves as a consultant as the client learns to reconceive the potentially anxiety-producing listening situation as a problem to be solved (Chermak & Musiek, 1997). Clients are taught to deploy executive processes in conjunction with the requisite auditory and language skills to resolve the message. They are instructed to analyze situations and generate a variety of potentially viable responses, recognizing and implementing the most effective response. Furthermore, they are helped to confront cognitive distortions (e.g., catastrophizing, jumping to conclusions), which may be sustaining unnecessary anxiety or fear (Hart & Morgan, 1993). Self-regulation procedures (described in the next section) are used to maintain and generalize the productive response (Goldfried & Davison, 1976). Cognitive problem solving is especially therapeutic when working with individuals with anxiety, fear, or phobias (Hart & Morgan, 1993) and has been used successfully in management of patients with tinnitus (Sweetow, 1986).

Perhaps the most important stage of problem solving, the process begins by familiarizing oneself with the nature of the problem (D'Zurilla, 1986). The second stage requires the generation of hypotheses regarding solutions to the problem. In the third stage, one evaluates the solution options, considers their utility and predicts possible costs or consequences, and selects the best one. The fourth stage is bifurcated. If a viable solution is found, it is implemented; if no solution is deemed tenable, the incubation phase begins during which no active effort is expended toward solving the problem (Halpern, 1984). Ironically, it is during this incubation phase that solutions often appear as an epiphany or *out of the blue* (Halpern, 1984, p. 163). A fifth stage in the process involves the monitoring and evaluation of one's performance in relation to solving the problem. Self-monitoring homework assignments are useful in measuring progress. Self-reinforcement for successful problem solving (e.g., spoken language understanding) should lead to enhanced self-efficacy and generalization of the process (Haaga & Davison, 1986). A flow chart illustrating cognitive problem solving in spoken language comprehension is presented in Figure 5–1.

In addition to self-instruction and self-monitoring, cognitive rehearsal is another useful problem-solving technique (Haaga & Davison, 1986). Mentally reviewing the listening task prior to completing it provides an opportunity to identify potential obstacles, solutions, and preventative steps so that listening may be successful (Chermak & Musiek, 1997).

Cognitive Strategy Training. Cognitive strategy training helps clients become more aware of their own cognitive processes and gain skills in deploying specific task strategies underlying effective performance (Brown & French, 1979; Whitman et al., 1984). Cognitive strategies may be trained following Meichenbaum and Goodman's (1971) five-step self-instruction program. Extended training of the strategy and feedback on the strategy's effectiveness are crucial to successful implementation of cognitive strategy training (Whitman et al., 1984).

Self-Regulation Procedures. Self-regulation training leads clients towards self-control through self-monitoring, self-evaluation, and self-reinforcement (Brown et al., 1981; Kanfer & Gaelick, 1991; Whitman et al., 1984). Training begins by increasing awareness of the behavior targeted for control and proceeds by teaching goal setting and self-monitoring skills for behavioral change (Whitman et al., 1984). Qualitative monitoring of performance involves the client noting factors such as attitude and emotional state, whereas quantitative monitoring measures successful performance (Chermak & Musiek, 1997). The client self-evaluates favorably if information obtained through self-monitoring matches his or her standards or listening comprehension goals. Self-reinforcement ensues, primarily from internal satisfaction and heightened motivation rather than self-administered reward (Kanfer & Gaelick, 1991).

Self-regulation training promotes effective listening by encouraging the listener to monitor comprehension processes to

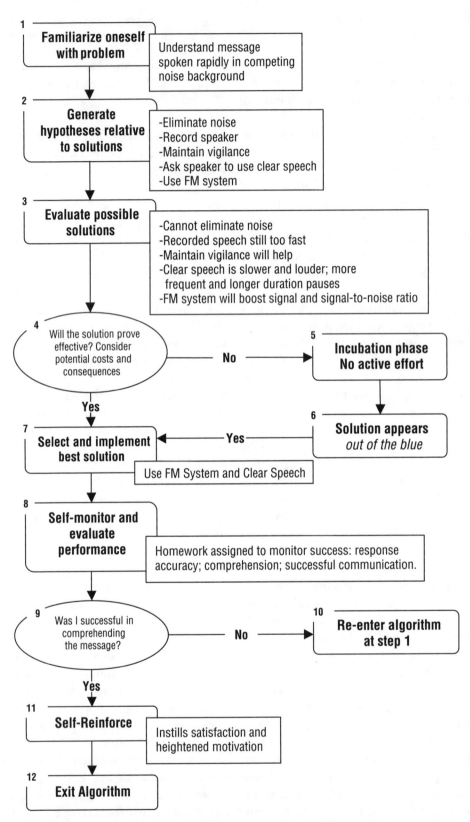

Figure 5–1. Cognitive problem solving in comprehending spoken language.

determine whether they are meeting his or her comprehension needs (Chermak & Musiek, 1997). When comprehension errors, disruptions, or inadequacies are detected, the listener learns to modify strategies to handle ambiguities, inconsistencies, or complexities that might otherwise compromise spoken language understanding (Danks & End, 1987).

Active Listening. Active listening emerges from information processing theory which suggests that skilled listeners actively deploy various bottom-up (e.g., segmenting, discriminating, and sequencing) and top-down strategies to monitor listening and extract information from the spoken message in discovering the speaker's message (Chermak & Musiek, 1997). Active listening training combines the techniques of essentially all the metacognitive strategies discussed above. The elements of active listening must be made explicit and practice opportunities provided for clients with (C)APD. These elements include: listening intently; showing interest through the use of eye contact, body language and posture; listening empathetically (i.e., placing yourself in the other's "shoes"); using closure, inferencing, deducing, and predicting skills; using communication repair strategies (e.g., requesting repetition, rephrasing, confirmations, etc.); ignoring background noise; and not giving up prematurely.

Reciprocal Teaching

The client and clinician alternate roles in reciprocal teaching, allowing the client to take the role of teacher as well as student (Casanova, 1989; Chermak, Curtis, & Seikel,, 1996; Palincsar & Brown, 1984). Reciprocal teaching lets clients anchor their knowledge of their execu-

tive processes by making explicit their knowledge and use of strategies; in addition, most clients enjoy heightened self-esteem and self-efficacy in reciprocal role-playing (Chermak & Musiek, 1997). Reciprocal teaching has produced demonstrated gains in reading comprehension, self-monitoring, memory, and health education, including hearing conservation (Aarnoutse et al., 1998; Brand-Gruwel et al., 1998; Chermak et al., 1996; Clarke, MacPherson, Holmes, & Jones, 1986; Palincsar & Brown, 1984, 1986; Palincsar & Klenk, 1992; Paris, Wixson, & Palincsar, 1986).

The following principles and procedures underlie reciprocal teaching: (1) modeling of the target behavior by the clinician-teacher, making the processing strategies overt, explicit and concrete; (2) contextual modeling of strategies; (3) verbal analysis of the strategies used by the client to comprehend the message, as well as corroboration of the message's content; (4) clinician feedback; and (5) transfer of responsibility for comprehension from the clinician to the client once competence is demonstrated by the client (Harris & Sipay, 1990).

Cognitive Style and Reasoning

Selecting the appropriate cognitive style is necessary to meet diverse processing demands and listening tasks (Chermak & Musiek, 1997). Skillfully matching the cognitive style with changing tasks requires reasoning: critically evaluating arguments, drawing inferences and conclusions, and generating and testing hypotheses (Nickerson, 1986). Effective listening requires reasoning to critically evaluate and ultimately reconstruct the messages we hear, as well as the flexibility to invoke the cognitive style that best meets changing task demands (Chermak & Musiek, 1997). Inflexible reasoning and sole reliance on any one cognitive style is ineffective in meeting the diverse processing demands of a complex linguistic signal often presented in challenging (and unfavorable) listening environments (e.g., noisy and reverberant). Dependence on a single cognitive style such as overreliance on literal interpretation, for instance, could lead to failure to comprehend figurative language such as metaphors, idioms, and proverbs (Bard, Shillcock, & Altmann, 1988; Marslen-Wilson & Tyler, 1980; Warren & Warren, 1970). Overreliance on the cognitive style of bottom-up processing could lead to failure to discern multiple meaning words (e.g., homonyms and heteronyms) and misunderstanding a message's content. Similarly, overreliance on top-down processing may cause schema inflexibility, biasing interpretation and impeding comprehension. (See Schema Theory and Use below.)

Spoken language is most efficiently comprehended through complementary cognitive styles. The model of central auditory processing outlined earlier in this chapter illustrates the necessity for the operation of complementary cognitive styles for spoken language comprehension. Accessing multiple cognitive styles is amplified for individuals with (C)APD whose deficient auditory processes render them less able to cope with degraded acoustic signals and for whom sole reliance on bottom-up processing would leave them extremely vulnerable to comprehension problems (Chermak & Musiek, 1997). Individuals with (C)APD should be trained to take advantage of specific information revealed through bottom-up processing (e.g., auditory segmentation, auditory discrim-

ination, pattern recognition), as well as more global information extracted from top-down processes that facilitate auditory and grammatical closure, inferencing, and recognition of conceptual nuances (Chermak & Musiek, 1997).

Although skilled listeners often unconsciously and automatically adjust their cognitive style to meet the processing demands of the task, less skilled listeners must be instructed to make these seamless transitions and reach a level of automaticity (Chermak & Musiek, 1997). Fortunately, cognitive style can be changed through training. For example, children become more reflective following training in the use of a verbal self-control strategy (Craighead, Wilcoxon-Craighead, & Meyers, 1978). Individuals with (C)APD may benefit from exercises that reveal the advantages of analysis and reflection prior to synthesizing information and converging on an interpretation of a complex message. Given the importance of cognitive style flexibility for spoken language comprehension, training individuals with (C)APD to vary their cognitive styles provides them the opportunity to become appropriately responsive listeners (Chermak & Musiek, 1997).

Deductive and Inductive Inferencing. Effective listening requires use of the full range of cognitive approaches to information processing and reasoning, including both deduction and induction and analysis and synthesis (Chermak & Musiek, 1997). Inductive inferencing involves generalization, reasoning from the particulars to the general; deductive inferencing involves reasoning from the general to the particular (Nickerson, 1986). Spoken language comprehension often requires that individuals infer information not specifically presented in the message, but which may be implied and induced or deduced from the available patterns of information. Inferencing skills can be developed through the context-derived vocabulary building technique described later in this chapter. Also useful are short stories requiring inferencing on the basis of perceptual information, logic, and/or evidence (see Gerber, 1993b). Attention to the appropriate use of diverse cognitive styles (e.g., divergent/convergent, impulsive/reflective, adaptive/innovative, synthetic/analytic, field dependent/field independent) should also be introduced in therapy (Chermak & Musiek, 1997).

Assertiveness Training

Assertiveness training empowers individuals and advances all intervention goals. Assertion can be defined as "self-expression through which one stands up for one's own basic human rights without violating the basic human rights of others" (Kelley, 1979, p. 14). Command of basic interpersonal and communication skills is necessary to assert effectively; however, motivation drives assertiveness, for without a desire to succeed and a positive cognitive *mindset*, one is not likely to assume the personal responsibility inherent to assertiveness (Chermak & Musiek, 1997). The goal of assertion is to attain personal effectiveness by communicating what one feels, thinks, and wants (Chermak & Musiek, 1997). Assertive behavior is self-enhancing and empowering, engendering good feelings about one's self, as well as furthering attainment of one's desired goals (Alberti & Emmons, 1978). Assertiveness can be learned (Bornstein, Bellack, & Hersen, 1977; Rehm, Fuchs, Roth, Kornblith, & Romano, 1979); however, self-confidence and self-esteem are prerequisite (Kelley, 1979).

Clinical experience indicates that successful treatment outcomes are correlated with a client's assertiveness (Chermak & Musiek, 1997). Because assertive clients tend to be more actively involved in planning and directing their own therapy, they tend to derive greater gains. Moreover, their higher motivation and positive mindset lead assertive clients to generalize new strategies and skills to everyday life contexts (Chermak & Musiek, 1997).

Assertion typically involves a verbal exchange, whereby the individual formulates and delivers an assertive message (Kelley, 1979). Nonverbal skills also influence message impact: the effectiveness of the assertion is influenced by the nonverbal aspects of the message's delivery, including paralinguistic elements (e.g., vocal intensity, intonation, rhythm), kinesics (e.g., facial expression, posture, gestures), and proxemics (e.g., distance between parties, seating arrangements) (Chermak & Musiek, 1997). Nonverbal cues can reinforce the verbal message and strengthen the effectiveness of that message. Assertiveness training techniques may involve modeling; guided practice; coaching; homework and self-management; readings; and small group discussion (Kelley, 1979).

Metacognition in the Classroom

Access to the communication in the classroom is crucial to academic success. In addition to the specific metacognitive strategies discussed above, audiologists and speech-language pathologists should alert teachers and students with (C)APD to the role of particular words (many of which are formal schemata) and phrases often used in the classroom that like schemata carry organizational, integrational, and predictive value. Ellis (1989) referred to these words as *alert words* and encouraged educators to make obvious to students their power to augment listening and participation in class discussions. The four word classes signal: (1) reasons (e.g., because, reasons, since, therefore); (2) examples (e.g., example, instance, sample, type, model); (3) comparisons (e.g., associated, contrast, differences, similarities, in relation to, opposite, parallel, on the other hand); (4) main idea (e.g., basically, in essence, in conclusion, in summary, key point, the most important,, the gist is); and (5) lists of important information (e.g., categories, characteristics, divisions, features, groups, kinds, parts, members, stages, ways).

Cognitive Training

Cognition refers to the automatic and unconscious processes (e.g., perceiving, recognizing, conceiving, judging, sensing, and reasoning) that underlie the activity of knowing (Nickerson, 1986). Cognition encompasses the acquisition, organization, and use of knowledge (Neisser, 1976). Cognitive processes allow the listener to transform, reduce, elaborate, store, recover, and use sensory input. Attention and memory are two primary and highly interdependent and interactive cognitive resources (de Fockert, Rees, Frith, & Lavie, 2001). Demonstrating increased reaction times, greater distracter interference, and increased activity in the prefrontal cortex under high working-memory loads, de Fockert et al. (2001) concluded that working memory maintains prioritization of rele-

vant information, reduces distraction, and modulates attention. In the same way, attention to a stimulus or task is essential to memory. Clearly, alerting a child in a classroom to *follow along* or *listen carefully* is an important first step toward improving a child's memory of the classroom presentation. (See section on Schema Theory and Use)

Attention

Attention is a multidimensional psychological construct, which when viewed from an information processing point of view includes sustained attention or vigilance, selective attention, and divided attention. Attention is fundamental to the coordination, organization and execution of human behavior (Sergeant, 1996). Attention is ubiquitous in perception, cognition, and learning. Demonstrating the powerful role of attention for learning, Solan, Shelley-Tremblay, Silverman, and Larson (2003) reported that 12 one-hour sessions of computer-assisted attention therapy improved reading comprehension in a group of adolescents with reading disabilities compared to the control group which showed no significant improvement in reading comprehension scores. The capacity for selective attention is fully developed in children by age 7 years of age, whereas sustained attention (i.e., vigilance) continues to develop throughout adolescence (McKay, Halperin, Schwartz, & Sharma, 1994).

Vigilance is a higher-order, supramodal process which serves acoustic signal processing (Farah, Wong, Monheit, & Morrow, 1989). Vigilance can be trained using procedures much like those employed in auditory or continuous performance tasks (Keith, 1994; Riccio, Reynolds, & Lowe, 2001). The individual is required to sustain attention to a continuous stream of auditory stimuli, such as environmental sounds, syllables, or words, and to respond (e.g., by raising a hand, tapping a table) when a particular stimulus is heard. Failure to detect the target stimulus reflects inattention. False positive errors (i.e., responding to a stimulus other than the target stimulus) may reflect impulsivity. Training auditory attention is discussed further in Chapter 4.

Memory

Exercises to strengthen memory should benefit individuals with (C)APD given the essential role of memory for spoken language processing and learning. Metamemory, or knowledge and awareness of one's own memory systems and strategies (Flavell & Wellman, 1977), provides one focus for memory improvement (Chermak & Musiek, 1997). A number of direct memory enhancement techniques provides a second group of approaches. Although some drugs have been shown to improve memory losses associated with neurodegenerative diseases such as Alzheimer's disease (Giacobini & Becker, 1989; Hock, 1995), pharmacologic therapies are not available yet nor recommended to enhance memory in individuals with (C)APD (Chermak & Musiek, 1997; Musiek & Hoffman, 1990). Given our still limited understanding of the neurochemistry of the auditory system (ASHA, 2005; Musiek & Oxholm, 2003) and the absence of a pharmacologic treatment for (C)APD, it is appropriate to consider the full range of behavioral interventions. (See Chapter 13 for emerging and future trends in intervention.)

Certainly, adults demonstrate a substantial understanding of metamemory (Flavell & Wellman, 1977). Children, however, gradually acquire knowledge and appreciation of retrieval cues and effective strategies for coding, organizing, and retrieving items in memory (Howe & Ceci, 1978). Most children begin to demonstrate some awareness of the limitations of memory and of factors affecting memory (e.g., realizing that they cannot remember all information with equal ease) by age 6 years (Kreutzer, Leonard, & Flavell, 1975) and by age 8 to 10 years, children demonstrate a conscious approach to encoding and retrieval, including becoming aware of mnemonics and their benefits (Cavanaugh & Perlmutter, 1982; Harris, 1978; Harris & Terwogt, 1978; Kail, 1990; Kreutzer et al., 1975).

Memory enhancement techniques and strategies discussed in this section include: mnemonics, auditory memory enhancement (AME), and mind mapping. Also discussed are a variety of specific approaches to target working memory, a specific and pervasive component of memory. External compensatory aids (e.g., prosthetic devices and cognitive orthotic devices) offer a relatively powerful and immediate means to augment memory; however, external devices should not be used to the exclusion of internal aids and repetitive practice (Chermak & Musiek, 1997). Internal strategies and repetitive practice are preferable to external aids because they require an individual's active control and self-regulation and are therefore more likely to be applied across settings and maintained over time (Borkowski et al., 1989; Guevremont, 1990). The reader is referred to Chermak and Musiek (1997), Harrell, Parente, Bellingrath, and Lisicia (1992), and Harris (1992) for discussion of external devices. In addition to the strategies and techniques presented here, the reader is reminded that memory can be enhanced through the influence of executive functions. (See Metacognitive Strategies above.)

Mnemonics

Mnemonics are *artificial* or contrived memory aids for organizing information that operate through the application of basic learning principles (e.g., association, organization, meaningfulness, attention) (Harris, 1992; Loftus & Loftus, 1976). Mnemonics can employ acronyms, rhymes, verbal mediators, visual imagery, and drawing, among other devices. They are consciously learned and used, and the majority are language-based. Mnemonic techniques and systems have been shown to improve memory in subjects of various ages, including preschool-aged children (Levin, 1976) and older adults (Treat, Poon, Fozard, & Popkin, 1977). Described below are elaboration, transformation, chunking, and coding, probably the four most frequently used mnemonic devices (Chermak & Musiek, 1997).

Elaboration entails assigning meaning to items to be remembered by recasting them in meaningful sentences, analogies, or acronyms. For example, the sentence "Richard Of York Gained Battles In Vain" is an example of elaboration in which the first letter of each word represents the first letter of the colors of the spectrum of light (i.e., red, orange, yellow, green, blue, indigo, and violet) (Chermak & Musiek, 1997). Another common example of an elaboration mnemonic is the sentence "Every Good Boy Does Fine," used to recall the notes on the treble staff lines (Chermak & Musiek, 1997). First-letter cueing to form acronyms aids memory for sequences. The acronym TORCH (i.e., toxoplasmosis, rubella, syphilis, cytomegalovirus, and herpes) represents the most common perinatal infections that raise the risk of morbidity, especially auditory morbidity. In the same manner, verbal chaining, or assembling items into sentences, may facilitate memory for otherwise unrelated items. The use of rhymes, such as the one beginning, "Thirty days hath September . . . " also demonstrates the power of elaboration to benefit memory for the odd distribution of days across the various months. Finally, paraphrasing and summarizing are two additional examples of elaborative techniques (Chermak & Musiek, 1997).

Transformation involves reconstituting complicated material into a more basic form that can be more easily remembered. For example, transforming Pythagoras' theorem regarding the relationships among the three sides of a right triangle into a simple equation $(a^2 + b^2 = c^2)$ gives the trigonometry student a concise means for storing complicated mathematical relationships. Some types of paraphrasing also may be considered transformations, and thus benefit memory (Chermak & Musiek, 1997).

Chunking entails organizing items into categories. Organizing a mental *to-do* list into office, home, and weekend is an example of chunking. In the same way, grouping telephone numbers into parts, a three-digit area code, three-digit exchange, and the final four digits into a calendar year also reflects a chunking operation (Chermak & Musiek, 1997).

Coding involves recasting the form in which information is presented. Creating mental images (e.g., real scenes or diagrams) or drawing pictures to capture information presented auditorily are examples of coding (Chermak & Musiek,

1997). Drawing may be a particularly useful coding technique for individuals experiencing spoken language processing difficulties because as a nonlinguistic mnemonic drawing activates the primary motor cortex of the right hemisphere and thereby applies bihemispheric processing to a verbal memory task (Musiek & Chermak, 1995).

Auditory Memory Enhancement (AME)

Musiek (1999) described the auditory memory enhancement procedure as an expansion and modification of the early work of Wittrock (1974). The frequent encouragement to *listen carefully* may inadvertently cause children with (C)APD to rely excessively on analytic processing such that they may not develop the complementary gestalt processing strategy (Musiek, 1999). Supporting this observation are findings that individuals with (C)APD have poor contour recognition, a gestalt feature, which is needed in acoustic pattern perception (Pinheiro & Musiek, 1985). The AME method stimulates the analytic-gestalt interface by encouraging imagery and spatial elaboration, as well as analytical listening (Musiek, 1999). The AME procedure promotes concept development and listening (reading) comprehension through the use of generative processes, interhemispheric transfer, and multimodal integration. The AME also provides a useful strategy for note taking and for interpreting complex auditory information and in this regard is similar to mind mapping techniques (discussed below), which employ drawings supplemented by words to enhance relationships and anchor concepts.

The three key steps in the AME procedure are: listening or reading (verbal/analytic), sketching (spatial/gestalt), and discussing or writing (Musiek, 1999). The choice of modality depends upon the individual's age and reading and writing capability. After listening (or reading) to several paragraphs or pages of information, the client is asked to sketch (within no more than 2–3 minutes) the main concept(s) presented (Musiek, 1999). The imposition of a time limit is key to the success of the procedure, as it forces the individual to reduce the main concept into its basic form and transfer from a verbal/analytic representation to a spatial/gestalt representation (Musiek, 1999). This transfer supports retention and access (Ashcraft, 1989; Wittrock, 1974). This process may be repeated until the entire story or other written material (e.g., journal article, newspaper article) is reviewed and sketched. In the final stage of this procedure, the client is asked to review the sketches and convey to the clinician, either orally or in writing, the entire story, including all the main concepts. Musiek (1999) described remedial steps if the individual experiences difficulty with the procedure. For example, if the client's sketch does not reflect the main concept, the clinician discusses the story with the client to help make the concept salient to the client. Following this discussion, the client is asked to resketch the story's main concept.

Engaging clients in sketching, a generative process, promotes retention of information (Wittrock, 1977). Transferring the analytic/verbal representation into a gestalt/spatial representation aids access and recall as a gestalt representation promotes the formulation of general concepts which are easier to remember than large quantities of analytic information (Hergenhan & Olsen, 1993). Also aiding memory is the involvement of multiple modalities, including the motor system (Musiek, 1999). Sketching activates the *visual-spatial sketch pad,* a subsystem of working memory, whereas the verbal information in its analytic form activates another working memory subsystem, the *phonologic loop* (Schacter & Tulving, 1994). The multiple representations (i.e., verbal, spatial, auditory, visual, somatic, and motor) should improve memory processes (Massaro, 1987). The transfer of analytic, verbal-based information (i.e., primarily left hemisphere) to a more gestalt representation (i.e., primarily right hemisphere) depends upon the use of mental imagery, which has been shown to enhance recall and information processing (as discussed above under mnemonics) (MacInnis & Price, 1987; Miller, 1956; Wittrock, 1974). The concurrent activation of analytic/verbal, gestalt/spatial, and motor processes galvanizes a larger neural network, with the attendant interactions, redundancies, and opportunities to guide memory and comprehension (Ashcraft, 1989).

Mind Mapping

Mind mapping is a visually based approach, involving the drawing of pictures, usually supplemented by words, as an alternative to note-taking or outlining (Margulies, 1991). These maps provide a nonlinear means of recording information and reflecting relationships among concepts and ideas. Like the AME procedure described above, mind mapping fosters retention and comprehension through the concurrent interplay of auditory, visual, somatic, and motor modalities, as well as activation of analytic/ verbal and gestalt/spatial processes and representations.

Encouraging students to use visual and auditory input for better comprehension is central to academic success; however, note taking (or mind mapping) precludes watching the teacher, forcing students with (C)APD to rely solely on their compromised auditory system for all information. Because these youngsters are often poor writers, their pedestrian note-taking skills exacerbate an already difficult situation as their transcription lags behind the spoken message (Chermak & Musiek, 1992). The resulting antagonism between writing and listening leads to division of attention; instead of summating information across auditory and visual modes, confusion ensues as attention is diverted from the already less than adequate auditory system (Chermak & Musiek, 1997). Providing lecture notes to youngsters with (C)APD prior to the class presentation, having another student take notes for them, or using a tape recorder for later transcription enables students with (C)APD to attend to and process both auditory and visual information (Chermak & Musiek, 1992). Similarly, supplementing verbal instructions with visual instructions and using computer-aided instruction and other audiovisual equipment benefits students with (C)APD. Concurrently, audiologists, speech-language pathologists, and teachers can collaborate to improve note-taking skills by encouraging students' use of prosodic cues and formal schemata (both discussed below), and metamemory strategies to gauge the relative importance of information, guide organization and outlining, and enhance retention. (See Chapter 8 for additional discussion of classroom and instructional modifications for students with (C)APD.)

Working Memory

Working memory involves the temporary storage of information used during reasoning and planning (Baddeley, 1995). It requires the storage of some information during processing of other information. Holding an address in mind while simultaneously retaining a sequence of travel directions or listening to a sequence of events while trying to understand the meaning are everyday examples of working memory. In contrast to short-term memory, working memory involves executive processing and manipulation in addition to simple storage of information. Working memory supports executive control and is crucial to problem solving (i.e., analysis and synthesis) (Barkley, 1997a, 1997b). Working memory modulates attention (de Fockert et al., 2001) and supports auditory processing, including auditory localization (Martinkauppi et al., 2002), auditory pattern processing (Zatorre et al., 2001), and speech recognition in noise (Salvi et al., 2002). Not unexpectedly, working memory demonstrates strong correlations with academics and language, including vocabulary, language acquisition, listening comprehension, reading comprehension, problem solving, and mathematics (Daneman & Blennerhasett, 1984; Daneman & Merikle, 1996).

Working memory deficits have been documented in individuals diagnosed with attention deficit hyperactivity disorder (ADHD), language impairment, learning disability, and those with histories of chronic otitis media (Daneman & Merikle, 1996). It is uncertain whether individuals diagnosed with (C)APD exhibit working memory deficits, although the common connection through chronic otitis media underscores the need for additional research into this potential association. Indeed, Mody, Schwartz, Gravel, and Ruben (1999) found poorer retention and recall of consonant-vowel syllables among subjects with positive histories of otitis media, which they attributed to underspecified coding of phonetic features in working memory. Working memory deficits likely result in difficulties maintaining relevant information simultaneously and integrating information, inefficient resource allocation, and listening comprehension deficits (Daneman & Blennerhasett, 1984).

Working memory can be exercised through a variety of activities, including formulating sentences, sentence combining or assembly, sentence completion, word associations, trail making, digit span, and verbal fluency. (Sentence completion also trains auditory closure.) Daneman and Carpenter (1980) designed a working memory span paradigm in which subjects listen to increasingly longer sets of sentences, and at the end of the set, they attempt to recall the final word of each sentence in the set. Ellis Weismer, Evans, and Hesketh (1999) described a rather standard approach to working memory in which subjects demonstrate comprehension by answering questions following a sentence, and demonstrate working memory by recalling the last word of each sentence after all the sentences in the series have been presented. Another common task that exercises working memory requires a client to answer a question about the set of rhyming words before reciting those words. For example, the clinician would present a series of rhyming words (e.g., fun, run, sun) and ask the client to recognize whether one or more words were among those on the list (e.g., was *bun* or *sun* presented) before recalling and reciting the rhyming words. Similarly, a client might be asked to order and recall a phoneme-number span (e.g., 4, /r/, 2, /m/) beginning with digits and following with the phonemes (e.g., 2, 4, /m/, /r/) (Baddeley 1986; Shallice & Vallar, 1990). Given the role of working memory in auditory processing, one can exercise working memory through formal and informal auditory training, including speech recognition in noise and time-compressed speech recognition, as well as through following auditory directives and reverse digit span recall (Chermak & Musiek, 1997). (See Chapter 4.)

Metalinguistic Strategies

Metalinguistic strategies comprise the final type of central resources training approaches. Metalinguistic strategies include: discourse cohesion devices, schema induction, auditory-verbal closure, segmentation (i.e., phonemic analysis and synthesis), and prosody.

Discourse Cohesion Devices

Discourse cohesion devices are linguistic forms that connect propositions into more complex messages (Halliday & Hasan, 1976; van Dijk, 1985). These devices allow speakers and listeners to more efficiently formulate and resolve messages. Cohesive devices establish relationships between ideas (e.g., causal relationships denoted by *because* or *so*) and build cohesive chains through the use of devices that are either explicit (e.g., pronouns and conjunctions) or must be inferred (e.g., ellipsis) (Chermak & Musiek, 1997). As illustrated in Table 5–3,

discourse cohesion devices include referents (e.g., pronouns); substitution (e.g., use of different terminology as coreferent); ellipsis (i.e., deleting rather than reiterating part of a message that can be inferred); definiteness (e.g., activating known versus new information); and conjunctions (e.g., words that connect and specify relationships across a message). In contrast to other cohesive devices, conjunctions specify relationships within and across propositions without presupposing other elements in the preceding or subsequent text.

Although discourse cohesion devices typically reduce verbiage and therefore increase efficiency of message transfer, they do so by placing additional cognitive (e.g., memory) and linguistic processing demands on the listener (Chermak & Musiek, 1997). Listeners must grasp precisely the relationships signaled by the cohesive devices to discern subtle semantic differences. Notwithstanding these additional demands, improved use of discourse cohesion devices should benefit listening and spoken language processing (Chermak & Musiek, 1997; McKenzie et al., 1981).

Schema Theory and Use

A schema is a metacognitive construct used to explain knowledge organization that is accessed when undertaking behavioral or cognitive tasks (Kintsch, 1988; Rumelhart, 1980). A schema is defined as "a structured cluster of concepts, a set of expectations, as well as an abstract and generic knowledge structure stored in memory that preserves the relations among constituent concepts and generalized knowledge about a text, event, message, situation, or object,

Table 5–3. Discourse Cohesion Devices[a]

Referents	
Pronouns	Isaac prepared dinner. *He* prepared *it*.
Pro-verbs	The blizzard enveloped the city. When it *did*, electrical lines were downed.
Comparatives	Alina dances with grace. *Similarly*, Isaac skis with agility and balance.
Substitution	The orchestra played a marvelous concert. The audience was surprised by the *musicians'* artistry.
Ellipsis	Isaac enjoys practicing his instrument. Alina does too. [Alina enjoys practicing too.]
Definiteness	The computer controlling the hybrid engine would not re-boot. The technician's utilities failed to correct *the* problem.
Conjunctions[b]	
Additive	A democratic nation must ensure security *and* freedom.
Adversative	*Although* he applied to many schools, none accepted him.
Causal	The CEO violated securities law; *therefore*, she was convicted and sent to prison.
Disjunctive	She chose to learn French *instead* of Spanish, despite Spanish being more useful.
Temporal	One should think *before* one speaks.

[a]This table provides examples of the major cohesion signaling devices. It is not an exhaustive listing of the various subtypes.

[b]In contrast to the other cohesive devices, conjunctions do not presuppose other elements in the preceding or subsequent text. Rather, they specify relationships within and across propositions.

thereby providing a framework to guide interpretation" (Chermak & Musiek, 1997, p. 194). A schema functions as a conceptual framework connecting interrelated ideas (Chermak & Musiek, 1997). Schema theory provides an explanation as to how knowledge and experience are mapped in the *mind* and how those representations facilitate comprehension and learning (Rumelhart, 1980, 1984).

Schemata have been invoked to explain one's ability to theorize, predict, infer, and make default assumptions about unmentioned aspects of a situation (Chermak & Musiek, 1997). "Schemata are employed in the process of interpreting sensory data (both linguistic and nonlinguistic), in retrieving information from memory, in organizing actions, in determining goals and subgoals, in allocating resources, and generally, in guiding the flow of processing in the system" (Rumelhart, 1980, pp. 33–34). By guiding processing, schemata serve an executive function (Chermak & Musiek, 1997). Although deploying schemata maximizes the best fit between data and structure, it does not guarantee message understanding (Rumelhart, 1980, 1984).

Schema activation demonstrates the complementary function of bottom-up (i.e., data-driven) and top-down (i.e., concept-driven) processing (Rumelhart, 1980). A schema provides top-down guidance to the listener; however, its activation is dependent on a match between its criterial features and descriptions yielded by lower level (i.e., bottom-up) analysis (Rumelhart, 1980). Through top-down processes the listener recognizes patterns and evidence supporting a schema and upholds the interpretation supported by the schema (Chermak & Musiek, 1997).

Children as young as 2 to 3 years demonstrate the use of formal schemata (e.g., *and*, *then*, and *because*) in their language as they develop awareness of spatial, temporal, and causal relationships (French & Nelson, 1985; Nippold, 1988). Development continues through adolescence to include more complex conjunctions (Nippold, 1988).

Content Schemata

Schemata function at two different levels. Formal schemata (discussed below) involve knowledge of discourse conventions and "give form or structure to experience" (Dillon, 1981, p. 51). Content or contextual schemata provide a generalized interpretation of the content of experience (Dillon, 1981). Also referred to as scripts, content schemata facilitate interpretation by organizing facts and establishing a framework that allows listeners to impose certain constraints on events, precepts, situations, and objects (Rumelhart, 1980).

Listeners use content schemata to interpret spoken messages (Chermak & Musiek, 1997). For example, listeners employ particular content schemata that stipulate the sequential stages of a common event. For example, having accessed a particular script, the listener anticipates that the story setting should precede the major actions of the characters, with a closing following the denouement (Chermak & Musiek, 1997).

Formal Schemata

Formal schemata are linguistic markers that organize, integrate, and predict relationships across propositions and thereby foster the cohesiveness and coherence of messages (Dillon, 1981). Formal schemata include conjunctions (i.e., additive [e.g., *and, furthermore*], adversative [e.g., *although, nevertheless, however*], causal [e.g., *because, therefore, accordingly*], disjunctive [e.g., *but, instead, on the contrary*], and temporal conjunctions [e.g., *before, after, subsequently*), as well as patterns of parallelism and correlative pairs (e.g., *not only/but also; neither/nor*).

Formal schemata do not specify meaning. As recurring patterns, however, they induce certain expectations, narrowing the range of possibilities and providing the skilled listener with direction in constructing meaning (Chermak & Musiek, 1997). By instantiating formal schemata, listeners gain insight as to the probable message structure and they use that knowledge as a framework to generate expectations about the organization and relationships among the content (Chermak & Musiek, 1997). Listeners must still construct the specific detail to fully understand the message.

The organizing function of formal schemata is most salient at the global level. This more global organizing function is represented by expressions such as *the first point*, *and finally*, and *in summary* (Chermak & Musiek, 1997). The addition of paralinguistic cues, including speaking rate, pauses, repetitions, and inflection, and nonverbal cues such as body posture, eye contact, facial expression, and hand gestures further potentiates the organizing function of these phrases for the listener (Buttrill, Niizawa, Biemer, Takahashi, & Hearn, 1989).

The integrative and predictive functions of formal schemata operate at local levels (Dillon, 1981). They focus listeners' attention on patterns that fuse and presage ideas and facilitate the construction of relationships between the ideas (Chermak & Musiek, 1992). For example, the causal conjunction *because* integrates two propositions and predicts the relationship between them (Chermak & Musiek, 1997). Similarly, *if-then* constructions activate schemata depicting either causation (prediction) or speculation (via the subjunctive conditional), thereby facilitating comprehension (Chermak & Musiek, 1997). The integrative function of formal schemata also reduces the processing required to comprehend complex sentences (Chermak & Musiek, 1997). For example, the suspensive construction in the sentence, "Children listen more effectively, despite the challenges imposed by competing noise, when deploying central resource strategies" is less likely to disrupt comprehension if a listener employs formal schematic knowledge. Finally, given their predictive function, formal schemata assist both literal and figurative interpretation, including inferencing, as discussed above under Cognitive Style and Reasoning.

In summary, formal schemata provide frameworks that facilitate the organi-zation, integration, and ultimately the comprehension of information. By providing extensive networks that link new stimuli with stored knowledge and expectation, they render particular perspectives salient, allow for efficient resource allocation and processing, and facilitate comprehension (Chermak & Musiek, 1997).

Clinical Application

Schemata influence listening comprehension. The ability to select and deploy appropriate schemata may account in part for differences between effective and ineffective listeners (Chermak & Musiek, 1992). Individuals with (C)APD and learning disabilities may experience difficulty processing schemata and other discourse cohesion devices (Liles, 1985, 1987; Wren, 1983). Lack of familiarity with the linguistic structure of a message leads to difficulty in determining what is important and relevant, as well as in deciphering the interrelationships among the information presented (Chermak & Musiek, 1997). This in turn leads to less efficient allocation of resources and to difficulties guiding the flow of processing in the system, both of which compromise message comprehension (Rumelhart, 1980). Because schema deployment depends not only on linguistic facility and cognition (e.g., memory), but also on executive functions (e.g., self-regulation and self-monitoring) and cognitive flexibility as well (Rumelhart, 1984), clinical approaches (discussed above) that enhance metacognitive knowledge and skills will also benefit schema use (Chermak & Musiek, 1997).

Exercises that emphasize recognizing and interpreting formal schemata should benefit individuals with (C)APD (Chermak & Musiek, 1992). Better able to elicit the appropriate formal schemata, the listener with (C)APD would invoke a generic framework that exposes relationships across propositions and thereby assists listening comprehension (Chermak & Musiek, 1997). In addition, because formal schemata often occur at phrase boundaries, they may help the listener parse larger and more complex messages into smaller units, promoting both comprehension and retention (Chermak & Musiek, 1997).

Schema Induction

Induction learning emphasizes the central role of discovery for learning and presupposes that induction is natural and that learners approach the learning situation with a predeveloped, perhaps innate, induction capability (Connell, 1988). As illustrated in Table 5–4, the induction procedure provides clients the opportunity to discover the functions and advantages of formal schemata for

Table 5–4. Clinical Illustration of Schema Induction

Objectives: To identify and produce causal conjunctions and constructions.[a]
Step 1   *Clinician:* "It snowed a lot last night. School was canceled. Why do you think school was canceled?" *Client:* "Because the roads are snowy. It's dangerous. If you drive on the road, you will have an accident."
Step 2   *Clinician:* "Yes, now let's listen to (look at[b]) what you said." (Clinician plays back client's response.) "Tell me which words tell you why school was canceled." *Client:* "Because I said *because.* I said *if* you drive on the road, you could have an accident." *Clinician:* "Yes, you are correct. *If* and *because* are the important words that prepare us for the reasons, the answers to the question *why.*"
Step 3   *Clinician:* "Listen to this short story and tell me if you recognize any of the same important words you just told me about."   Mom and Dad tell me that I should sleep well every night. They say that if I sleep well, then I will be more alert in school. If I am more alert, then I will earn better grades. If I earn better grades, then I will be more successful. I will sleep well because I want to be successful.
Step 4   *Clinician:* "Did you recognize any of the important words?" *Client:* "You said that mom and dad said *if* I sleep well and *if* I am alert." *Clinician:* "Yes. You are correct. Did you hear any other important key words?" (Clinician may play back the story if the client has difficulty recalling additional words.) *Client:* "Yes, the boy said he will sleep well *because* he wants to be successful."
Step 5   *Clinician:* "Now, I want you to tell me a short story using these important key words and I will try to identify them and explain their function to you.[c]

continues

Table 5–4. *continued*

Objectives: To produce and identify temporal conjunctions.[d]

Step 1   *Clinician:* "Tell me what you do when you get up in the morning."
Client: "First I get out of bed. Then I brush my teeth. Finally, I get dressed.

Step 2   *Clinician:* "Now, let us listen to (look at) what you said." (Clinician plays back client's description.) "Tell me the important key words you said to let me know that you began by getting out of bed."
Client: "I said, *first* I get out of bed."
Clinician: "Yes, that word *first* certainly gave me a big clue. Now tell me which important word you said so that I would know what happened in the end."
Client: "I said *finally*, I get dressed."
Clinician: "Yes, that is correct."

---

[a]The reader will note variations in the sequence of activities supporting the two different objectives. For the first objective (to identify and produce causal conjunctions and constructions), clients listen to a story that is likely to lead them to produce causal conjunctions and constructions. The clinician then asks the client to identify the causal conjunctions/constructions and explain their function. The last step, illustrating reciprocal teaching, requires that the client generate a story, which the clinician then analyzes. In the second series of steps supporting the production and identification of temporal conjunctions, the client first produces the organizational words and then identifies them and explains their function. The clinician may then proceed to tell the client a story and ask the client to identify the temporal conjunctions and explain their function. The reader will recognize yet other variations on this induction sequence.

[b]The clinician may wish to exploit the advantage of bisensory processing by using audiovisual presentations. Audiotaping and visual aids (e.g., pictures for younger children and written transcripts for older clients) should improve the effectiveness of this procedure.

[c]This step begins a reciprocal teaching sequence wherein the client assumes the teacher's role and thereby promotes metacognitive control.

[d]This truncated sequence begins with the client generating a story. The clinician may expand this sequence by generating stories for the client to examine.

listening comprehension. The clinician's goal is to facilitate the client's recognition of the patterns that exist in the message and to explain these patterns so that they may be used to support message comprehension, as well as message formulation (Chermak & Musiek, 1997). To achieve these outcomes, the clinician structures the message so that information necessary to induce the rules governing the patterns are salient to the listener (Connell, 1988).

Although the discovery aspect of the inductive method can be engaging and effective, it may be too difficult for some clients. Even the most basic conjunctions (e.g., *and, then, because*) may prove too difficult to decipher when presented in the context of the inductive method to young clients, those with more severe (C)APD, and those with associated cognitive, language, or peripheral hearing problems (Chermak & Musiek, 1997). If prompting, rephrasing, and modeling prove ineffective, it may be necessary to suspend the strict inductive approach and revert to an approach that more directly draws the client's attention to the formal schemata (Chermak & Musiek, 1997). Chermak and Musiek (1997) offered several modifications of the approach outlined in Table 5–4 for clients who cannot contextually extract the meaning of formal schemata. One alternative approach to underscoring schematic contrast is to focus on minimal pairs (e.g., (1) *I eat because I am hungry* contrasted with *I eat because I am satisfied*; (2) *I sleep because I am tired* vs. *I sleep, but I am tired*; (3) *Before I go to school, I get dressed* vs. *Before I go to school, I eat dinner;* (4) *I sleep because I am tired vs. I sleep, but I am awake;* (5) *I get dressed before I go to school* vs. *I get dressed after I go to school*). Sentence pairs that contrast conjunctions (#2, #5) present greater challenge than pairs involving only one conjunction (#1, #3). Pairs with contrasting conjunctions also serve to transition to another conjunction in a training sequence. Sentence pairs in which both the conjunction and the predicate phrase vary concurrently (#4) are inherently more difficult than sentence pairs in which either the conjunction (#5) or the predicate phrase is altered (#1, #3). The semantic absurdities resulting from inappropriate use of a conjunction (and/or predicate phrase) intrigue youngsters while providing an opportunity to examine the rule and then return to the induction approach with more confidence and knowledge at some later time (Chermak & Musiek, 1997). Another alternative to the direct induction approach involves asking clients to paraphrase conjoined sentences by incorporating conjunctions (e.g., *The exams were graded./Scores*

were posted is conjoined as *After the exams were graded, the scores were posted* or *Before the scores were posted, the exams were graded.*)

Closure

Listeners employ several levels of closure to complete and make whole an incomplete message. Auditory closure refers to the most basic type of closure in which a listener recognizes a whole word despite the absence of certain elements. Listeners achieve auditory closure by filling in the gaps in the acoustic sound stream, in part by taking advantage of the inherent acoustic redundancies due to coarticulation and parallel transmission of the acoustic-phonetic information (Liberman et al., 1967). Auditory-verbal closure refers to the ability to use spoken contextual (i.e., primarily semantic) information to facilitate message recognition. Grammatic closure, perhaps the most sophisticated type of closure, denotes the ability to invoke syntactic rules to complete phrases or sentences despite missing words or morphemes (e.g., filling in the verb form *is* versus *are* to conjugate with the subject *he*). Listeners use context and language knowledge, inductive and deductive reasoning, and auditory and grammatic closure to derive the meaning of words and messages.

Practice recognizing (low-redundancy) speech that is distorted or degraded (e.g., filtered, compressed, interrupted, or presented in noise, competing messages, or reverberation) offers a direct approach to developing auditory and auditory-verbal closure skills. This approach is elaborated as a component of auditory training in Chapter 4.

Vocabulary Building and Construction of Meaning

Deficits in word knowledge have been reported in individuals with (C)APD and learning disabilities, including limited vocabulary, restrictions in word meaning, difficulties with multiple meaning words, difficulties with comprehension of conjunctions, and deficits in interpreting figurative language (Ferre & Wilber, 1986; Gajar, 1989; Hoskins, 1983; Houck & Billingsley, 1989; Johnson & Myklebust, 1967; Keith & Novak, 1984; Mann, 1991; Matkin & Hook, 1983; Snider, 1989; Willeford & Burleigh, 1985; Wren, 1983). Given the central role vocabulary serves in spoken language comprehension (Perfetti, 1985; Samuels, 1987; Stanovich, 1993; Sticht & James, 1984; Wiig, Semel, & Crouse, 1973), central resources training for (C)APD should incorporate vocabulary building from both a quantitative and a qualitative or semantic network perspective. By focusing on semantic relationships as well as lexicon, the network perspective broadens vocabulary building to foster the larger goal of the construction of meaning (Chermak & Musiek, 1997). Context-derived vocabulary building, word derivation, flexibility with multiple meaning words, and inferencing are among the procedures recommended for extending the breadth and depth of vocabulary knowledge. Concurrently, several of these procedures also promote auditory closure skills that are especially important to resolving messages in unfavorable listening environments.

Context-Derived Vocabulary Building

Linguistic context reduces uncertainty and can be used to derive word meaning and thereby expand vocabulary and enhance message comprehension (Miller & Gildea, 1987). The listener must invoke auditory-verbal, as well as grammatic closure in some instances, to resolve vocabulary (Chermak & Musiek, 1992). Like sentence completion tasks, as well as the Cloze procedure employed in reading instruction, context-derived vocabulary building encourages listeners to delve into their linguistic and world knowledge to ascertain specific word meaning and ultimately comprehend the auditory message (Gerber, 1981).

In many cases context establishes word meaning; however, relying on context may not always prove effective because some contexts are ambiguous, misleading, or simply uninformative (Miller & Gildea, 1987). For example, the context surrounding the unknown word *alighted* in the sentence "The bird alighted on the perch" is sufficiently informative to enable a listener with basic vocabulary knowledge to derive its meaning. In contrast, the relatively uninformative context preceding the unknown word *magnanimity* in the sentence "The man spoke about magnanimity" does not provide sufficient information to clarify meaning. Nonetheless, deducing word meaning from context may be more effective than consulting a dictionary, which requires considerable sophistication if the user is to select the intended meaning from the multiple listings of alternative meanings in dictionaries (Miller & Gildea, 1987).

In constructing sentences for context-derived vocabulary building, the clinician embeds an unknown word in the context of rather concrete, known vocabulary that provides sufficient contextual cues to enable the client to deduce the meaning of the new vocabulary word. Task difficulty can be modified by altering the number and quality of contextual cues.

Developing auditory-verbal closure skills while emphasizing the important comprehension cues provided by context also may be accomplished through the use of sentence material like that incorporated in the Speech Perception in Noise (SPIN) test (Bilger, Neutzel, Rabinowitz, & Rzeczkowski, 1984; Kalikow, Stevens, & Elliott, 1977). The listener is required to identify the final word of sentences that are preceded by phrases providing high or low test-word predictability. High predicatability sentences contain high levels of context or *clue words* (e.g., *The watchdog gave a warning growl*.). Low predictability sentences contain little context from which the final target word can be deduced (e.g., *I had not thought about the growl*.).

Construction of Meaning

Examining the relationship between root words and derivations (e.g., able/disability, know/knowledge, spirit/inspire, revise/revision) fosters word knowledge and vocabulary expansion (Chermak & Musiek, 1997). Multiple meaning words (e.g., block, fly, hard, menu, spring) and homophones (e.g., night/knight, fowl/foul, muscle/mussel, medal/meddle) encourage facility and flexibility in comprehension (Gerber, 1993a) while providing opportunities to expand semantic networks and increase vocabulary (Chermak & Musiek, 1997). Multiple meaning words placed in context can also serve as material for context-derived vocabulary building. For example, the sentence "When *spring* arrives, I *spring* to my feet to walk leisurely along the *spring* that flows beside the trail" serves several instructional goals: to learn word meaning, expand semantic networks, and use context to determine meaning (Chermak

& Musiek, 1997). In the same way, heteronyms (e.g., project/project, object/object, record/record, digest/digest), words spelled identically but pronounced with different stress patterns, afford an excellent vehicle for building vocabulary while also focusing on the role of prosody (i.e., temporal distinctions cued by stress) in spoken language comprehension (Musiek & Chermak, 1995). Finally, in addition to exercises directed toward construction of literal meaning, efforts also may be focused on expanding figurative language. Use of metaphors, similes, slang, sarcasm, idioms, and proverbs provide additional opportunities to build semantic networks (Nippold, 1991; Nippold & Fey, 1983).

Segmentation

Phonologic awareness, the explicit awareness of the sound structure of language, includes the recognition that words are comprised of syllables and phonemes (Catts, 1991). Listeners use phonologic awareness to segment words into their constituent sound elements (Lewkowitz, 1980). Segmentation training (i.e., phonemic analysis) exercises temporal processing, albeit within the context of phonologic awareness. Beyond temporal processing, such training should benefit reading and language processing, given the increasing evidence of the causal linkages between phonologic processing ability and reading skill, as well as spoken language comprehension (Adams, 1990; Ball & Blachman, 1991; Stanovich, 1993; Wagner & Torgesen, 1987). The cognitive and linguistic demands inherent to phonologic awareness activities must be considered carefully, however, as the development of phonologic awareness varies among children (Bradley & Bryant, 1985; Catts, 1991). (The reader is referred to Catts [1991] for an excellent review of phonologic awareness and segmentation training.) Other metalinguistic approaches that dually train temporal processing within the context of central resources training (i.e., following directives and resolving prosodic cues) are discussed below.

Auditory Discrimination

Auditory discrimination is one of the most fundamental central auditory processing skills underlying spoken language comprehension (Chermak & Musiek, 2002). The ability to perceive acoustic similarities and differences between sounds is essential to segmentation skills, which require the listener to recognize the acoustic contrasts among contiguous phonemes (Chermak & Musiek, 1997). In this way, auditory discrimination is fundamental to phonemic analysis and phonemic synthesis. Auditory discrimination and phonemic segmentation are so crucial to spoken language comprehension that treatment programs for (C)APD have been designed around them (Sloan, 1986). (See Chapter 4 for additional discussion of auditory discrimination.)

Phonemic Analysis and Phonemic Synthesis

Phonemic analysis and phonemic synthesis (i.e., sound blending) provide two reciprocal approaches to phonologic awareness and segmentation training (Chermak & Musiek, 1997). The primary goal of phonemic analysis is to develop phonemic encoding and decoding skills using either multisyllabic nonsense sequences (Lindamood & Lindamood, 1975) or single syllables and multisyl-

labic words (Sloan, 1986). The listener identifies which sound is heard and its position in the syllable or word.

Several commercially available treatment programs provide extensive activities to strengthen auditory discrimination and phonemic analysis, including Sloan's (1986) treatment program and the Lindamood Phoneme Sequencing Program for Reading, Spelling, and Speech (LiPS) (formerly Auditory Discrimination in Depth [ADD]) training program (Lindamood & Lindamood, 1975). Recognizing the linkage among central auditory processing, language learning, and language use, Sloan's (1986) four-part program develops skills in auditory discrimination, sound analysis, and sound-symbol (phoneme-grapheme) association and applies these skills to reading and spelling words. Similarly, the LiPS program develops auditory discrimination for sameness, difference, number, and order of speech sounds, as well as sound-symbol association encoding (spelling) and decoding (reading) skills as prerequisite, and complementary, to reading programs.

Other programs targeting phonemic synthesis stress the blending of discrete phonemes into the correctly sequenced, coarticulated sound patterns. The Phonemic Synthesis program developed by Katz and Harmon (1982) is an example of a program designed to promote mastery of sequential phoneme blending skills. (See Chermak and Musiek [1997] for additional discussion of approaches to syllabic segmentation and blending.)

Prosody

In contrast to segmental analysis, prosody involves the suprasegmental aspects of spoken language. Prosody refers to the dynamic melody, timing, rhythm, and amplitude fluctuations of fluent speech. Prosodic information is integral to spoken language processing at a number of levels. Prosody links phonetic segments (Goldinger, Pisoni, & Luce, 1996). Prosody guides attention to the more instructive parts of a message (Cutler & Fodor, 1979; Cutler & Foss, 1977). Furthermore, prosody provides information about the lexical, semantic, and syntactic content of the spoken message (Goldinger, Pisoni, & Luce, 1996; Studdert-Kennedy, 1980).

A number of approaches may be useful in targeting perception of prosody in the context of spoken language (Chermak & Musiek, 1997). As mentioned above in the section on vocabulary building and the construction of meaning, heteronyms require focus on prosody (specifically accent or stress pattern) to resolve semantic distinctions. Ambiguous phrases also can be used to draw attention to prosodic detail while training context-derived vocabulary building skills (Chermak & Musiek, 1992). For example, durational contrasts and context allow the listener to disambiguate sentences with identical surface structure (e.g., *The girl saw the boy with the binoculars* that she purchased for a bird-watching expedition./*The girl saw the boy with the binoculars* that she hoped to purchase for herself some day.).

Intonation is used as an aid to resolve ambiguous messages where prosody changes meaning. As illustrated by Musiek and Chermak (1995), the sentence, "Look out the window," can be parsed and interpreted differently depending on the speaker's intonation and timing. It could mean "Look out!, the window," Look!, Out the window," or simply the simple imperative statement "Look out the window." In a similar manner, tempo-

rally cued sentences (e.g., "The judge went to the *fairgounds* for a divorce" versus "The judge said he saw *fair grounds* for a divorce) (Cole & Jakimik, 1980, p. 159) also may serve to instill an appreciation in the listener for the use of prosody and segmentation knowledge (as well as context) in resolving messages (Chermak & Musiek, 1997). Parsing of words and phrases based on duration and juncture (e.g., nitrate vs. night rate, it sprays vs. it's praise) and reading poetry and noting the location of the emphasis and stress in sentences and words also promote this appreciation and may improve perception of prosody (Chermak & Musiek, 1997). (The reader is referred to Cole and Jakimik [1980] who present a series of temporally cued sentence pairs that contrast one- versus two-word segmentation of the same phoneme sequence.)

Central Resources Training with Preschool Aged Children

Early identification and diagnosis of (C)APD in children is crucial given the potential adverse impact of (C)APD for communication, academic achievement, and social function (ASHA, 2005; Bellis, 2003; Bellis & Ferre, 1999; Musiek & Chermak, 1995; Willeford, 1985). Unfortunately, few tests with sufficiently documented sensitivity and specificity for (C)APD are available for young children, rendering diagnosis of (C)APD difficult at best (Chermak & Musiek, 1997). Nonetheless, it is prudent to involve preschool children suspected of, or at risk for, (C)APD (e.g., children with histories of recurrent and persistent otitis media with effusion; prematurity and low birth weight; prenatal drug exposure; associated developmental disorders) in programs designed to promote development of auditory perceptual skills. (See Chapters 6 and 7 of Volume I of this Handbook for discussion of screening for (C)APD, and considerations when testing young children, respectively.)

Central resource training for children at risk for and suspected of (C)APD should emphasize the principles of natural language learning (Norris & Damico, 1990). An enriched language environment involving activities that engage young children and provide natural opportunities for listening and communication fosters the development of auditory perceptual and auditory-language skills (Chermak & Musiek, 1997). For example, repetition of daily routines creates a sense of familiarity, allowing the child to focus attention on new auditory information. Collaboration between speech and hearing professionals, preschool teachers, and families maximizes the transfer of skills to daily routines and other settings (Chermak, 1993).

Because listening supports learning, providing optimal listening environments is pivotal to the success of early intervention (or prevention) efforts (Chermak & Musiek, 1997). Strategies used to enhance the acoustic signal and the listening environment for individuals with hearing impairment also are appropriate for children suspected of, or at risk for, (C)APD. In addition to auditory strategies, maximizing access to visual information (e.g., pictures, facial expression, gestures and other nonverbal cues) supports and reinforces auditory information and thereby enhances the saliency of the acoustic signal (Chermak & Musiek, 1997). Strategies to enhance

the acoustic signal and the listening environment, including personal FM and sound-field technology are described in Chapters 3, 7, and 8.

A number of activities are outlined below that provide opportunities to reinforce good listening skills through bottom-up (e.g., discriminating sounds) and top-down processes (e.g., being read to) and may be used with older children, as well as with preschool aged children. Activities are described that promote a number of emerging processes and skills, including selective attention, metalinguistic skills (e.g., auditory-verbal closure), resolution of prosodic cues, multisensory integration, vocabulary building, following directions, inferencing skills, executive function (e.g., planning and self-regulation), and comprehension. (See Chapter 4 for discussion of additional activities that develop listening skills in young children.)

Listening to Stories

Reading aloud to children promotes concept learning, vocabulary building, and practice in vigilance and selective listening (Musiek & Chermak, 1995). If one's focus is to encourage selective listening, target words, for which the child is instructed to monitor and signal the occurrence (e.g., by raising their hands each time a word is read that represents an animal), should be designated before beginning the story. The child might also be encouraged to listen for subtle prosodic cues (e.g., intonation, stress), while focusing on target words. Posing comprehension questions at the end of the story promotes listening for meaning (i.e., comprehension) while still exercising targeted or selective listening

(Chermak & Musiek, 1997). Questions can be formulated around a story grammar (e.g., where and when did events in the story take place [setting]; what did the main character do [action]; what happened as a result of the main character's action [consequences]). A combination of questions that require tracking of the story context as well as the designated target words promotes auditory closure and comprehension (Chermak & Musiek, 1997). Concurrently, multisensory integration can be encouraged by allowing the child to examine the accompanying pictures and words as the story is read aloud (Chermak & Musiek, 1997). Having the caregiver and the child jointly elaborate on the pictures in a book or sections of the text that are of particular interest to the child fosters vocabulary development and reading skills (Ninio, 1980; Teale, 1984, Wells, 1985).

Following Directions

Following directions engages a number of central resources, including attention and working memory, as well as basic central auditory processes, most notably temporal processing. In addition to providing real, everyday functional contexts in which the child must follow sequenced directives to successfully complete a task, games can be organized that require the child to follow directions presented auditorily (e.g., *Simon Says*) (Musiek & Chermak, 1995). To augment reauditorization and transference to a motor activity (for directives requiring some motor task), the child can be required to repeat the directive before acting (Chermak & Musiek, 1997). A variety of other games (e.g., *Telephone*) requiring children to repeat (in sequence) what they have heard to other people, as well as barrier games in which the child must follow directions presented auditorily to create something (e.g., building or drawing) or to replicate a configuration of objects on the other side of the barrier without the benefit of visual cues also are effective activities to promote listening.

Chermak and Musiek (1997) outlined a range of directives of varying complexity and difficulty. Oral directives may be made more complex by inserting adjective sequences, prepositions, and a number of facts, or by using more sophisticated linguistic concepts (e.g., use of *suspensive* phrasing such as "Point to the pictures of animals, but only if they live on farms, after you point to the pictures of toys").

Inferencing

Activities that require the drawing of inferences can be entertaining and appropriate for younger clients. The context-derived vocabulary building technique (discussed above) can be used to develop inferencing skills, as well as build vocabulary and develop auditory-verbal closure skills (Chermak & Musiek, 1997). Young children can be encouraged to draw inferences on the basis of information (i.e., *clues*) presented in stories and in poetry read aloud. Clinicians should discuss with children their inferences and the processes they deployed to externalize and strengthen their reasoning strategies (Chermak & Musiek, 1997). In addition to promoting cognitive style flexibility, inferencing also challenges memory, as stored knowledge is essential to the inferencing process (Chermak & Musiek, 1997).

Executive Function

By age 5 years, children have begun to develop metacognitive knowledge and executive strategies (Kreitler & Kreitler, 1987). As these strategies underlie attention and listening comprehension, activities to reinforce and cultivate these strategies are worthwhile (Chermak & Musiek, 1997). Preschool aged children have developed metacognitive message evaluation skills and respond well to self-regulation training that involves asking questions and evaluating message ambiguity (Pratt & Bates, 1982). Short scenarios can provide contexts for follow-up questions that require planning knowledge and thereby develop executive strategies (Kreitler & Kreitler, 1987), as illustrated in the following scenario.

> Isaac and Alina were both planning birthday parties for the same day. Both children wanted their parties at the arts and crafts center in the local mall. The management agreed to allow both parties to run concurrently; however, the children would have to share the facilities. If you were Alina or Isaac, how would you plan your party so that you did not interfere with the other child's celebration?

Metalinguistic Skills and Vocabulary Building

A number of activities promote the development of metalinguistic skills in preschool aged children, including rhyme play and *knock-knock* jokes (van Kleeck, 1994). For example, emerging metalinguistic skills enable preschool aged children to appreciate the word play (duration and juncture variations) and humor of the following *knock-knock* jokes: "Knock, knock. Who's there? Pasture. Pasture who? It's *past your* bedtime." and "Knock, knock. Who's there? Gladys. Gladys who? *Gladys we can be* to wish you a happy birthday!" In the same way, auditory-verbal closure skills can be developed in young children by omitting phrase and sentence final words in familiar nursery rhymes and songs (e.g., "Twinkle, twinkle little *star*," "Little Bo Peep has lost her *sheep*"). Word games (e.g., Mad Gab™) that involve duration, juncture, and segmentation skills (e.g., resegment "amen ask hurt" to form a meaningful phase "a mini skirt") engage the young child while training central resources. Other classic word games (e.g., Password™) take advantage of semantic relationships to build vocabulary.

Central Resources Training for Adults and Older Adults

Age is one of the most significant sources of individual variability. The individual's response to the variety of developmental, situational, environmental, social, and economic factors influencing that individual at various periods throughout life is dynamic (Chermak & Musiek, 1997). Just as children experience increasing and more complex central auditory processing demands as they face more intellectually and linguistically challenging academic and social situations, the central auditory processing demands facing the older adult in retirement differ from the demands he or she confronted as a young, ambitious professional (Chermak & Musiek, 1997). However, in contrast to children with (C)APD who may never have developed efficient processing skills, older adults with (C)APD are experiencing loss or disruption of processing functions that were previously intact (Chermak & Musiek, 1997). Moreover, the older adult with (C)APD typically presents a complex clinical profile due to the difficulties caused by comorbid conditions, including peripheral hearing loss and cognitive deficits, as well as the diminished plasticity of the central nervous system. Older adults also may present differences in cognitive style that may affect processing outcomes. For example, finding that older adults required longer duration segments to correctly identify monosyllabic word targets, Craig, Kim, Rhyner, and Chirillo (1993) concluded that older adults may impose greater lexical restraint than younger adults, displaying less flexible lexical searching behavior. Also exacerbating older adults' difficulties understanding spoken language are differences in decision-making strategies and reduction in the overall speed of processing (Craig et al., 1993). All the aforementioned factors may complicate efforts to alleviate the central auditory processing deficits experienced by older adults. (The reader is referred to Bellis' Chapter 13 in Volume I of this Handbook for an in-depth review of the aging auditory system and factors contributing to older adults' speech understanding difficulties.)

Clinical Profile

Estimates of (C)APD in older adults range from 23% to 76% (Cooper & Gates, 1991; Golding, Carter, Mitchell, & Hood, 2004; Stach, Spretnjak, & Jerger, 1990). (C)APD is seen in older adults due to aging, or associated with neurologic diseases,

disorders and insults, including neurodegenerative diseases (Baran & Musiek, 1991; Bellis, Nicol, & Kraus, 2000; Jerger, Moncrieff, Greenwald, Wambacq, & Seipel, 2000; Musiek & Gollegly, 1988; Musiek, Gollegly, Lamb, & Lamb, 1990; Pichora-Fuller & Souza, 2003; Tremblay, Piskosz, & Souza, 2003; Willott, 1999; Woods & Clayworth, 1986). Approximately one in three adults 65 years of age and older present with peripheral hearing loss (Ries, 1994).

Although peripheral hearing loss, particularly at the high frequencies, accounts for some of the difficulties older adults experience understanding speech in competing noise backgrounds, other factors including CANS changes and/or senescent changes in cognition may also contribute to reduced speech understanding in noise among older adults (CHABA Working Group on Speech Understanding and Aging, 1988; Pichora-Fuller & Souza, 2003). A substantial body of research has demonstrated that age-related decline in spoken language comprehension cannot be explained on the basis of peripheral hearing loss or cognitive decline alone (Chmiel & Jerger, 1996; Chmiel, Jerger, Murphy, Pirozzolo, & Tooley-Young, 1997; Jerger, 1992; Jerger, Jerger, Oliver, & Pirozzolo, 1989; Jerger, Jerger, & Pirozzolo, 1991; Jerger, Stach, Pruitt, Harper, & Kirby, 1989). (C)APD may account for the decline in spoken language comprehension unexplained by these other peripheral and cognitive factors (Chermak & Musiek, 1997).

Following an extensive literature review, Bellis (Chapter 13, Volume I of this Handbook) concludes that older adults experience a variety of central auditory processing deficits due to aging that exacerbate the speech understanding difficulties attributed to peripheral auditory dysfunction and that can lead to speech understanding difficulties even in the absence of peripheral hearing loss. Moreover, noting the absence of correlation between degree of cognitive deficit and perceived self-assessment of hearing handicap in older listeners, Bellis also concludes that the speech understanding difficulties of older adults cannot be explained completely or even primarily by cognitive decline. In contrast, positive correlations between perceived degree of hearing handicap and CANS status (Fire, Lesner, & Newman, 1991) underscore both the impact of (C)APD in compromising spoken language understanding and the value of intervention to improve central processing function.

Neurophysiology of (C)APD in Older Adults

A neurobiologic disorder is suspected in the majority of youngsters with (C)APD, possibly involving inefficient interhemispheric transfer of auditory information and/or lack of appropriate hemispheric lateralization, atypical hemispheric asymmetries, imprecise synchrony of neural firing, or other factors (Jerger et al., 2002; Kraus et al., 1996; Moncrieff, Jerger, Wambacq, Greenwald, & Black, 2004). In contrast, the central auditory processing deficits of older adults are acquired, resulting from accumulated damage or deterioration to the CANS due to neurologic diseases, disorders and insults, including neurodegenerative diseases, which may or may not involve fairly circumscribed and identifiable lesions of the CANS (Baran & Musiek, 1991; Musiek & Gollegly, 1988; Musiek et al., 1990), or from the aging process (e.g., less synchrony and time-locking, slower refractory

periods, decreased central inhibition, and interhemispheric transfer deficits) (Bellis et al., 2000; Jerger et al., 2000; Pichora-Fuller & Souza, 2003; Tremblay et al., 2003; Willott, 1999; Woods & Clayworth, 1986).

Neuroplasticity and Aging

Neural reorganization and recovery of function following injury or disease is less likely in older adults due to the reduction in brain plasticity associated with aging, as well as the slow, but sustained loss of neurons that begins in adolescence and continues throughout the aging process (Kolb, 1995). In fact, neural reorganization (e.g., tonotopic reorganization of frequency maps) may actually *cause* or exacerbate perceptual difficulties for some older adults (Willott, 1999). Although young children may benefit from a great degree of brain plasticity, they do not present the wealth of language and world knowledge or the metacognitive knowledge acquired by the older adult, all of which, if intact, can mitigate the impact of (C)APD (Chermak & Musiek, 1997). Conversely, decline in an older adult's central resources can exacerbate the impact of the (C)APD.

Implications for Intervention

Intervention to alleviate some of the central auditory processing deficits common to the aging process often is complicated by several factors, including diminished plasticity and comorbid peripheral hearing loss and cognitive deficits. There is little doubt that peripheral deficits and cognitive decline or differences potentially exacerbate the effects of (C)APD

(Chermak & Musiek, 1997). Management must begin by considering amplification, as the primary complaint of the older adult with (C)APD is difficulty understanding spoken language in the presence of background noise, as well as the frequent co-occurrence of peripheral hearing loss in this population (Chmiel & Jerger, 1996; Stach et al., 1990). Hearing aids and personal hearing assistive technology (e.g., personal frequency modulation [FM] systems) should be fitted in advance of intervention directed toward the (C)APD. The remote microphone technology employed in FM systems is more effective than hearing aids in reducing background competition, which interferes with the older adult's ability to understand spoken language (Stach et al., 1990; Stach, Loiselle, Jerger, Mintz, & Taylor, 1987). When fitting hearing aids to older adults with mixed peripheral and central hearing problems, consideration should be given to the possibility that a monaural fitting may be more effective than a binaural fitting due to interhemispheric transfer problems (Bellis et al., 2000; Jerger et al., 2000; Strouse Carter, Noe, & Wilson, 2001).

The intervention program should also include communication repair strategies and auditory-visual speech perception training (i.e., speechreading), particularly when the older adults presents with both peripheral and central auditory disorders. Home-based therapy programs may be particularly appropriate for older adults. One such program designed specifically for adults with peripheral hearing impairment, LACE™ (Listening and Communication Enhancement), trains auditory-visual communication via an interactive computer program (Sweetow & Henderson-Sabes, 2004). The development of strategies to enhance utilization of central (i.e., compensatory) resources discussed in this chapter is essential to ensure that the older adult takes optimum advantage of linguistic and other top-down skills and strategies during listening. Intact, central resources provide tremendous opportunity to mitigate the consequences of the (C)APD in the older adult.

Remedial efforts to acquire or recover normal (or equivalent) function in children should prove successful due to the inherent plasticity of their developing brains. In contrast, due to the reduced plasticity inherent to their mature central nervous system, intervention for older adults (and adults) often focuses more (although not exclusively) on compensation rather than recovery of function (ASHA, 1996). Nonetheless, remedial approaches may still succeed, for example, with adults and older adults who have sustained acute brain insults where opportunity presents for spontaneous recovery and stimulation-induced recovery of function (ASHA, 1996). Likewise, as elaborated earlier in this chapter, intervention for children should be comprehensive, including central resources (i.e., compensatory strategies) training to scaffold skills not completely responsive to treatment or remediation, as well as to provide bridging strategies during periods of (re)learning (Chermak & Musiek, 1997).

The prognosis for effective implementation of compensatory or remedial strategies is determined in large part by the source of the (C)APD (i.e., circumscribed lesion or pervasive and diffuse neuropathology). An older adult suffering from aphasia is likely to benefit less from (C)APD therapies than an otherwise normal older adult with presbycusis who is experiencing (C)APD as a result of an aging CANS (ASHA, 1996). Differences in intellectual, cognitive, linguistic, and psychosocial state will influence treatment outcomes across individuals, and must, therefore, be taken into consideration in planning and delivering intervention. Key to successful outcomes with older adults, as with children, is the collaborative involvement of family, other communicative partners, and related professionals in the comprehensive intervention program.

Summary

Given the pivotal role of audition for communication and learning, as well as the frequent comorbidity of (C)APD with cognitive, attention, language, and related deficits, comprehensive intervention is essential to address the clinical and functional deficit profile frequently associated with (C)APD. Although the complex organization of the brain, involving interactive and interfacing sensory, cognitive, and linguistic networks leads to more heterogeneous deficit profiles, that organization also provides treatment and management opportunities. To achieve the ultimate goals of improved listening ability and spoken language comprehension, comprehensive intervention must include central resources training with an emphasis on self-regulation of listening strategies. Coupling auditory training with central resources knowledge, skills, and strategies training helps listeners structure auditory input and orchestrate information processing. Moreover, coupling direct auditory skills training with central resources training empowers clients to invoke complementary strategies to meet the variety of processing demands and listening tasks. This approach should provide a powerful intervention program likely to lead to generalization of skills across settings. A growing body of research has demonstrated the effectiveness of auditory training (see Chapter 4) and the potential of metacognitive training to improve listening and reduce spoken language comprehension deficits. Nonetheless, additional research is needed to confirm these encouraging findings. Such research should involve subjects diagnosed with (C)APD (rather than learning disabilities or language impairment with characteristics suggestive of [C]APD) and employ a robust battery of tests to obtain the high levels of evidence (e.g., randomized controlled trials; meta-analysis of randomized controlled trials) needed to demonstrate intervention effectiveness and efficacy.

References

Aarnoutse, C. A. J., Van Den Bos, K. P., Kees, P., & Brand-Gruwel, S. (1998). Effects of listening comprehension training on listening and reading. *Journal of Special Education, 32*(2), 115–126.

Adams, M. J. (1990). *Beginning to read: Thinking and learning about print.* Cambridge, MA: MIT Press.

Adelman, H. S., & Taylor, L. (1983). Enhancing motivation for overcoming learning and behavior problems. *Journal of Learning Disabilities, 16,* 384–392.

Agnew, J. A., Dorn, C., & Eden, G. F. (2003). Effect of intensive training on auditory processing and reading skills. *Brain and Language, 88,* 21–25.

Ahissar, M., & Hochstein, S. (1993). Attentional control of early perceptual learning. *Proceedings of the National Academy of Science, 90*(12), 5718–5722.

Alberti, R. E., & Emmons, M. L. (1978). *Your perfect right* (3rd ed.). San Luis Obispo, CA: Impact.

American Speech-Language-Hearing Association. (1996). Central auditory processing: Current status of research and implications for clinical practice. *American Journal of Audiology, 5*(2), 41–54.

American Speech-Language-Hearing Association. (2005). *(Central) auditory processing disorders.* Available at http://www.asha.org/members/deskref-journals/deskref/default.

Aoki, C., & Siekevitz, P. (1988). Plasticity in brain development. *Scientific American, 259*(6), 56–64.

Ashcraft, M. H. (1989). *Human memory and cognition.* Glenview, IL: Scott, Foresman.

Baddeley, A. (1986). *Working memory.* Oxford: Oxford University Press.

Baddeley, A. (1995). Working memory. In M. Gazzaniga (Ed.), *The cognitive neurosciences* (pp. 755–764). Cambridge, MA: MIT Press.

Ball, E. W., & Blachman, B. A. (1991). Does phoneme segmentation training in kindergarten make a difference in early word recognition and developmental spelling. *Reading Research Quarterly, 26,* 49–66.

Baran, J. A., & Musiek, F. E. (1991). Behavioral assessment of the central auditory nervous system. In W. F. Rintelmann (Ed.), *Hearing assessment* (pp. 549–602). Austin, TX: Pro-Ed.

Bard, E. G., Schillcock, R. C., & Altmann, G. T. M. (1988). The recognition of words after their acoustic offsets in spontaneous speech: Effects of subsequent context. *Perception and Psychophysics, 44*(5), 395–408.

Barkley, R. A. (1997a). Behavioral inhibition, sustained attention, and executive functions: Constructing a unifying theory of ADHD. *Psychological Bulletin, 121*(1), 65–94.

Barkley, R. A. (1997b). *ADHD and the nature of self-control.* New York: The Guildford Press.

Bartoli, J., & Botel, M. (1988). *Reading/learning disability: An ecological approach.* New York: Teachers College Press.

Bellis, T. J. (2003). *Assessment and management of central auditory processing disorders in the educational setting* (2nd ed.). Clifton Park, NY: Delmar Learning.

Bellis, T. J., & Ferre, J. M. (1999). Multidimensional approach to the different diagnosis of central auditory processing disorders in children. *Journal of the American Academy of Audiology, 10,* 319–328.

Bellis, T. J., Nicol, T., & Kraus, N. (2000). Aging affects hemispheric asymmetry in the neural representation of speech sounds. *Journal of Neuroscience, 20,* 791–797.

Bilger, R. C., Neutzel, J. M., Rabinowitz, W. M., & Rzeczkowski, C. (1984). Standardization of a test of speech perception in noise. *Journal of Speech and Hearing Research, 27,* 32–48.

Bloom, B. (1956). *Taxonomy of educational objectives handbook I: Cognitive domain.* New York: McKay.

Borkowski, J. G., & Burke, J. E. (1996). Theories, models, and measurement of executive functioning: An information processing perspective. In G. R. Lyon & N. A. Krasnegor (Eds.), *Attention, memory, and executive function* (pp. 235–261). Baltimore: Paul H. Brookes.

Borkowski, J. G., Estrada, M. T., Milstead, M., & Hale, C. (1989). General problem-solving skills: Relations between metacognition and strategic processing. *Learning Disability Quarterly, 12,* 57–70.

Borkowski, J. G., Johnston, M. B., & Reid, M. K. (1987). Metacognition, motivation, and controlled performance. In S. J. Ceci (Ed.), *Handbook of cognitive, social, and neuropsychological aspects of learning disabilities* (Vol. 2, pp. 147–174). Hillsdale, NJ: Lawrence Erlbaum.

Borkowski, J. G., Weyhing, R. S., & Carr, M. (1988). Effects of attributional retraining on strategy-based reading comprehension in learning-disabled students. *Journal of Educational Psychology, 80,* 46–53.

Bornstein, M. R., Bellack, A. S., & Hersen, M. (1977). Social-skills training for unassertive children: A multiple-baseline analysis.

Journal of Applied Behavior Analysis, *10*, 183-195.

Bos, C., & Filip, D. (1982). Comprehension monitoring skills in learning disabled and average students. *Topics in Learning Disabilities, 2*, 79-85.

Bradley, L., & Bryant, P. (1985). Rhyme and reason in reading and spelling. *International Academy for Research in Learning Disabilities Monograph Series, No. 1.* Ann Arbor: University of Michigan Press.

Brand-Gruwel, S., Aarnoutse, C. A. J., & Van Den Bos, K. P. (1998). Improving text comprehension strategies in reading and listening settings. *Learning and Instruction, 8*(1), 63-81.

Brophy, J. E. (1981). Teacher praise: A functional analysis. *Review of Educational Research, 51*, 5-32.

Brown, A. L., Bransford, J., Ferrara, R. A., & Campione, J. C. (1983). Learning, remembering, and understanding. In J. Flavell & E. M. Markman (Eds.), *Carmichael's manual of child psychology.* (Vol. 1, pp. 77-166). New York: John Wiley & Sons.

Brown, A. L., Campione, J., & Barclay, C. R. (1979). Training self-checking routines for estimating test readiness: Generalization for list learning to prose recall. *Child Development, 50*, 501-512.

Brown, A. L., Campione, J. C., & Day, J. D. (1981). Learning to learn: On training students to learn from texts. *Educational Researcher, 10*, 14-21.

Brown, A. L., & French, L. (1979). The zone of potential development: Implications for intelligence testing in the year 2000. *Intelligence, 2*, 46-53.

Bryan, T. (1991). Social problems and learning disabilities. In B.Y. L. Wong (Ed.), *Learning about learning disabilities* (pp. 195-229). San Diego, CA: Academic Press.

Butkowski, I. S., & Willows, D. M. (1980). Cognitive-motivational characteristics of children varying in reading ability: Evidence for learned helplessness in poor readers. *Journal of Educational Psychology, 72*, 408-422.

Buttrill, J., Niizawa, J., Biemer, C., Takahashi, C., & Hearn, S. (1989). Serving the language learning disabled adolescent: A strategies-based model. *Language, Speech, and Hearing Services in Schools, 20*, 185-203.

Casanova, U. (1989). Being the teacher helps students learn. *Instructor, 98*(9), 12-13.

Catts, H. W. (1991). Facilitating phonological awareness: Role of speech-language pathologists. *Language, Speech, and Hearing Services in Schools, 22*, 196-203.

Cavanaugh, J. C., & Perlmutter, M. (1982). Metamemory: A critical examination. *Child Development, 53*, 11-28.

Chapin, M., & Dyck, D. G. (1976). Persistence in children's reading behavior as a function of N length and attribution retraining. *Journal of Abnormal Psychology, 85*, 511-515.

Chermak, G. D. (1993). Dynamics of collaborative consultation with families. *American Journal of Audiology, 2*(3), 38-43.

Chermak, G. D. (Ed.). (2002). Management of auditory processing disorders. *Seminars in Hearing, 23*(4).

Chermak, G. D., Curtis, L., & Seikel, J. A. (1996). The effectiveness of an interactive hearing conservation program for elementary school children. *Language, Speech, and Hearing Services in Schools, 27*(1), 29-39.

Chermak, G. D., Hall, J. W., & Musiek, F. E. (1999). Differential diagnosis and management of central auditory processing disorder and attention deficit hyperactivity disorder. *Journal of the American Academy of Audiology, 10*, 289-303.

Chermak, G. D., & Musiek, F. E. (1992). Managing central auditory processing disorders in children and youth. *American Journal of Audiology, 1*, 61-65.

Chermak, G. D., & Musiek, F. E. (1997). *Central auditory processing disorders: New perspectives.* San Diego, CA: Singular Publishing Group.

Chermak, G. D., & Musiek, F. E. (2002). Auditory training: Principles and approaches for remediating and managing auditory processing disorders. *Seminars in Hearing*, *23*(4), 297–308.

Chmiel, R., & Jerger, J. (1996). Hearing aid use, central auditory disorder, and hearing handicap in elderly persons. *Journal of the American Academy of Audiology*, *7*, 190–202.

Chmiel, R., Jerger, J., Murphy, E., Pirozzolo, G., & Tooley-Young, C. (1997). Unsuccessful use of binaural amplification by an elderly person. *Journal of the American Academy of Audiology*, *8*, 1–10.

Clarke, J., MacPherson, B., Holmes, D., & Jones, R. (1986). Reducing adolescent smoking: A comparison of peer-led, teacher-led, and expert interventions. *Journal of School Health*, *98*(2), 92–96.

Clifford, M. M. (1978). Have we underestimated the facilitative effects of failure? *Canadian Journal of Behavioral Science*, *10*, 308–316.

Cole, R., & Jakimik, J. (1980). A model of speech perception. In R. Cole (Ed.), *Perception and prediction of fluent speech* (pp. 133–160). Engelwood Cliffs, NJ: Lawrence Erlbaum.

Committee on Hearing, Bioacoustics, and Biomechanics (CHABA) Working Group on Speech Understanding and Aging. (1988). Speech understanding and aging. *Journal of the Acoustical Society of America*, *83*, 859–893.

Connell, P. J. (1988). Induction, generalization, and deduction: Models for defining language generalization. *Language, Speech, and Hearing Services in Schools*, *19*(3), 282–291.

Cooper, J. C., Jr., & Gates, G. A. (1991). Hearing in the elderly—The Framingham Cohort, 1983–1985: Part II. Prevalence of central auditory processing disorders. *Ear and Hearing*, *12*, 304–311.

Craig, C. H., Kim, B. W., Rhyner, P. M. P., & Chirillo, T. K. B. (1993). Effects of word predictability, child development, and aging on time-gated speech recognition performance. *Journal of Speech and Hearing Research*, *36*, 832–841.

Craighead, W. E., Wilcoxon-Craighead, L., & Meyers, A. (1978). New directions in behavior modification with children. In M. Hersen, R. Eisler, & P. Miller (Eds.), *Progress in behavior modification* (Vol. 6, pp. 159–201). New York: Academic Press.

Cutler, A., & Fodor, J. A. (1979). Semantic focus and sentence comprehension. *Cognition*, *7*, 49–59.

Cutler, A., & Foss, D. J. (1977). On the role of sentence stress in sentence processing. *Language and Speech*, *20*, 1–10.

Damico, J. S., Augustine, L. E., & Hayes, P. A. (1996). Formulating a functional model of attention deficit hyperactivity disorder for the practicing speech-language pathologist. *Seminars in Speech and Language*, *17*(1), 5–20.

Daneman, M., & Blennerhasset, A. (1984). How to assess the listening comprehension skills of prereaders. *Journal of Educational Psychology*, *76*, 1372–1381.

Daneman, M., & Carpenter, P. A. (1980). Individual differences in working memory and reading. *Journal of Verbal Learning and Verbal Behavior*, *19*, 450–466.

Daneman, M., & Merikle, P. (1996). Working memory and language comprehension: A meta-analysis. *Psychonomic Bulletin and Review*, *3*(4), 422–433.

Danks, J. H., & End, L. J. (1987). Processing strategies for reading and listening. In R. Horowitz & S. J. Samuels (Eds.), *Comprehending oral and written language* (pp. 271–294). San Diego, CA: Academic Press.

de Fockert, J., Rees, G., Frith, C., & Lavie, N. (2001). The role of working memory in visual selective attention. *Science*, *291*, 1803–1806.

Dillon, G. L. (1981). *Constructing texts*. Bloomington: Indiana University Press.

Duranti, A., & Goodwin, C. (1990). *Rethinking context: Language as an interactive phenomenon*. Cambridge, UK: Cambridge University Press.

Dweck, C. S. (1975). The role of expectations and attributions in the alleviation of learned helplessness. *Journal of Personality and Social Psychology, 31*, 674–685.

Dweck, C. S. (1977). Learned helplessness and negative evaluation. *The Educator, 14*, 44–49.

D'Zurilla, T. J. (1986). *Problem-solving therapy: A social competence approach to clinical intervention.* New York: Springer.

Ehri, L. C., Nunes, S. R., Willows, D. M., Schuster, B. V., Yaghoub-Zadeh, Z., & Shanahan, T. (2001). Phonemic awareness instruction helps children learn to read: Evidence from the National Reading Panel's Meta-Analysis. *Reading Research Quarterly, 36*(3), 250–287.

Elbert, T., Pantev, C., Wienbruch, C., Rockstroh, B. & Taub, E. (1995). Increased cortical representation of the fingers of the left hand in string players. *Science, 270*, 305–306.

Ellis, E. (1989). A metacognitive intervention for increasing class participation. *Learning Disabilities Focus, 5*(1), 36–46.

Ellis, E. S., & Friend, P. (1991). Adolescents with learning disabilities. In B. Y. L. Wong (Ed.), *Learning about learning disabilities* (pp. 506–561). San Diego, CA: Academic Press.

Ellis, E. S., Lenz, B. K., & Sabornie, E. J. (1987). Generalization and adaptation of learning strategies to natural environments—Part 2: Research into practice. *Remedial and Special Education, 8*(2), 6–23.

Ellis Weismer, S., Evans, J., & Hesketh, L.J. (1999). An examination of verbal working-memory capacity in children with specific language impairment. *Journal of Speech, Language, and Hearing Research, 42*, 1249–1260.

Fabricius, W. V., & Hagen, J. W. (1984). Use of causal attributions about recall performance to assess metameory and predict strategic memory behavior in young children. *Developmental Psychology, 20*, 975–987.

Farah, M. J., Wong, A. B., Monheit, M. A., & Morrow, L. A. (1989). Parietal lobe mechanisms of spatial attention: Modality-specific or supramodal? *Neuropsychologia, 27*(4), 461–470.

Ferre, J. M., & Wilber, L. A. (1986). Normal and learning disabled children's central auditory processing skills: An experimental test battery. *Ear and Hearing, 7*, 336–343.

Fire, K. M., Lesner, S. A., & Newman, C. (1991). Hearing handicap as a function of central auditory abilities in the elderly. *American Journal of Otolaryngology, 122*, 105–108.

Flavell, J. H. (1976). Metacognitive aspects of problem solving. In L. B. Resnick (Ed.), *The nature of intelligence* (pp. 231–235). Hillsdale, NJ: Lawrence Erlbaum Associates.

Flavell, J. H. (1981). Cognitive monitoring. In W. P. Dickson (Ed.), *Children's oral communication skills* (pp. 35–60). New York: Academic Press.

Flavell, J. H., & Wellman, H. M. (1977). Metamemory. In R. V. Kail & J. W. Hagan (Eds.), *Perspectives on the development of memory and cognition* (pp. 3–33). Hillsdale, NJ: Lawrence Erlbaum.

French, L., & Nelson, K. (1985). *Young children's knowledge of relational terms.* New York: Springer-Verlag.

Gaffan, D. (2005). Widespread cortical networks underlie memory and attention. *Science, 309*, 2172–2173.

Gajar, A. H. (1989). A computer analysis of written language variables and a comparison of compositions written by university students with and without learning disabilities. *Journal of Learning Disabilities, 22*, 125–130.

Gerber, A. (1981). Remediation of language processing problems of the school-age child. In A. Gerber & D. N. Bryen (Eds.), *Language and learning disabilities* (pp. 159–215). Baltimore: University Park Press.

Gerber, A. (1993a). Intervention: Preventing or reversing the failure cycle. In A. Gerber (Ed.), *Language-related learning disabilities: Their nature and treatment* (pp. 323–393). Baltimore: Paul H. Brookes.

Gerber, A. (Ed.). (1993b). *Language-related learning disabilities: Their nature and treatment.* Baltimore: Paul H. Brookes.

Giacobini, E., & Becker, R. (1989). Present progress and future development in the therapy of Alzheimer's disease. *Progress in Neuropsychopharmacology and Biological Psychiatry, 13*, 1121-1154.

Gibson, J. J. (1966). *The senses considered as perceptual systems.* Boston: Houghton Mifflin.

Gillon, G. T. (2005). Facilitating phoneme awareness development in 3 and 4-year-old children with speech impairment. *Language, Speech, and Hearing Services in Schools, 36*(4), 308-324.

Goldfried, M. R., & Davison, G. C. (1976). *Clinical behavior therapy.* New York: Holt, Rinehart & Winston.

Golding, M., Carter, N., Mitchell, P., & Hood, L. (2004). Prevalence of central auditory processing (CAP) abnormality in an older Australian population: The Blue Mountains hearing study. *Journal of the American Academy of Audiology, 15*, 633-642.

Goldinger, S. D., Pisoni, D. B., & Luce, P. A. (1996). Speech perception and spoken word recognition: Research and theory. In N. J. Lass (Ed.), *Principles of experimental phonetics* (pp. 277-327). St. Louis: Mosby.

Gopal, K., Bishop, C., & Carney, L. (2004a). Auditory measures in clinically depressed individuals. II. Auditory evoked potentials and behavioral speech tests. *International Journal of Audiology, 43*, 499-505.

Gopal, K., Carney, L., & Bishop, C. (2004b). Auditory measures in clinically depressed individuals. I. Basic measures and transient otoacoustic emissions. *International Journal of Audiology, 43*, 493-498.

Grafman, J., & Litvan, I. (1999). Evidence for four forms of neuroplasticity. In J. Grafman & Y. Christen (Eds.), *Neuronal plasticity: Building a bridge from the laboratory to the clinic* (pp. 131-139). New York: Springer-Verlag.

Graham, S., & Harris, K. R. (2003). Students with LD and the process of writing: A meta-analysis of SRSD studies. In L. Swanson, K. R. Harris, & S. Graham (Eds.), *Handbook of research on learning disabilities* (pp. 323-344). New York: Guilford Press.

Griffiths, H., & Craighead, E. W. (1972). Generalization in operant speech therapy for misarticulation. *Journal of Speech and Hearing Disorders, 37*, 485-492.

Guevremont, D. (1990). Social skills and peer relationship training. In R. A. Barkley (Ed.), *Attention-deficit hyperactivity disorder: A handbook for diagnosis and treatment* (pp. 540-572). New York: Guilford Press.

Haaga, D. A., & Davison, G. C. (1986). Cognitive change methods. In F. H. Kanfer & A. P. Goldstein (Eds.), *Helping people change: A textbook of methods* (pp. 236-282). New York: Pergamon Press.

Hallahan, D. P., & Kneedler, R. D. (1979). *Strategy deficits in the information processing of learning-disabled children* (Technical Report No. 6). Charlottesville: University of Virginia Learning Disabilities Research Institute.

Halliday, M. A. K., & Hasan, R. (1976). *Cohesion in English.* London: Longman.

Halpern, D. F. (1984). *Thought and knowledge: An introduction to critical thinking.* Hillsdale, NJ: Lawrence Erlbaum.

Harrell, M., Parente, F., Bellingrath, E. G., & Lisicia, K. A. (1992). *Cognitive rehabilitation of memory: A practical guide.* Gaithersburg, MD: Aspen.

Harris, A. J., & Sipay, E. R. (1990). *How to increase reading ability* (9th ed.). New York: Longman.

Harris, J. E. (1992). Ways to help memory. In B. Wilson & N. Moffat (Eds.), *Clinical management of memory problems* (pp. 56-82). San Diego, CA: Singular Publishing Group.

Harris, K., Reid, R., & Graham, S. (2004). Self-regulation among students with LD and ADHD. In B. Y. L. Wong (Ed.), *Learning about learning disabilities* (3rd ed., pp.167-195). San Diego, CA: Elsevier Academic Press.

Harris, P. L. (1978). Developmental aspects of memory: A review. In M. M. Gruneberg, P. E. Morris, & R. N. Sykes (Eds.), *Practical aspects of memory* (pp. 369-377). London: Academic Press.

Harris, P. L., & Terwogt, M. M. (1978). How does memory write a synopsis. In M. M. Gruneberg, P. E. Morris, & R. N. Sykes

(Eds.), *Practical aspects of memory* (pp. 385–392). London: Academic Press.

Hart, K. J., & Morgan, J. R. (1993). Cognitive-behavioral procedures with children: Historical context and current status. In A. J. Finch, W. M. Nelson, & E. S. Ott (Eds.), *Cognitive-behavioral procedures with children and adolescents* (pp. 1–24). Boston: Allyn & Bacon.

Hassamannova, J., Myslivecek, J., & Novakova, V. (1981). Effects of early auditory stimulation on cortical areas. In J. Syka & L. Aitkin (Eds.), *Neuronal mechanisms of hearing* (pp. 355–359). New York: Plenum Press.

Hayes, E. A., Warrier, C. M., Nichol, T. G., Zecker, S. G., & Kraus, N. (2003). Neural plasticity following auditory training in children with learning problems. *Clinical Neurophysiology, 114,* 673–684.

Hergenhahn, B. R., & Olson, M. H. (1993). *An introduction to theories of learning.* Englewood Cliffs, NJ: Prentice-Hall.

Hock, F. J. (1995). Therapeutic approaches for memory impairments. *Behavioral Brain Research, 66,* 143–150.

Hoskins, B. (1983). Semantics. In C. Wren (Ed.) *Language learning disabilities* (pp. 85–111). Rockville, MD: Aspen Systems.

Houck, C. K., & Billingsley, B. S. (1989). Written expression of students with and without learning disabilities: Differences across the grades. *Journal of Learning Disabilities, 22,* 561–572.

Howe, M. J. A., & Ceci, S. J. (1978). Why older children remember more: Contributions of strategies and existing knowledge of developmental changes in memory. In M. M. Gruneberg, P. E. Morris, & R. N. Sykes (Eds.), *Practical aspects of memory* (pp. 393–400). London: Academic Press.

Jacob, J. E., & Paris, S. G. (1987). Children's metacognition about reading: Issues in definition, measurement and instruction. *Educational Psychology, 22*(3/4), 255–278.

Jerger, J. (1992). Can age-related decline in speech understanding be explained by peripheral hearing loss? *Journal of the American Academy of Audiology, 3,* 33–38.

Jerger, J., Jerger, S., Oliver, T., & Pirozzolo, F. (1989). Speech understanding in the elderly. *Ear and Hearing, 10*(2), 79–89.

Jerger, J., Jerger, S., & Pirozzolo, F. (1991). Correlational analysis of speech audiometric scores, hearing loss, age, and cognitive abilities in the elderly. *Ear and Hearing, 12*(2), 103–109.

Jerger, J., Moncrieff, D., Greenwald, R., Wambacq, I., & Seipel, A. (2000). Effect of age on interaural asymmetry of event-related potentials in a dichotic listening task. *Journal of the American Academy of Audiology, 11,* 383–389.

Jerger, J., Stach, B., Pruitt, J., Harper, R., & Kirby, H. (1989). Comments on "Speech understanding and aging." *Journal of the Acoustical Society of America, 85*(3), 1352–1354.

Jerger, J., Thibodeau, L., Martin, J., Mehta, J., Tillman, G., Greenwald, R., Britt, L., Scott, J., & Overson, G. (2002). Behavioral and electrophysiologic evidence of auditory processing disorder: A twin study. *Journal of the American Academy of Audiology, 13,* 438–460.

Jirsa, R. E. (1992). The clinical utility of the P3 AERP in children with auditory processing disorders. *Journal of Speech and Hearing Research, 35,* 903–912.

Johnson, D. J., & Myklebust, H. R. (1967). *Learning disabilities: Educational principles and practices.* New York: Grune & Stratton.

Kail, R. V. (1990). *The development of memory in children.* New York: W. H. Freeman.

Kalikow, D. N., Stevens, K. N., & Elliott, L. L. (1977). Development of a test of speech intelligibility in noise using sentence materials with controlled word predictability. *Journal of the Acoustical Society of America, 61*(5), 1337–1351.

Kalil, R. E. (1989). Synapse formation in the developing brain. *Scientific American, 261*(6), 76–85.

Kanfer, F. H., & Gaelick, L. (1991). Self-management methods. In F. H. Kanfer & A. P. Goldstein (Eds.), *Helping people change: A textbook of methods* (4th ed., pp. 305-360). Needham Heights, MA: Allyn & Bacon.

Katz, J., & Harmon, C. (1982). *Phonemic synthesis*. Allen, TX: Developmental Learning Materials.

Keith, R. W. (1994). *ACPT: Auditory continuous performance test*. San Antonio, TX: Psychological Corporation.

Keith, R. W., & Novak, K. K. (1984). Relationships between tests of central auditory function and receptive language. *Seminars in Hearing*, *5*(3), 243-250.

Kelley, C. (1979). *Assertion training: A facilitator's guide*. San Diego, CA: University Associates.

Kendall, P. C., & Braswell, L. (1982). Cognitive-behavioral self-control therapy for children. A components analysis. *Journal of Consulting and Clinical Psychology*, *50*, 672-689.

Kennedy, B. A., & Miller, D. J. (1976). Persistent use of verbal rehearsal as a function of information about its value. *Child Development*, *47*, 566-569.

Kintsch, W. (1988). The role of knowledge in discourse comprehension: A construction-integration model. *Psychological Review*, *95*, 163-182.

Kistner, J. A., Osborne, M., & LeVerrier, L. (1988). Causal attributions of learning-disabled children: Developmental patterns and relation to academic progress. *Journal of Educational Psychology*, *80*, 82-89.

Koegel, L. K., Koegel, R. L., & Ingham, J. C. (1986). Programming rapid generalization of correct articulation through self-monitoring procedures. *Journal of Speech and Hearing Disorders*, *51*, 24-32.

Kolb, B. (1995). *Brain plasticity and behavior*. Mahwah, NJ: Lawrence Erlbaum.

Kotsonis, M. E., & Patterson, C. J. (1980). Comprehension monitoring skills in learning disabled children. *Developmental Psychology*, *16*, 541-542.

Kraus, N., & Disterhoff, J. F. (1982). Response plasticity of single neurons in rabbit auditory association cortex during tone-signalled learning. *Brain Research*, *246(2)*, 205-215.

Kraus, N., McGee, T., Carrell, T., King, C., Tremblay, K., & Nicol, T. (1995). Central auditory system plasticity associated with speech discrimination training. *Journal of Cognitive Neuroscience*, *7*(1), 25-32.

Kraus, N., McGee, T. J., Carrell, T. D., Zecker, S. D., Nicol, T. G., & Koch, D. B. (1996). Auditory neurophysiologic responses and discrimination deficits in children with learning problems. *Science*, *273*, 971-973.

Kreitler, S., & Kreitler, H. (1987). Plans and planning: Their motivational and cognitive antecedents. In S. L. Friedman, E. K. Scholnick, & R. R. Cocking (Eds.), *Blueprints for thinking: The role of planning in cognitive development* (pp. 110-178). New York: Cambridge University Press.

Kreutzer, M. A., Leonard, C., & Flavell, J. H. (1975). An interview study of children's knowledge about memory. *Monographs of the Society for Research in Child Development*, *40* (Serial No. 159), 1-58.

Lenz, B. K. (1984). *The effect of advance organizers on the learning and retention of learning disabled adolescents within the context of a cooperative planning model*. Final research report submitted to the U.S. Department of Education, Special Education Services. Lawrence: University of Kansas.

Levin, J. R. (1976). What have we learned about maximizing what children learn? In J. R. Levin, & V. L. Allen (Eds.), *Cognitive learning in children* (pp. 105-134). New York: Academic Press.

Lewkowitz, N. (1980). Phonemic awareness training: What to teach and how to teach it. *Journal of Educational Psychology*, *72*, 686-700.

Liberman, A. M., Cooper, F. S., Shankweiler, D., & Studdert-Kennedy, M. (1967). Perception of the speech code. *Psychological Review*, *74*, 431-461.

Licht, B., & Kistner, J. A. (1986). Motivational problems of learning-disabled children: Individual differences and their implications for treatment. In J. K. Torgesen & B. Y. L. Wong (Eds.), *Psychological and educational perspectives on learning disabilities* (pp. 225-255). San Diego, CA: Academic Press.

Licht, B., Kistner, J., Ozkaragoz, T., Shapiro, S., & Clausen, L. (1985). Causal attributions of learning disabled children: Individual differences and their implications for persistence. *Journal of Educational Psychology*, 77, 208-216.

Liles, B. Z. (1985). Cohesion in the narratives of normal and language disordered children. *Journal of Speech and Hearing Research*, 28, 123-133.

Liles, B. Z. (1987). Episode organization and cohesive conjunctions in narratives of children with and without language disorders. *Journal of Speech and Hearing Research*, 30, 185-196.

Lindamood, C., & Lindamood, P. (1975). *Auditory discrimination in depth* (Rev. ed.). Austin, TX: Pro-Ed.

Lloyd, J. (1980). Academic instruction and cognitive behavior modification: The need for attack strategy training. *Exceptional Education Quarterly*, 1, 53-64.

Lodico, M. G., Ghatala, E. S., Levin, J. R., Pressley, M., & Bell, J. A. (1983). The effects of strategy-monitoring training on children's selection of effective memory strategies. *Journal of Experimental Child Psychology*, 35, 263-277.

Loftus, G. F., & Loftus, E. F. (1976). *Human memory: The processing of information*. Hillsdale, NJ: Lawrence Erlbaum.

Maag, J. W., & Reid, R. (1996). Treatment of attention deficit hyperactivity disorder: A multi-modal model for schools. *Seminars in Speech and Language*, 17(1), 37-58.

MacInnis, D., & Price, L. (1987). The role of imagery in information processing: Review and extensions. *Journal of Consumer Research*, 13, 473-491.

Mann, V. (1991). Language problems: A key to early reading problems. In B. Y. L. Wong (Ed.), *Learning about learning disabilities* (pp. 130-162). San Diego, CA: Academic Press.

Margulies, N. (1991). *Mapping inner space*. Tucson, AZ: Zephyr Press.

Marler, J. A., Champlin, C. A., & Gillam, R. B. (2002). Auditory memory for backward masking signals in children with language impairment. *Psychophysiology*, 39(6), 767-780.

Marslen-Wilson, W. D., & Tyler, L. K. (1980). The temporal structure of spoken language understanding. *Cognition*, 8, 1-71.

Martinkauppi, S., Rama, P., Aronen, H. J., Korvenoja, A., & Carolson, S. (2002). Working memory of auditory localization. *Cerebral Cortex*, 10, 889-898.

Massaro, D. W. (1975a). Language and information processing. In D. W. Massaro (Ed.), *Understanding language: An information-processing analysis of speech perception, reading, and psycholinguistics* (pp. 3-28). New York: Academic Press.

Massaro, D. W. (1975b). *Understanding language: An information-processing analysis of speech perception, reading, and psycholinguistics*. New York: Academic Press.

Massaro, D. W. (1976). Auditory information processing. In W. K. W. Estes (Ed.), *Handbook of learning and cognitive processes: Vol. 4: Attention and memory* (pp. 275-320). Hillsdale, NJ: Lawrence Erlbaum.

Massaro, D. W. (1987). *Speech perception by ear and eye: A paradigm for psychological inquiry*. Hillsdale, NJ: Lawrence Erlbaum.

Masterton, R. B. (1992). Role of the central auditory system in hearing: The new direction. *Trends in Neuroscience*, 15, 280-285.

Matkin, N., & Hook, P. (1983). A multidisciplinary approach to central auditory evaluations. In E. Lasky & J. Katz (Eds.), *Central auditory processing disorders* (pp. 223-342). Baltimore: University Park Press.

Mattingly, I. G. (1972). Reading, the linguistic process, and linguistic awareness. In J. F. Kavanaugh & I. G. Mattingly (Eds.), *Language by ear and by eye: The relationship between speech and reading* (pp. 133-148). Cambridge: MIT Press.

McKay, K. E., Halperin, J. M., Schwartz, S. T., & Sharma, V. (1994). Developmental analysis of three aspects of information processing: Sustained attention, selective attention and response organization. *Developmental Neuropsychology*, *10*, 121–132.

McKenzie, G. G., Neilson, A. R., & Braun, C. (1981). The effects of linguistic connectives and prior knowledge on comprehension of good and poor readers. In M. Kamil (Ed.), *Directions in reading: Research and instruction* (pp. 215–218). Rochester, NY: National Reading Conference.

McReynolds, L. V. (1989). Generalization issues in the treatment of communication disorders. In L. V. McReynolds & J. E. Spradlin (Eds.), *Generalization strategies in the treatment of communication disorders* (pp. 1–12). Philadephia: B.C. Decker.

Medway, F. J., & Venino, G. R. (1982). The effects of effort feedback and performance patterns on children's attributions and task persistence. *Contemporary Educational Psychology*, *7*, 26–34.

Meichenbaum, D. (1986). Cognitive-behavior management. In F. H. Kanfer & A. P. Goldstein (Eds.), *Helping people change: A textbook of methods* (3rd ed., pp. 346–380). New York: Pergamon Press.

Meichenbaum, D., & Goodman, J. (1971). Training impulsive children to talk to themselves: A means of developing self-control. *Journal of Abnormal Psychology*, *77*, 115–126.

Merzenich, M., Grajski, K., Jenkins, W., Recanzone, G., & Peterson, B. (1991). Functional cortical plasticity: Cortical network origins of representations changes. *Cold Spring Harbor Symposium on Quantitative Biology*, *55*, 873–887.

Merzenich, M., Jenkins, W., Johnston, P., Schreiner, C., Miller, S.L., & Tallal, P. (1996). Temporal processing deficits of language-learning impaired children ameliorated by training. *Science*, *271*, 77–80.

Merzenich, M., Schreiner, C., Jenkins, W., & Wang, X. (1993). Neural mechanisms underlying temporal integration, segmentation, and input sequence representations: Some implications for the origin of learning disabilities. *Annals of the New York Academy of Science*, *682*, 1–22.

Miller, G. A. (1956). The magical number seven, plus or minus two: Some limits on our capacity for processing information. *Psychological Review*, *63*, 81–97.

Miller, G. A., & Gildea, P. M. (1987). How children learn words. *Scientific American*, *257*, 94–99.

Miller, G. L., & Knudsen, E. I. (2003, February). Adaptive plasticity in the auditory thalamus of juvenile barn owls. *Journal of Neuroscience*, *23*(3), 1059–1065

Miller, R. L., Brickman, P., & Bolen, D. (1975). Attribution versus persuasion as a means for modifying behavior. *Journal of Personality and Social Psychology*, *31*, 430–441.

Mody, M., Schwartz, Gravel, J. S., & Ruben, R. J. (1999). Speech perception and verbal memory in children with and without histories of otitis media. *Journal of Speech, Language, and Hearing Research*, *42*, 1069–1079.

Moncrieff, D., Jerger, J., Wambacq, I., Greenwald, R., & Black, J. (2004). ERP evidence of a dichotic left-ear deficit in some dyslexic children. *Journal of the American Academy of Audiology*, *15*, 518–534.

Moncrieff, D., & Musiek, F. (2002). Interaural asymmetries revealed by dichotic listening tests in normal and dyslexic children. *Journal of the American Academy of Audiology*, *13*, 428–437.

Moore, D. R. (1993). Plasticity of binaural hearing and some possible mechanisms following late-onset deprivation. *Journal of the American Academy of Audiology*, *4*(5), 227–283.

Morley, B. J., & Happe, H. K. (2000). Cholinergic receptors: Dual roles in transduction and plasticity. *Hearing Research*, *147*, 104–112.

Moynahan, E. D. (1978). Assessment and selection of paired associate strategies: A developmental study. *Journal of Experimental Child Psychology*, *26*, 257–266.

Murdock, J. Y., Garcia, E. E., & Hardman, M. L. (1977). Generalizing articulation training with trainable mentally retarded subjects. *Journal of Applied Behavior Analysis, 10*, 717-733.

Musiek, F. E. (1999). Habilitation and management of auditory processing disorders: Overview of selected procedures. *Journal of the American Academy of Audiology, 10*, 329-342.

Musiek, F. E., Baran, J. A., & Pinheiro, M. L. (1992). P300 results in patients with lesions of the auditory areas of the cerebrum. *Journal of the American Academy of Audiology, 3*, 5-15.

Musiek, F. E., Baran, J. A., & Shinn, J. (2004).Assessment and remediation of an auditory processing disorder associated with head trauma. *Journal of the American Academy of Audiology, 15*(2), 117-132.

Musiek, F. E., Bellis, T. J., & Chermak, G. D. (2005). Nonmodularity of the CANS: Implications for (central) auditory processing disorder. *American Journal of Audiology, 14*, 128-138.

Musiek, F. E., & Chermak, G. D. (1995). Three commonly asked questions about central auditory processing disorders: Management. *American Journal of Audiology, 4*(1), 15-18.

Musiek, F. E., & Gollegly, K. (1988). Maturational considerations in the neuroauditory evaluation of children. In F. Bess (Ed.), *Hearing impairment in children* (pp. 231-252). Parkton, MD: York Press.

Musiek, F. E., Gollegly, K., Lamb, L., & Lamb, P. (1990). Selected issues in screening for central auditory processing of dysfunction. *Seminars in Hearing, 11*, 372-384.

Musiek, F. E., & Hoffman, D. W. (1990). An introduction to the functional neurochemistry of the auditory system. *Ear and Hearing, 11*(6), 395-402.

Musiek, F. E., & Oxholm, V. (2003). Central auditory anatomy and function. In L. M. Luxon, J. M Furman, A. Martini, & D. C. Stephens (Eds.), *Textbook of audiological medicine* (pp. 517-572). London: Taylor and Francis Group.

Neisser, U. (1976). *Cognition and reality*. San Francisco: W. H. Freeman.

Nickerson, R. S. (1986). *Reflections on reasoning*. Hillsdale, NJ: Lawrence Erlbaum.

Ninio, A. (1980). Picture-book reading in mother-infant dyads belonging to two subgroups in Israel. *Child Development, 51*, 587-590.

Nippold, M. A. (1988). The literate lexicon. In M. Nippold (Ed.), *Later language development* (pp. 29-47). Boston: College-Hill Press.

Nippold, M. A. (1991). Evaluating and enhancing idiom comprehension in language-disordered students. *Language, Speech, and Hearing Services in Schools, 22*, 100-106.

Nippold, M. A., & Fey, S. H. (1983). Metaphoric understanding in preadolescents having history of language acquisition difficulties. *Language, Speech, and Hearing Services in Schools, 14*, 171-180.

Norris, J. A., & Damico, J. S. (1990). Whole language in theory and practice: Implications for language intervention. *Language, Speech, and Hearing Services in Schools, 21*(4), 212-220.

Olswang, L. B., & Bain, B. (1994). Data collection: Monitoring children's treatment progress. *American Journal of Speech-Language Pathology, 3*(3), 55-66.

Palincsar, A. S., & Brown, A. L. (1984). Reciprocal teaching of comprehension fostering and comprehension monitoring activities. *Cognition and Instruction, 1*, 117-175.

Palincsar, A. S., & Brown, A. L. (1986). Interactive teaching to promote independent learning from text. *Reading Teacher, 39*, 771-771.

Palincsar, A. S., & Brown, A. L. (1987) Enhancing instructional time through attention to metacognition. *Journal of Learning Disabilities, 20*, 66-75.

Palincsar, A. S., & Klenk, L. (1992). Fostering literacy learning in supportive contexts. *Journal of Learning Disabilities, 25*(4), 211-225.

Paris, S. G., & Myers, M. (1981). Comprehension monitoring, memory, and study strategies of good and poor readers. *Journal of Reading Behavior, 13*, 5-22.

Paris, S. G., Newman, R. S., & McVey, K. A. (1982). Learning the functional significance of mnemonic actions: A microgenetic study of strategy acquisition. *Journal of Experimental Child Psychology, 34*, 490-509.

Paris, S. G., Wixson, K. K., & Palincsar, A. S. (1986). Instructional approaches to reading comprehension. In E. Z. Rothkopf (Ed.), *Review of research on education* (Vol. 13, pp. 91-218). Washington, DC: American Educational Research Association.

Pearl, R. A. (1982). LD children's attributions for success and failure: A replication with a labeled LD sample. *Learning Disability Quarterly, 5*, 173-176.

Pearson, P. D., & Fielding, L. (1982). Research update: Listening comprehension. *Language Arts, 59*(9), 617-629.

Perfetti, C. A. (1985). *Reading ability*. New York: Oxford University Press.

Perfetti, C. A., & McCutchen, D. (1982). Speech processes in reading. *Speech and Language Advances in Basic Research and Practice, 7*, 237-269.

Phillips, D., Hall, S., Harrington, I., & Taylor, T. (1998). "Central" auditory gap detection: A spatial case. *Journal of the Acoustical Society of America, 103*, 2064-2068.

Phillips, D., Taylor, T., Hall, S., Carr, M., & Mossop, J. (1997). Detection of silent intervals between noises activating different perceptual channels: Some properties of "central" auditory gap detection. *Journal of the Acoustical Society of America, 101*, 3694-3705.

Pichora-Fuller, M. K., Schneider, B.A., & Daneman, M. (1995). How young and old adults listen to and remember speech in noise. *Journal of the Acoustical Society of America, 97*(1), 593-608.

Pichora-Fuller, M., & Souza, P. (2003). Effects of age and age-related hearing loss on the neural representation of speech cues. *Clinical Neurophysiology, 114*, 1332-1343.

Pinheiro, M., & Musiek, F. (1985). *Assessment of central auditory dysfunction: Founda-tions and clinical correlates.* Baltimore: Williams & Wilkins.

Poplin, M.S. (1988a). Holistic/constructivist principles of the teaching/learning process: Implications for the field of learning disabilities. *Journal of Learning Disabilities, 21*, 401-416.

Poplin, M. S. (1988b). The reductionist fallacy in learning disabilities: Replicating the past by reducing the present. *Journal of Learning Disabilities, 21*, 389-400.

Poremba, A., Saunders, R.C., Crane, A. M., Cook, M., Sokoloff, L., & Mishkin, M. (2003). Functional mapping of the primate auditory system. *Science, 299*, 568-571.

Pratt, M., & Bates, K. (1982). Young editors: Preschoolers' evaluation and production of ambiguous messages. *Developmental Psychology, 18*(1), 30-42.

Pressley, M. (1982). Elaboration and memory development. *Child Development, 53*, 296-309.

Pressley, M., Borkowski, J. G., & O'Sullivan, J. T. (1984). Memory strategy instruction is made of this: Metamemory and durable strategy use. *Educational Psychologist, 19*, 94-107.

Pressley, M., Johnson, C. J., & Symons, S. (1987). Elaborating to learn and learning to elaborate. *Journal of Learning Disabilities, 20*, 76-91.

Pressley, M., & Levin, J. R. (1987). Elaborative learning strategies for the inefficient learner. In S. J. Ceci (Ed.), *Handbook of cognitive, social and neuropsychological aspects of learning disabilities* (Vol. 2, pp. 175-212). Hillsdale, NJ: Lawrence Erlbaum.

Recanzone, G. H., Schreiner, C.E., & Merzenich, M. M. (1993). Plasticity in the frequency representation of primary auditory cortex following discrimination training in adult owl monkeys. *Journal of Neuroscience, 13*, 87-103.

Rehm, L. P., Fuchs, C. Z., Roth, D. M., Kornblith, S. J., & Romano, J. M. (1979). A comparison of self-control and assertion skills treatments of depression. *Behavior Therapy, 10*, 429-442.

Reid, L. (1992). Improving young children's listening by verbal self-regulation: The effect of mode of rule presentation. *Journal of Genetic Psychology, 153*(4), 447–461.

Reid, M. K., & Borkowski, J. G. (1987). Causal attributions of hyperactive children: Implications for training strategies and self-control. *Journal of Educational Psychology, 76,* 225–235.

Riccio, C. A., Reynolds, C. R., & Lowe, P. A. (2001). *Clinical applications of continuous performance tests.* New York: John Wiley & Sons.

Ries, P. W. (1994). Prevalence and characteristics of persons with hearing trouble: United States. National Center for Health Statistics, *Vital Statistics, 24,* 188.

Ringel, B. A., & Springer, C. J. (1980). On knowing how well one is remembering: The persistence of strategy use during transfer. *Journal of Experimental Child Psychology, 29,* 322–333.

Robertson, D., & Irvine, D. R. F. (1989). Plasticity of frequency organization in auditory cortex of guinea pigs with partial unilateral deafness. *Journal of Comparative Neurology, 282,* 456–471.

Rumbaugh, D. M., & Washburn, D. A. (1996). Attention and memory in relation to learning: A comparative adaptation perspective. In G. R. Lyon & N. A. Krasnegor (Eds.), *Attention, memory, and executive function* (pp. 199–220). Baltimore: Paul H. Brookes.

Rumelhart, D. E. (1980). Schemata: The basic building blocks of cognition. In R. Spiro, B. Bruce, & W. Brewer (Eds.), *Theoretical issues in reading comprehension* (pp. 33–58). Hillsdale, NJ: Lawrence Erlbaum.

Rumelhart, D. E. (1984). Understanding understanding. In J. Flood (Ed.), *Understanding reading comprehension* (pp. 1–20). Newark, DE: International Reading Association.

Russo, N., Nicol, T., Zecker, S., Hayes, E., & Kraus, N. (2005). Auditory training improves neural timing in the human brainstem. *Behavioural Brain Research, 156,* 95–103.

Sahley, T. L., Musiek, F. E., & Nodar, R. H. (1996). Naloxone blockage of (-) pentazocine-induced changes in auditory function. *Ear and Hearing, 17,* 341–353.

Sahley, T. L., & Nodar, R. H. (1994). Improvement in auditory function following pentazocine suggests a role for dynorphins in auditory sensitivity. *Ear and Hearing, 15*(6), 422–431.

Salvi, R. J., Lockwood, A. H., Frisina, R. D., Coad, M. L., Wack, D. S., & Frisina, D. R. (2002). PET imaging of the normal human auditory system: Responses to speech in quiet and in background noise. *Hearing Research, 170,* 96–106.

Samuels, S. J. (1987). Factors that influence listening and reading comprehension. In R. Horowitz & S.J. Samuels (Eds.), *Comprehending oral and written language* (pp. 295–325). San Diego, CA: Academic Press.

Schacter, D. L., & Tulving, E. (1994). *Memory systems.* Cambridge, MA: MIT Press.

Schunk, D.H. (1982). Effects of effort attributional feedback on children's perceived self-efficacy and achievement. *Journal of Educational Psychology, 74,* 548–556.

Sergeant, J. (1996). A theory of attention: An information processing perspective. In G. R. Lyon, & N. A. Krasnegor (Eds.), *Attention, memory, and executive function* (pp. 57–70). Baltimore: Paul Brookes.

Shallice, T., & Vallar, G. (1990). The impairment of auditory-verbal short-term storage. In G. Vallar & T. Shallice (Eds.), *Neuropsychological impairments of short-term memory* (pp. 11–53). New York: Cambridge University Press.

Sloan, C. (1986). *Treating auditory processing difficulties in children.* San Diego, CA: College-Hill Press.

Snider, V. E. (1989). Reading comprehension performance of adolescents with learning disabilities. *Learning Disability Quarterly, 12,* 87–96.

Solan, H. A., Shelley-Tremblay, J., Silverman, M., & Larson, S. (2003). Effect of attention therapy on reading comprehension. *Journal of Learning Disabilities, 36*(6), 556–563.

Speece, D., McKinney, J., & Appelbaum, M. (1985). Classification and validation of behavioral subtypes of learning disabled children. *Journal of Educational Psychology*, *77*, 67-77.

Stach, B., Loiselle, L., Jerger, J., Mintz, S., & Taylor, C. (1987). Clinical experience with personal FM assistive listening devices. *Hearing Journal, 10*(5), 24-30.

Stach, B., Spretnjak, M., & Jerger, J. (1990). The prevalence of central presbycusis in a clinical population. *Journal of the American Academy of Audiology, 1*(2), 109-115.

Stanovich, K. E. (1993). The construct validity of discrepancy definitions of reading disability. In G. R. Lyon, D. B. Gray, J. F. Kavanaugh, & N. A. Krasnegor (Eds.), *Better understanding learning disabilities* (pp. 273-307). Baltimore: Paul H. Brookes.

Sticht, T. G., & James, J. H. (1984). Listening and reading. In P. D. Pearson (Ed.), *Handbook of reading research* (pp. 293-317). New York: Longman.

Stokes, T. F., & Baer, D. M. (1977). An implicit technology of generalization. *Journal of Applied Behavior Analysis, 10*, 349-367.

Stone, C. A., & Wertsch, J. V. (1984). A social interactional analysis of learning disabilities remediation. *Journal of Learning Disabilities, 17*, 194-199.

Strouse Carter, A., Noe, C., & Wilson, R. (2001). Listeners who prefer monaural to binaural hearing aids. *Journal of the American Academy of Audiology, 12*, 261-271.

Studdert-Kennedy, M. (1980). Speech perception. *Language and Speech, 23*, 45-66.

Suiter, M. L., & Potter, R. E. (1978). The effects of paradigmatic organization on recall. *Journal of Learning Disabilities, 11*, 247-250.

Swanson, H. L. (1987). Information processing theory and learning disabilities: A commentary and future perspective. *Journal of Learning Disabilities, 20*, 155-166.

Swanson, H. L. (1989). Strategy instruction: Overview of principles and procedures for effective use. *Learning Disability Quarterly, 12*, 3-15.

Swanson, H. L. (1993). Learning disabilities from the perspective of cognitive psychology. In G. R. Lyon, D. B. Gray, J. F. Kavanagh, & N. A. Krasnegor (Eds.), *Better understanding learning disabilities* (pp. 199-228). Baltimore: Paul H. Brookes.

Swanson, T. J., Hodson, B. W., & Schommer-Aikins, M. (2005). An examination of phonological awareness treatment outcomes for seventh-grade poor readers from a bilingual community. *Language, Speech, and Hearing Services in Schools, 36*(4), 336-345.

Sweetow, R. W. (1986). Cognitive aspects of tinnitus patient management. *Ear and Hearing, 7*(6), 390-396.

Sweetow, R. W., & Henderson-Sabes, J. H. (2004). The case for LACE, individualized listening and auditory communication enhancement training. *The Hearing Journal, 57*(3), 32-40.

Syka, J. (2002). Plastic changes in the central auditory system after hearing loss, restoration of function, and during learning. *Physiological Reviews, 82*, 601-636.

Tallal, P., Miller, S., Bedi, G., Byma, G., Wang, X., Nagarajan, S. S., Schreiner, C., Jenkins, W. M., & Merzenich, M. M. (1996). Language comprehension in language-learning impaired children improved with acoustically modified speech. *Science, 271*, 81-84.

Teale, W. H. (1984). Reading to young children: Its significance for literacy development. In H. Goelman, A. A. Oberg & F. Smith (Eds.), *Awakening to literacy* (pp. 110-121). London: Heinemann Educational Books.

Thiebaut de Shotten, M., Urbanski, M., Duffau, H., Volle, E., Ley, R., Dubois, B., & Bartolomeo, P. (2005). Direct evidence for a parietal-frontal pathway subserving spatial awareness in humans. *Science, 309*, 2226-2228.

Thomas, A., & Pashley, B. (1982). Effects of classroom training on LD students' task persistence and attributions. *Learning Disability Quarterly, 5*, 133-144.

Torgesen, J. K. (1979). Factors related to poor performance on rote memory tasks in reading-disabled children. *Learning Disability Quarterly, 2,* 17–23.

Torgesen, J. K. (1980). Conceptual and educational implications of the use of efficient task strategies by learning disabled children. *Journal of Learning Disabilities, 13,* 364–371.

Torgesen, J. K., & Houck, G. (1980). Processing deficiencies in learning disabled children who perform poorly on the digit span task. *Journal of Educational Psychology, 72,* 141–160.

Treat, N. J., Poon, L. W., Fozard, J. L., & Popkin, S. J. (1977, August). *Toward applying cognitive skill training to memory problems.* Paper presented at the meeting of the American Psychological Association, San Francisco, CA.

Tremblay, K., & Kraus, N. (2002). Auditory training induces asymmetrical changes in cortical neural activity. *Journal of Speech, Language, and Hearing Research, 45,* 564–572.

Tremblay, K., Kraus, N., Carrell, T., & McGee, T. (1997). Central auditory system plasticity: Generalization to novel stimulation following listening training. *Journal of the Acoustical Society of America, 102,* 3762–3773.

Tremblay, K., Kraus, N., & McGee, T. (1998). The time course of auditory perceptual learning: Neurophysiological changes during speech-sound training. *NeuroReport, 9,* 3557–3560.

Tremblay, K., Kraus, N., McGee, T., Ponton, C., & Otis, B. (2001). Central auditory plasticity: Changes in the N1-P2 complex after speech-sound training. *Ear and Hearing, 22*(2), 79–90.

Tremblay, K., Piskosz, M., & Souza, P. (2003). Effects of age and age-related hearing loss on the neural representation of speech cues. *Clinical Neurophysiology, 114,* 1332–1343.

Ungerleider, L.G. (1995). Functional brain imaging studies of cortical mechanisms for memory. *Science, 270,* 769–775.

van Dijk, T. A. (1985). Semantic discourse analysis. In T. A. van Dijk (Ed.), *Handbook of discourse analysis. Vol. 2: Dimensions of discourse* (pp. 103–136) London: Academic Press.

Van Kleeck, A. (1994). Metalinguistic development. In G. P. Wallach & K. G. Butler (Eds.), *Language learning disabilities in school-age children and adolescents* (pp. 53–98). New York: Charles E. Merrill.

Wagner, R. K., & Torgesen, J. K. (1987). The nature of phonological processing and its causal role in the acquisition of reading skills. *Psychological Bulletin, 101,* 192–212.

Warren, R. M., & Warren, R. P. (1970). Auditory illusions and confusions. *Scientific American, 223,* 30–36.

Warrier, C. M., Johnson, K. L., Hayes, E. A., Nicol, T., & Kraus, N. (2004). Learning impaired children exhibit timing deficits and training-related improvements in auditory cortical responses to speech in noise. *Experimental Brain Research, 157,* 431–441.

Watson, C. S., & Foyle, D. C. (1985). Central factors in the discrimination and identification of complex sounds. *Journal of the Acoustical Society of America, 78,* 375–380.

Weaver, C. (1985). Parallels between new paradigms in science and in reading and literary theories: An essay review. *Research in the Teaching of English, 19*(3), 298–316.

Weaver, C. (1993). Understanding and educating students with attention deficit hyperactivity disorder: Toward a system theory and whole language perspective. *American Journal of Speech-Language Pathology, 2*(3), 78–89.

Weinberger, N. M., & Diamond, D. M. (1987). Physiological plasticity in auditory cortex: Rapid induction by learning. *Progress in Neurobiology, 29,* 1–55.

Wells, G. (1985). Preschool literacy-related activities and success in school. In D. R. Olson, N. Torrance, & A. Hildyard (Eds.), *Literacy, language, and learning* (pp. 229–255). Cambridge: Cambridge University Press.

Whitman, T. L., Burgio, L., & Johnson, M. B. (1984). Cognitive behavioral interventions with mentally retarded children. In A. Meyers & W. E. Craighead (Eds.), *Cognitive behavior therapy with children* (pp. 193–227). New York: Plenum Press.

Wible, B., Nicol, T., & Kraus, N. (2005). Correlation between brainstem and cortical auditory processes in normal and language-impaired children. *Brain, 128,* 417–423.

Wiens, J. W. (1983). Metacognition and the adolescent passive learner. *Journal of Learning Disabilities, 16,* 144–149.

Wiig, E. H., Semel, E. M., & Crouse, M. A. B. (1973). The use of morphology by high risk and learning disabled children. *Journal of Learning Disabilities, 6*(7), 457–465.

Willeford, J. A. (1985). Assessment of central auditory disorders in children. In M. L. Pinheiro & F. E. Musiek (Eds.), *Assessment of central auditory dysfunction* (pp. 239–257). Baltimore: Williams & Wilkins.

Willeford, J. A., & Burleigh, J. M. (1985). *Handbook of central auditory processing disorders in children.* Orlando, FL: Grune & Stratton.

Willott, J. F. (1999). *Neurogerontology: Aging and the nervous system.* New York: Springer.

Willott, J. F., Aitken, L. M., & McFadden, S. L. (1993). Plasticity of auditory cortex associated with sensorineural hearing loss in adult mice. *Journal of Comparative Neurology, 329*(3), 402–411.

Wilson, C. C., Lanza, J. R., & Barton, J. S. (1988). Developing higher level thinking skills through questioning techniques in the speech and language setting. *Language,* *Speech, and Hearing Services in Schools, 19,* 428–431.

Wittrock, M. C. (1974). Learning as a generative process. *Educational Psychology, 11,* 87–95.

Wittrock, M. C. (1977). *The human brain.* Englewood Cliffs, NJ: Prentice-Hall.

Wong, B. Y. L. (1987). How do the effects of metacognitive research impact on the learning disabled individual? *Learning Disability Quarterly, 10,* 189–195.

Wong, B. Y. L. (1991). The relevance of metacognition to learning disabilities. In B. Y. L. Wong (Ed.), *Learning about learning disabilities* (pp. 232–261). San Diego: Academic Press.

Wong, B. Y. L., & Jones, W. (1982). Increasing metacomprehension in learning-disabled and normally-achieving students through self-questioning training. *Learning Disability Quarterly, 5,* 228–240.

Wong, G. L. (1993). Comparing two modes of teaching a question-answering strategy for enhancing reading comprehension: Didactic and self-instruction. *Journal of Learning Disabilities, 26*(4), 270–279.

Woods, D. L., & Clayworth, C. C. (1986). Age-related changes in human middle latency auditory evoked potentials. *Electroencephalography and Clinical Neurophysiology, 65,* 297–303.

Wren, C. T. (1983). *Language and learning disabilities: Diagnosis and remediation.* Rockville, MD: Aspen.

Zatorre, R. J. (2001). Neural specialization for tonal processing. *Annals of the New York Academy of Sciences, 930,* 193–210

CHAPTER 6

COMPUTER-BASED AUDITORY TRAINING (CBAT) FOR (CENTRAL) AUDITORY PROCESSING DISORDERS

LINDA M. THIBODEAU

Auditory training techniques have been advocated for a variety of communication difficulties. Over the years, many techniques have been developed for use with persons with hearing loss (Carhart, 1960; Goldstein, 1939; Sweetow & Palmer, 2005; Wedenberg, 1951). More recently, efforts have been devoted to development of auditory-based computerized programs for children with language disorders (Merzenich et al., 1996; Tallal et al., 1996; Zwolan, McDonald Connor, & Kileny, 2000). Strong support for performance changes made possible through computer-based auditory training (CBAT) stems from investigations of neural plasticity in animals (Galvan & Weinberger, 2002; Kilgard & Merzenich, 1998b; Recanzone,

Schreiner, & Merzenich, 1993). With the accumulating evidence documenting improved neurophysiologic representation of acoustic stimuli, as well as improved listening and related functions in children and adults following targeted auditory training, several CBAT programs have been developed for individuals with auditory, language, and learning disorders (e.g., Hayes, Warrier, Nicol, Zecker, & Kraus, 2003; Jirsa, 1992; Kraus, McGee, Carrell, King, Tremblay, & Nicol, 1995; Merzenich et al., 1996; Musiek, Baran, & Shinn, 2004; Russo, Nicol, Zecker, Hayes, & Kraus, 2005; Schopmeyer, Mellon, Dobaj, Grant, & Niparko, 1998; Tallal et al., 1996; Tremblay & Kraus, 2002; Tremblay, Kraus, Carrell, & McGee, 1997; Tremblay, Kraus, & McGee, 1998; Tremblay, Kraus, McGee, Ponton, & Otis, 2001; Warrier et al., 2004). Like other training protocols,

CBAT should be evaluated according to the principles of evidence-based practice (EBP), as explained in Chapter 2.

The primary purpose of this chapter is to provide a framework for the evaluation of CBAT so that researchers and practitioners may address the important variables that may impact outcomes and influence EBP studies. At this time, there have been only two Level 3, randomized, controlled clinical trials with relatively large subject pools that have been conducted to determine the effectiveness of various types of computer-based training programs designed for children with language impairments and/or reading difficulty (Gillam et al., 2005; Rouse & Krueger, 2004). Therefore, the information presented in this chapter should be viewed only as a guide for the evaluation of available programs, and not as an endorsement of any particular program.

Critical evaluation of CBAT requires consideration of the reason for training, the process of training, and how the participants react to the training. First, there must be some rationale for the type of training and what is being trained. For example, is the training designed to address increased attention or to refine temporal processing? Consistent with a specific rationale, several training factors such as type of stimuli, schedule of training, and method of delivery may gain importance relative to others. Once the training factors have been prioritized, then the appropriate CBAT program may be selected. Even though all the optimal features may be in place, there may still be other factors as to how the training is conducted that will influence success, such as reinforcement and motivation.

The second purpose of this chapter is to provide a review of some of the cur-

rently available CBAT methods. Typically, a speech-language pathologist or audiologist selects the CBAT program and determines the treatment plan, including frequency of treatment and duration of sessions. In some cases, CBAT programs are selected by educational administrative personnel who are responsible for curriculum decisions. This review of currently available CBAT programs may be used as a guide to compare important features that may impact success. All currently available CBAT programs involve some degree of linguistic processing and, therefore, actually may be considered computer-based *auditory-language* training. However, the broader term CBAT will be used to represent all the levels possible for training, which may include verbal and nonverbal stimuli.

The final purpose of the chapter is to review research that supports the effectiveness of CBAT and to provide suggestions for future studies. This is an exciting time for the application of CBAT as computers are becoming more readily available in schools, the home, and even in vehicles which, in turn, allows greater access to effective training techniques.

Parameters of CBAT

Most are in agreement that auditory training can be an effective intervention for children with (central) auditory processing disorder ([C]APD) (Chermak & Musiek, 2002). As the term implies, such training requires some form of auditory input which could be naturally or electronically produced. In order to propose a model to support the use of CBAT, there are three areas to consider: meaningfulness of the stimuli, active versus passive interaction, and frequency of training. Animal and human research underlying auditory training principles and CBAT discussed in this chapter are elaborated in Chapter 4.

Meaningfulness of the Stimuli

Stimuli for auditory training vary along two dimensions: natural versus synthetic, and speech versus nonspeech. The easiest stimuli to produce quickly, of course, are natural speech and these stimuli are likely the most meaningful to most individuals, particularly children. Synthetic speech, however, allows for more accurate control of parameters such as duration and intensity. Natural, nonspeech sounds (e.g., environmental sounds) are used less frequently, perhaps because of the lack of or reduced cognitive association evoked to maintain interest. The final category, synthetically produced, nonspeech signals such as tones or noise bursts would be least interesting. However, these nonspeech signals can be easily manipulated for targeted training of basic perceptual features and auditory processes that correspond to speech and language processes. An example of training with such nonspeech stimuli would be the use of frequency sweeps that are analogous to second-formant transitions. Historically, the stimuli for auditory training have evolved from primarily natural speech to synthetically generated stimuli that have become increasingly accessible with improvements in technology and easier access to the Internet. The application of these four types of auditory stimuli will be reviewed with respect to their use in auditory training programs.

Natural Speech Stimuli

Human speech is the typical input for naturally produced auditory stimuli. Perhaps the earliest formal auditory training programs that involved natural speech were those designed to enhance communication skills of persons with hearing loss (Carhart, 1960; Wedenberg, 1951). These programs generally involved a hierarchy of skills moving from awareness, to discrimination, to identification, and finally to comprehension. Depending on the age of the child and residual hearing, the parent or teacher would provide activities involving vocabulary that was meaningful to the child at that time. For example, a child would be more inclined to focus on a same/different auditory discrimination task involving animal names following a trip to the zoo. Although natural speech stimuli have been widely used in auditory training, there are no studies documenting the benefits of a particular non-CBAT program with children with hearing loss. Walden and colleagues have demonstrated the benefits of auditory training, however, using natural speech with adults with hearing loss (Montgomery, Walden, Schwartz, & Prosek, 1984; Walden, Erdman, Montgomery, Schwartz, & Prosek, 1981).

Synthetic Speech Stimuli

Auditory training specifically designed for children with (C)APD often involves a dimension of speech processing requiring central integration, such as dichotic listening, phonemic synthesis, and/or temporal processing. Training in these areas requires more precise stimulus control, which is enabled through the use of synthetic speech or nonspeech signals. By controlling acoustic aspects of the stimuli, graduated difficulty may be introduced; however, this may be offered at the expense of using less interesting and less meaningful stimuli for the client.

Tallal and colleagues explored auditory training with synthetic speech based on the theory that children with language disorders are unable to process the rapid fluctuations of frequency information in speech and, therefore, miss important cues for perception (Merzenich et al., 1996; Tallal et al., 1996). They created CBAT programs in which children were presented synthetic speech with modified acoustic cues to aid recognition. For example, recognition training might begin using speech tokens with second-formant transitions with durations twice that found in normal speech. As the child responds correctly, the transitions can be shortened gradually to normal values.

Natural Nonspeech Stimuli

Environmental sounds are the most common natural, nonspeech stimuli that have been used in auditory training. In the early stages of training, programs for children with hearing loss often include discrimination and identification of common environmental sounds such as those produced by telephones, car horns, dogs, alarm clocks, and so forth.

Although not specifically designed for remediation of communication disorders, the Suzuki method of learning music, which involves training with naturally produced, nonspeech stimuli, has implications for the rationale to use CBAT. This intensive auditory-based program designed for music instruction involves daily listening to recordings of songs played on the instrument that is being learned (Suzuki, 1981, 1983). Suzuki reasoned that, just as children did not learn to read printed letters before they learned to speak, children can learn to play music prior to learning how to read printed musical notation. Similarly, he recognized that children learn to communicate by hearing the speech of their parents on a daily basis and proposed that it is logical, therefore, to expect that children could learn to play an instrument through repetitive listening to a hierarchy of songs with guided instruction. (See the discussion of music in auditory training in Chapters 4 and 13.)

Synthetic Nonspeech Stimuli

The use of nonspeech stimuli allows for more precise training in discrete frequency, intensity, or temporal domains. These alterations of the stimulus characteristics are easily accomplished in CBAT. Because of the lack of inherent meaningfulness, such stimuli are typically accompanied by attractive pictures that relate to some aspect of the training. For example, Tallal and colleagues (1996) include synthetic, nonspeech stimuli in the Fast ForWord® training in a game presented in a circus setting. It includes specific training exercises on frequency sweeps that are analogous to rapid formant transitions in speech. Although results of some studies have been interpreted as support for this type of training for children with language impairments (Rouse & Krueger, 2004; Temple et al., 2003; Troia & Whitney, 2003), recent evidence suggests that the improvements may not be the result of the characteristics of the nonspeech, synthetic stimuli but rather are related to other features of the auditory training program (Gillam et al., 2005), as discussed below.

Nonspeech, synthetic stimuli also have been used to specifically retrain cortical processing of frequency-specific stimuli following reorganization resulting from hearing loss. Research with animals with noise-induced hearing loss has shown that regions of the cortex that responded to specific frequency stimuli are reorganized to respond to other frequencies when there is no input at the former frequencies as a result of hearing loss (Eggermont & Komiya, 2000; Robertson & Irvine, 1989). In fact, frequency-specific response regions on the cortex actually expand over time such that areas that are no longer stimulated become responsive to sounds in frequency regions where there is no hearing loss (Irvine, 2000; Robertson & Irvine, 1989). It has been proposed that with intensive training with frequencies reintroduced in the hearing loss region, cortical reorganization can return toward the pre-hearing-loss state (Willott, 1996). See discussions of plasticity in Chapters 1, 4, and 5 of this volume and in Chapters 3 and 4 of Volume I of this Handbook.)

Based on the findings with animals, Scott and Thibodeau examined the possibility that training with frequency-specific stimuli might result in speech recognition benefits for adults with hearing loss (Scott & Thibodeau, 2006). Adults with high-frequency hearing loss were provided amplification that restored high-frequency audibility. They then participated in two weeks (one hour daily) of discrimination training with frequency-sweep stimuli modeled after second-formant transitions. Although there was no change in consonant-vowel-consonant (CVC) identification following training, there was a significant improvement in sentence recognition in noise and self-report of benefit. It is possible that, despite

the audibility of the signal, the damaged cochlea continued to pass on to the central auditory nervous system a distorted signal, thereby limiting improvements possible in CVC identification. It is important to note that this training involved nonspeech, nonmeaningful stimuli with very limited graphic feedback.

Focused (Active) Versus Unfocused (Passive) Experience

The rationale for CBAT must also include consideration of the role of attention in training. Much acoustic information is processed without attention seemingly focused on particular stimuli. For example, one may recall hearing a radio commercial when asked about it even though there was no specific task to record information or respond to that information. Throughout a typical day, there are numerous unfocused (i.e., passive) auditory events that are processed by the auditory system, but not necessarily acknowledged unless circumstances require specific recall of that information. Research with guinea pigs, rats, and monkeys has shown that, for measurable cognitive reorganization to occur following training with tones, some form of focused or active attention through pairing electrical stimulation with acoustic stimuli or through conditioned discrimination training is required (Galvan & Weinberger, 2002; Kilgard & Merzenich, 1998a; Recanzone et al., 1993).

Perhaps the most common example of unfocused or passive auditory training in humans is the process of learning language by a normally developing infant. By 12 months of age, infants show discrimination patterns specific to the language to which they have been exposed auditorily (Kuhl & Meltzoff, 1996). Another common, unfocused, passive auditory training experience occurs when listeners with hearing impairment receive hearing aids or cochlear implants. Adjustment to the new sound provided by the assistive technology occurs over time as the individual continually acquires more auditory experience. This is referred to as acclimatization and can occur over six weeks to two years (Cox & Alexander, 1992; Gatehouse, 1992, 1993; Horwitz & Turner, 1997; Tyler & Summerfield, 1996).

Unlike this passive (unfocused) auditory stimulation, auditory training with focused attention employs various techniques that require the listener to actively direct attention to specific information in the stimuli. For example, pairing a visual stimulus with an auditory stimulus that is made progressively more difficult in a discrimination task or providing a reward for attending increases the likelihood of active, focused attention. Typically, focused auditory attention involves selection of specific stimuli for training (e.g., nonspeech gap detection or speech comprehension of stories). Stemming from findings with animals, research with humans has shown that, as a result of brain plasticity, the cognitive processes that underlie perception of certain acoustic cues can be trained. Improvements in perception following focused auditory attention have been shown for adults with hearing aids (Walden et al., 1981), children with cochlear implants (Zwolan et al., 2000), and children with language impairments (Tallal et al., 1996). Unfortunately, although these studies show improvements, the specific acoustic ability that was trained is unknown, in part, because of the lack of carefully defined control groups.

Although a program may be designed for focused attention training, if the tasks are not engaging because of excessive difficulty level or lack of redundancy, attention to the task may be lost. What may have been intended as a focused attention task may become an unfocused attention task. Unlike traditional therapy, where a clinician immediately recognizes the need to redirect a child's attention by changing tasks or reinforcement, a child may progress through CBAT with only the minimal attention needed to press the response key to advance the game, unbeknownst to the clinician or parent. In this situation, the child is probably not truly focusing auditory attention to the task. In experiments with animals, training with unfocused attention has been shown to be less effective (Kilgard & Merzenich, 1998b); therefore, allowing a child to progress through CBAT in the absence of true, focused auditory attention could result in an undesirable attention pattern that could affect performance on other training tasks, as was suggested by Friel-Patti et al. (2001) after reviewing performance of a child with language impairment.

Friel-Patti et al. (2001) described a subject who participated in the CBAT program Fast ForWord for 31 days, yet he did not meet the criterion of 90% completion on five of the seven exercises. In fact, his performance increased over the first 10 days on all tasks except one, a nonspeech, frequency-sweep discrimination task. His performance on that task never rose above 5% completion over the 31 training days. Performance on three of the six remaining tasks either reached a plateau (30% and 70% performance level) or declined during the final 10 days of training. In the same way, two other children showed declines in performance near the end of training. It was concluded that the temporal processing system was bombarded with stimuli that could not be discriminated by the children and therefore they were operating at an unsuccessful level, which may have created interference. In other words, the tasks might have interfered with each other as the children responded "with limited and increasingly stressful resources" (Friel-Patti, DesBarres, & Thibodeau, 2001). See Chapter 4 for discussion of passive listening studies with animals in enriched as well as ambient, everyday acoustic environments.

Frequency of Training

The typical treatment model for children with communication disorders is therapy two or three times per week (Gillam et al., 2005). This is somewhat constrained by the service delivery model in the public schools where caseloads are so large that students cannot be seen every day. Research by Tremblay and colleagues have demonstrated, however, that intensiveness of training is crucial to successful outcomes. They reported that nine, 20-minute training sessions over five days resulted in significantly improved discrimination of voice onset time cues in synthetic speech by adults with normal communication (Tremblay, Kraus, Carrell, & McGee, 1997). Interestingly, changes in the mismatched negativity potential (MMN) occurred after only four consecutive days of training in all 10 subjects, and significant behavioral changes in speech discrimination occurred in 9 of the 10 listeners (with additional training) on day 10 (Tremblay, Kraus, & McGee, 1998).

Also demonstrating the importance of frequency of training, Russo, Nicol, Zecker, Hayes, and Kraus (2005) found that children who had difficulties encoding the acoustic features of speech showed improvements following intensive training with Earobics relative to control subjects who received no training. Specifically, measures were made of neural timing in the brainstem in response to the presentation of the syllable "da." Children in the training group showed improved stimulus encoding precision relative to the controls. The authors concluded that the training resulted in improvements in neural synchrony concomitant with improvements in perceptual, academic, and cognitive measures. This research suggests that with frequent auditory training, the ability to code information into auditory patterns that may facilitate perception may be enhanced.

In summary, research suggests that the impact of auditory training for language processing can be enhanced through the use of meaningful stimuli. Moreover, employing tasks that direct one's attention to specific aspects of the stimulus and which are presented frequently over a concentrated time period are more likely to result in improved outcomes.

Processing Models of CBAT

A number of theories and models to test those theories continue to evolve to account for the complex processes involved in auditory perception, speech perception, and spoken language processing. Among these models are those that focus on bottom-up versus top-down processing; interactive and parallel processes versus autonomous and serial processes; passive, nonmediated single factor theories versus active, mediated dual factor theories; and reliance on either feature detection, template matching, filtering, or other means of analyzing relevant dimensions of auditory stimuli (Borden, Harris, & Raphael, 2003; Jusczyk, & Luce, 2002; Kent & Read, 2002). Commonly accepted is that auditory-language processing involves multiple sources of information and interactive and parallel networks broadly activated across the brain (ASHA, 1996; Chermak & Musiek, 1997).

Although no specific model completely explains the benefits derived from auditory training, several comments are in order relative to the individual with (C)APD, who, typically, experiences difficulty in the actual coding and organization of the auditory stimulus. Regardless of whether feature detection, template matching, or filtering is used to analyze relevant dimensions of stimuli, individuals with (C)APD, and particularly children with (C)APD, are likely to have less extensive experience and fewer *data sets* (e.g., stores of acoustic templates with associated meaning) and are more likely to experience difficulty attending to acoustic events, which results in the coding of fewer acoustic features. All this reduces the probability that acoustic matches will be made and meaning subsequently extracted from the signal. An individual with (C)APD may compensate for these limitations in quiet, but have considerable difficulty under challenging conditions of noise, reverberation, rapid speech, and so forth. Interfering noise compromises one's ability to store the acoustic trace accurately. It is as if the sharp edges on a complex geometric design become fuzzy. Anything that

reduces the distinctiveness of the signal will reduce the accuracy with which the acoustic information is stored and consequently the probability that meaning can be derived. What is unique to CBAT is that the stimuli can be manipulated to strengthen the acoustic templates deciphered at the periphery as well as the neural networks required for cognitive processing. This occurs through the repetitive presentations of acoustic information in a focused-listening task that is experienced frequently (i.e., several times a week) by children who are motivated to attend due to the interesting and rewarding graphics of the CBAT.

Benefits of CBAT

Although the three principles described above (i.e., meaningfulness of the stimuli, focused training, and intensity of treatment) can be accomplished via traditional therapy, CBAT offers several advantages relative to these principles and thereby facilitates training. These advantages include stimulus control, hierarchy of activities, and the inherently interesting vehicle that computers offer to engage children in intensive training.

Precise Stimulus Control

Through the use of synthetic speech and nonspeech stimuli, precise acoustic features can be manipulated and presented in a graduated sequence of difficulty. For example, if the child's *template* for the word "hotdog" did not include a brief silent interval between the stop consonants /t/ and /d/, then training to recognize small gaps would be productive so that when "hotdog" or other similar two-syllable words are presented, the templates may be refined to include this brief silence between syllables. Training may begin with noise bursts with easily perceptible gaps and through precise digital manipulation the gap duration could be altered in a sequential manner. This is known as an adaptively controlled paradigm where the difficulty level is based on the response to the previous stimulus. For example, if a gap is correctly detected, then the next trial would have a smaller duration gap. If the response to that trial is incorrect, the next gap would be longer in duration to facilitate perception. A typical adaptive gap detection paradigm involves stimulus manipulation so that the participant can correctly detect the gap with 70% accuracy. This type of graduated training could not be accomplished via natural speech, despite repeated presentations of the stimulus word. If the participant is not able to detect that silence, then no amount of repetition of that same interval would facilitate perception.

An example of manipulating the stimulus in the frequency domain that is possible in CBAT involves the perception of second-formant transitions. If the participant is unable to hear the difference between "bad" and "dad," it is likely that he or she is not discriminating differences between second-formant transitions that cue the difference between the bilabial and alveolar placement. Repeatedly presenting stimuli that the participant cannot discriminate will not strengthen the accuracy of internal auditory representations. Training should begin with stimuli incorporating large changes in frequency that are greater than that which occur in real speech (Thibodeau, Friel-Patti, & Britt, 2001). Initially, the participant should be

able to discriminate these large changes with about 70% accuracy. This 70% level allows for a balance between challenging and successful performance. Once accuracy rate improves beyond 70%, the change in frequency should be slightly reduced and training continued toward the 70% accuracy rate. As has been accomplished by Tallal and colleagues, the use of CBAT allows precise manipulation of the signal in an adaptive manner so that the acoustic differences are increased until 70% performance is reached. Subsequently, frequency differences are decreased gradually until participants are able to discriminate frequency differences characteristic of normal speech (Merzenich et al., 1996).

Access to Levels and Games

Another advantage of CBAT is the easy access to an appropriate training level that the digital format provides. Because the selection of the stimulus to be presented can be chosen based on the previous response (i.e., adaptive training), training becomes more efficient as the participant does not have to sit through either multiple trials where there is no success or where trials are too easy and the participant achieves 100% success. Furthermore, to maintain interest CBAT also easily allows the clinician to hold the training objective constant while changing the game scene. For example, rather than continue selecting a balloon that corresponds to a change in frequency, the scene may change after 3 minutes so that the child is listening for the monkey that made a different sound. Variety helps to maintain the child's attention and continue practicing to strengthen the auditory representation.

Youth's Interest in Computers

Children are surrounded by electronic images today more than ever. It may not be surprising that one third of children under 6 years of age (36%) have a television in their bedroom (Rideout, Vandewater, & Wartella, 2003). More than 25% of these children have a video recorder/player or digital video disk player, 10% have a video game player, and 7% have a computer in their bedroom. The latest trend is large-screen televisions luring youth to the couch to view action-filled reality shows. The scenes may range from youth programs with a potpourri of three-minute scenes to adult programs with scenes of adventure and survival. In addition, these images can be taken almost anywhere through portable digital video players. Children enjoy electronic entertainment while riding in the car, sitting at siblings' sporting evens, or even while waiting for a haircut. Such frequent visual input potentially conditions children to expect entertaining electronic input regularly. In fact, much of their communication with friends occurs without auditory input, as they exchange information electronically through text messaging on mobile phones or instant messaging on computers.

With the increase in access to computers in the schools, home, doctors' offices, coffee shops, movie theaters, and so forth, children are increasingly comfortable with electronic communication and some may choose it as a form of recreation rather than physical activity. Children are also accessing their favorite music via the computer because there is convenient access to downloading songs for a nominal price. Computers then are used to exchange favorite music among friends through software that allows burning of compact disks. With the advent of networking software for local area networks (LAN) and associated interactive games, students are even planning weekend social events around their computers by having LAN parties. Teens gather with their laptops or personal computers and compete with one another through interactive, challenging games.

With the increased exposure, availability, and utility of computers, it is logical to consider their application for remediation of communication disorders. It is doubtful that this will be a passing trend, as computers continue to expand in capability while costs decline. The challenge will be to develop training software compatible with technology, with its fast-paced upgrades, that can be conveniently accessed. For example, complex interactive software may exceed the storage and memory capabilities of the typical home or clinic computer and therefore require Internet resources to function completely. Moreover, within a few years, CBAT software, hardware, or both can become obsolete and require totally different digital signal access, storage, and encoding.

Convenience of Training

Computers are available not only in educational settings, but in most homes. According to a U.S. survey (Rideout et al., 2003), 73% of homes with young children have a computer. More than a third (39%) of 4- to 6-year-olds use a computer several times a week. With regard to computer games, one in four (25%) play several times a week or more (Rideout et al., 2003). Children are even accessing media while driving in cars. It is conceivable that some form of auditory training could take place while on a daily commute or while traveling. Furthermore, hotels are often equipped with Internet access that might also facilitate intensive training regardless of a family's schedule.

Standardization of Training

The use of CBAT allows consistency in training because the stimuli and activities are controlled by the computer. In some instances, this could be a disadvantage because the child's attention may wander with less human interaction. However, to facilitate comparison across clinics and training protocols, the consistent format is attractive. Another argument to support the standardization of training is the benefits for training large groups. If a standardized set of activities can be helpful for a large number of children, then administration can be streamlined and cost effectiveness maximized. However, as discussed below under Treatment Outcomes, Efficacy, and Effectiveness, a review of the research shows that gains are made often by only some children on only a subset of the outcome measures. It will continue to be important, therefore, to assess the needs of an individual child throughout training to ensure that he or she is engaged in the process and continuing to make progress.

Design of CBAT

Training Areas

One of the first decisions that must be made, of course, is the purpose of the training. Table 6–1 provides a list of auditory skills or processes that have been suggested for training children with (C)APD. No single CBAT program addresses all of these areas; therefore, a combination of programs may be necessary to comprehensively address the processing deficits. Although a global auditory training program may be attractive, most software developers have based the training tasks on the perceived needs of a particular population, such as children with hearing impairment (Otokids), language impairments (Fast ForWord), and attention deficit hyperactivity disorder (Brain Train). There has been much crossover, however, in the application of available training programs. This may result in significant problems if the training tasks designed for one group are too difficult for another, which may be counterproductive and lead to frustration. Moreover, overgeneralized use of software with populations not originally intended to

Table 6–1. Areas of Training for Children with (C)APD

Training Area	Possible Stimuli	Software
Awareness	Nonspeech or Speech	Otto's World Earobics Brain Train
Memory	Nonspeech or Speech	Brain Train Earobics Fast ForWord Learning Fundamentals

continues

Table 6–1. *continued*

Training Area	Possible Stimuli	Software
Temporal Processing, Including Sequencing	Nonspeech or Speech	Fast ForWord Earobics
Localization	Nonspeech or Speech	None
Auditory Discrimination	Nonspeech or Speech	Fast ForWord Otto's World
Auditory Pattern Perception	Nonspeech or Speech	Brain Train Earobics Fast ForWord Learning Fundamentals
Phonologic Awareness	Speech	Conversation Made Easy Earobics Fast ForWord Foundations in Speech Perception Learning Fundamentals
Auditory Synthesis	Speech	Learning Fundamentals Earobics
Dichotic Processing (Binaural Integration)	Nonspeech or Speech	None
Identification	Nonspeech or Speech	Brain Train Earobics Fast ForWord Sound and Beyond
Degraded Speech Recognition (Filtered Speech, Compressed Speech, Speech-In-Competition/Noise, Auditory Closure)	Speech	Conversation Made Easy Earobics Learning Fundamentals
Binaural Interaction	Nonspeech or Speech	None
Binaural Separation	Nonspeech or Speech	None
Comprehension	Speech	Brain Train Conversation Made Easy Earobics Fast ForWord Learning Fundamentals
Auditory Vigilance	Nonspeech or Speech	Brain Train Learning Fundamentals

be trained with that software can lead to inefficient and ineffective treatment. For example, children with hearing impairment may not have the frequency resolution capabilities to successfully complete the easiest level of the frequency-sweep discrimination task of the program Fast ForWord, which was designed for children with language impairments who have normal hearing sensitivity. It is crucial, therefore, to know the intended audience, and if synthetic stimuli are used, to review the acoustic characteristics of the stimuli at the easiest and most difficult levels. Tasks that are either too difficult or too easy can lead to lack of attention and consequently less training benefit (Prensky, 2001). Similarly, cognitive, visual, and verbal skills required for use of particular CBAT must be considered.

Type of Training Stimuli

The next consideration in designing CBAT might be the choice of stimuli. The four possibilities, including speech versus nonspeech and natural versus synthetic, were described above under Meaningfulness of Stimuli. All the areas listed in Table 6–1 could be trained using speech stimuli, either natural or synthetic. Depending on the hierarchy of training, discussed in the next section, synthetic stimuli may be necessary to precisely control the difficulty of the task. Interestingly, most of the skill areas listed in Table 6–1 could also be trained with nonspeech stimuli, either natural or synthetic. Although many programs use primarily natural speech, there is no research to support the benefits of training with natural speech versus synthetic nonspeech.

Table 6–1 lists sample software for school-aged children using each of the stimulus types for each training area.

The choices are more limited, of course, to train comprehension with nonspeech, natural stimuli. For such a task, natural environmental sounds (e.g. fire truck, violin music, alarm clock) could be presented. Recognition could be trained by requiring the client to choose a picture that corresponds to the source. To train comprehension of these sounds, the client would be asked to associate the sound with the meaning the sound conveys by choosing a picture that corresponds to an associated event (e.g., people running from a house with flames, people walking into a concert hall, someone laying in bed with stretched out arms, respectively). Research by Gillam and colleagues (2005) suggests that children with language impairments experience equal gains in expressive and receptive language regardless of whether natural speech, synthesized speech, or nonspeech tokens are used as training stimuli. Given Gillam's findings, the clinician might prefer to use nonspeech stimuli in CBAT to more precisely target the underlying auditory skills without introducing potential confounding variables of speech and language.

Regardless of the type of stimulus used, the clinician must assess the fidelity of the signal presented to the participant. The fidelity of the acoustic representation of stimuli, whether they are brief stimuli or intentionally distorted (e.g., filtered, time-compressed, presented in noise) stimuli, is essential to train efficiently and effectively toward the treatment goals. Poor fidelity can result from poor transducers (i.e., earphones and speakers) or poor signal processing itself.

Training Hierarchy

By definition, training implies a hierarchy of tasks. The challenge in CBAT is to determine the optimal starting and difficulty levels within a program. Naturally, the age of the listener is a determining factor, but even within an age group, there can be a wide range of abilities. Diagnostic test findings should provide some guidance in this determination. Ideally, the CBAT would include a "pre-training" assessment to determine the optimal starting levels so that the participant can begin training with relatively high success and gradually move toward more challenging activities. Without this feature, it becomes the responsibility of the audiologist or speech-language pathologist administering the CBAT to determine if the starting level chosen is appropriate to provide initial success required to maintain interest and motivation. As mentioned in the section on Frequency of Training, there is some evidence to suggest that if children are asked to perform tasks that are too difficult, overall attention may decline and result in reduced outcomes.

Irrespective of any particular software, an overall training hierarchy is proposed stemming from Garstecki's work with adults with hearing loss (Garstecki, 1982). In his scheme of auditory-visual training, he proposed starting at the easiest level to be successful and moving through the hierarchy of increasingly more difficult tasks until a plateau in performance is reached (i.e., when no further increases in performance are made despite continued training). Garstecki's hierarchy included four variables: (1) message type— unrelated sentences to related sentences; (2) competing noise type—multispeaker, babble, single noise, quiet; (3) competing noise level— negative to positive ratio; and (4) use of situational cues—no background cues, relevant visual background cues. Table 6–2 illustrates the hierarchy matrix as applied to variables in auditory processing. One might start training with no noise, natural speech, and many picture cues relating to the stimuli. The most difficult task would be training with synthetic, nonspeech stimuli, with multitalker babble at −10 signal-to-noise ratio (SNR) with no picture cues. Generally,

Table 6–2. Hierarchy of Training

	Very Easy	Easy	Difficult	Very Difficult
Stimuli	Natural Speech	Synthetic Speech	Natural Nonspeech	Nonspeech Synthetic
Competing Noise	No Noise	Single Noise	Two Talker Babble	Multitalker Babble
Noise Level	N/A	+10 SNR	0 SNR	−10 SNR
Situation Cues	Pictures present	Pictures precede task	Single word cue	No Cue

one progresses through the matrix one cell at a time, rather than increasing difficulty on several dimensions concurrently.

Adaptive Difficulty Levels

Another significant decision that must be made in designing CBAT is whether the activities will be presented at fixed difficulty level or whether the software will adapt based on the participant's response. As mentioned above, programs that operate at a fixed level might be too easy. This is not as detrimental, however, as starting an activity that might have 20 presentations that are too difficult, thereby discouraging the participant and jeopardizing motivation and persistence on task. Nonetheless, the benefit of having an adaptive program is that the task can continually adjust to more difficult levels as the participant answers correctly. Typically, if the participant answers incorrectly, the next presentation is at an easier level; if the child answers correctly, the next presentation could be at a more difficult level. That is known as *one up, one down*, or *simple up/down* and allows the participant to perform at an accuracy rate of about 50%. This may actually be frustrating for some children and it might be better to train with a *two down, one up* adaptive procedure which results in performance with 70% accuracy (Levitt, 1978). With this tracking rule, a child must respond correctly to two consecutive trials before the difficulty level of the next trial is increased. After every incorrect response, the difficulty level is lowered so the next trial will likely be completed successfully. This *two down, one up* procedure allows greater accuracy (70% vs. 50%) and may be considered more enjoyable by some children.

Reinforcement

To increase accuracy of performance, feedback must be provided regarding performance accuracy. In the absence of feedback, the participant is less likely to focus on a particular aspect of the signal that would foster continued accurate performance. Indeed, feedback can be reinforcing and reinforcement has been used successfully to increase learning in children with learning disabilities and mental retardation (Dawson, Hallahan, Reeve, & Ball, 1980; De Csipkes, Smouse, & Hudson, 1975). The reinforcement provided in CBAT typically includes some type of animation that occurs following a certain number of correct responses. The more interesting and novel the animation, the more likely the child will maintain motivation to perform successfully. As the task difficulty increases, reinforcement becomes even more important to maintain attention.

A distinction should be made between reinforcement and feedback. When participants receive some information regarding their performance, they are receiving feedback. Such information is critical to any learning experience. Depending on the form of the information, the feedback also may be considered positive reinforcement, which will likely increase the desired behavior. In CBAT, the goal is to provide positive reinforcement that will encourage the child to persist on task despite increasing difficulty.

Feedback in the form of positive reinforcement may be one of the major factors that maintains participants' engagement in a computer game, an engaged state that facilitates learning. Digital, game-based learning engages the participant through a hierarchy of experiences that cause enjoyment (Prensky, 2001). Prensky proposed that there are a series of relationships that occur through game-based learning that result in motivation to continue. He stated that because games are a form of *fun* they give the participant enjoyment and pleasure. Games are also a form of *play*, which may result in intense and passionate involvement. With rules that provide structure, games have goals that motivate the participant to continue. As the activities move toward the goals, there are outcomes and feedback which cause motivation and learning. When games are adaptive, the participant is allowed to perform at the optimum level and achieve a sense of *winning*, which adds to ego gratification. Games that present competition or challenge may spark creativity and problem-solving. Finally, games convey events in a storylike format can evoke positive emotions (e.g., enjoyment) that perpetuates the cycle of relationships. For participants with (C)APD who are offered this series of experiences through CBAT, one would expect their interest to persist and learning to increase relative to non-computer based strategies where the relationships between reinforcement, goals, and *winning* are less apparent. See Chapter 5 for further discussion of the role of feedback and reinforcement for effective intervention.

Operating Format

When designing software, it is necessary to consider how the program will run on the computer. The choices are to run from a CD ROM, from an installed version stored on the computer's hard drive, or from some combination of these two approaches. Most programs are designed to be installed and run independently of the CD ROM. When the CD ROM is required during training, less data are stored on the hard drive, but loading the software is required each time it is used, which may be time consuming. This would also be inconvenient if the software were to be used in multiple locations.

Factors That May Influence Success

Treatment Schedule

The scheduling of training includes the time of day training is offered, the length of each training session, and the duration and frequency of training. As with any intervention program, it is optimal to offer training at a time of day when the participant is most alert. As mentioned previously, the frequency and duration of training are important factors. It is optimal to conduct the CBAT at approximately the same time each day as this helps to facilitate relatively equivalent attention across days and to reduce variability in performance (Gillam et al., 2005). Depending on the time of day and the duration of training that is offered, it may be necessary to have snacks available to help maintain attention.

Several programs recommend a 30- to 90-minute training session three to five times per week, a training regimen in sharp contrast to the typical quantity and frequency with which children receive speech-language and hearing services in schools (Gillam et al., 2005). In contrast, some studies show improvements with as little as 15 minutes of training, two times per week (Segers & Verhoeven, 2003). Gillam reported significantly greater gains achieved by children with specific language impairments when the therapy was provided daily for 90 minutes compared to the gains achieved by children who were served in traditional models (Gillam et al., 2005). Most CBAT is recommended for a period of at least 4 to 6 weeks (e.g., Earobics© and Fast For-Word). When the training is frequent, the child becomes more accustomed to a routine of attending for a certain time period. The experience of attending becomes more familiar and requires less effort with training. It has been shown that frequent auditory training results in increased attention span and ability to complete a complex task (e.g., persever-ance) (Scott, 1992).

Auditory Environment

Given the nature of auditory training, it is critical that the child be able to con-centrate on the training signals and not be distracted by ambient signals. The use of headphones is often recommended to reduce ambient sounds, particularly when there is more than one training station in a room. In the group situation, there also should be a system for asking a question by raising an indicator to alert the clinician, parent, or other monitor to come to that station.

An FM system is another tool to help participants focus attention on the CBAT signal. The FM system may be useful in CBAT to enhance the signal from the computer relative to the surrounding classroom noise. By connecting the sig-nal from the sound output jack of the computer to the audio input on the FM transmitter, the child may hear the audi-tory signal more readily, yet still be able to hear some sounds in the classroom, unlike headphones which would block most of the environmental sounds. As mentioned above in the section on hier-archy of training, moving from an ideal

SNR to less favorable conditions during training will facilitate carryover into the -tions are rare. See Chapter 7 for dis-cussion of FM technology and signal enhancement.

Motivation

Motivation may be internal or external. Internal motivation is based on a desire from within oneself to accomplish a task because it is interesting, arouses plea-sure, or enhances self-esteem. For exam-ple, when a child receives an animated scene to indicate completion of a train-ing level, the child feels a sense of accomplishment, which may lead to feel-ings of greater self-worth. A sense of pleasure may also result from knowing that accomplishing a level means the end of training is near. Hence, motivation may be facilitated by advising the partic-ipants at the beginning of training about the number of training levels or games to be accomplished during that session.

Although CBAT typically is designed with interesting graphics and visual rein-forcement, maintaining a child's atten-tion during lengthy training periods may require external motivators. Reinforcers may be needed not only for the individual session but also to motivate the child to return week after week. These external motivators may be as simple as some recognition for completion of the training sequence each day to more elaborate re-wards after completing each five-minute segment. Tangible, nonsticky, reinforcers may be given at frequent intervals to maintain motivation, particularly when tasks are more difficult. Small prizes also may be offered for reaching criterion per-formance each day of the week. Having children share their progress with an interested adult (besides the clinician) on a daily basis also may contribute to their motivation to perform well. Whatever the schedule of reinforcement, reinforcers will be more effective when the participant understands in advance the critical steps needed to obtain them. See Chapters 4 and 5 for further discussion of the role of motivation for effective intervention.

Factors to Consider in Selecting CBAT

Differentiating Software for Training

As a teacher, parent, or clinician considers offering CBAT, there are many factors to examine prior to selecting software. First, the purpose of the training should be determined. If there are specific language concepts to be trained, software that includes activities that focus on these language concepts should be considered. If phonemic processing skills are of concern, for example, software that includes discrimination training of phonemic differences is desirable. Memory and attention skills are indirectly exercised in all CBAT programs. Some programs increase focus on attention and memory by requiring an additional task to be performed before responding, or by adding noise to the task to compete for attention. Table 6–1 provides some guidance as to the specific areas of central auditory processing particular software is designed to train.

Option to Train with a Home Computer

To increase the frequency of training, it may be desirable to have the option for CBAT in the home. The price of computers has dropped such that many families have systems that meet the minimum requirements of the most sophisticated programs. The challenge for training at home is to control distractions and provide time for focused training without interruptions. When training is conducted in a clinic or school, the child is usually there for the sole purpose for training. When CBAT is conducted in the home, a regular time should be set aside to minimize interruptions caused by carpools, television, or visits from friends. For the older child, it will be paramount to restrict *Instant Messaging* or chat room access during training because so many teens are accustomed to multitasking by typing messages to several people while ostensibly doing homework on the computer. Such attempts at multitasking would likely detract from the older child's attention to the CBAT and therefore diminish benefit derived.

Because home computers are often shared by multiple users for multiple reasons, the designated training time must be communicated to all members who can plan their computer use accordingly. Furthermore, during home training, there must be a system for accountability to the monitoring professional. If a certain program is recommended for training so many minutes each day, a record keeping log should be provided that can be monitored weekly.

System Requirements

Most software comes with a description of the computer hardware requirements for effective operation. These should always be consulted prior to installation to avoid lengthy and/or unnecessary troubleshooting. An overview of computer requirements for Fast ForWord serves as an example (Table 6–3).

Manufacturers will list the minimal requirements because, typically, the software is *backward* compatible for a few

Table 6–3. Hardware Requirements for Operating Fast ForWord® Training Programs

Operating Systems	Windows 98SE Windows 2000 Professional Service Pack 4 Windows XP Home or Professional Service Pack 2 or later
Processor	500 MHz Intel or AMD Processor
Memory	256 MB RAM or higher
CD-ROM Drive	8× or faster
Video Card/Monitor	Maximum supported resolution of 800 × 600 with thousands of colors
Sound Card	Any Creative Labs or 100% compatible sound card, including Sound Blaster 16 (or 32), PCI 64, or 16-bit VIBRA series products *Note:* Integrated sound cards are not recommended
Mouse	Any Microsoft or compatible mouse (required)
Keyboard	Any Microsoft or compatible keyboard (required)
Hard drive space needed for installation	1. Approximately 40 MB for a one-product installation 2. Approximately 10 MB for each additional installation 3. Optional space for installing multimedia content: 100 MB for Fast ForWord Language Basics 510 MB for Fast ForWord Language 460 MB for Fast ForWord Middle and High School 410 MB for Fast ForWord Language to Reading 100 MB for Fast ForWord to Reading Prep 360 MB for Fast ForWord to Reading 1 310 MB for Fast ForWord to Reading 2 175 MB for Fast ForWord to Reading 3 300 MB for Fast ForWord to Reading 4 250 MB for Fast ForWord to Reading 5
Hard drive space needed to run the product	1. 1 MB per participant, per product for backup creation 2. 1 MB per participant, per product for entire machine archive 3. 1 MB per participant, per session to expand files and creation of data files
Internet connection, if needed	56 k.p.s. or faster *Note:* Direct connection is recommended *Note:* Internet connection is required for Progress Tracker

Source: Adapted from www.scilearn.com.

years. If a program was written to function with the most recent, common operating system, it will typically also work with the previous one or two versions. However, newer operating systems that are developed after the generation of CBAT software may not be compatible. After checking the operating system requirements, one must consider processor and memory requirements. Typically, if the operating system requirements are met, processing and memory requirements for video and sound cards also are acceptable. Programs may require quite different amounts of hard drive space, however, depending on the graphics involved. The hard drive storage requirements for Fast ForWord programs range from 140 megabytes for a single program to approximately 3 gigabytes for the entire set of programs (see Table 6–3). One should also consider whether the program requires a CD ROM inserted in the drive to operate the program or if all the games are stored on the hard drive. CBAT developers often require CD ROM-dependent operation to minimize licensing abuse and to reduce memory requirements during operation.

Some programs require an additional hard disk space for each participant or provide the option to assign an external memory option (e.g., floppy disk, zip disk, flash memory) for storage of individual performance. This may be a significant negative factor if the program is to be used with a large group of students because the initial assignment of data storage media and the daily access to individual disks may be quite time consuming. Some CBAT programs require an Internet connection so that participant performance may be compiled into training reports which store data and show progress across sessions. Requiring Inter-

net access may be a limiting factor in selecting a CBAT program, particularly when the primary concern is individual training rather than planning for a large group of users (e.g., students).

Considerations for CBAT in Schools

The use of CBAT in the schools has been addressed in previous sections regarding interfacing with FM systems, avoiding distracting ambient noise, and group training arrangements. There are three other important considerations, however, which involve the actual installation of the software, licensing, and interfacing with the current service delivery options.

An important consideration for CBAT in schools is knowing how many students will use the software. Multiple site licenses will be more cost-effective for large group applications. Prior to adding software to school-based computers that may be part of a network, technical support for the network should be consulted regarding installation requirements. In many cases, there are designated personnel to manage software installations to be sure that compatibility requirements are met. As mentioned above, CD ROM-dependent software may be more difficult to manage as young children or busy teachers have to organize data disks or software CD's for training sessions.

Schools must also consider how CBAT will be implemented in relation to the regular curriculum and special services. Will the use of the CBAT be a supplement to the traditional therapy? If FM systems are provided, will the training be offered at a time when the transmitter can be interfaced with the computer for a given student? Finally, as discussed above, can

CBAT be made available in schools consistent with an intensive therapy schedule as required for maximum effectiveness?

CBAT Software Comparison

In general, CBAT programs have all been designed to strengthen some aspect of auditory processing or auditory-language processing, whether it is discrimination of nonspeech sounds or comprehension of directions through interesting graphics paired with auditory stimuli. The programs differ in the levels of instruction, the specific training areas, response reinforcement, and how they operate relative to the computer hardware. They range in price from $99 for a single CD ROM for one type of program to over $3,000 for a site license for a set of training programs. The more expensive programs typically have more complex adaptive training reflecting more sophisticated algorithms (e.g., Fast ForWord). Such complexity often requires considerable consumer support for troubleshooting and interpretation, which is a factor that adds to the program costs.

CBAT programs also vary in their hardware requirements. Table 6–4 provides basic information for 10 auditory-language training software programs that are currently available (with the exception of the program Foundations of Speech Perception, which is no longer sold but is included for comparison because it is still in use). The random access memory or RAM requirements for the programs listed in Table 6–4 are typically 32 MB, but they range from requiring 8 MB for Foundations of Speech Perception to 256 MB for Sound and Beyond™. The

required hard drive storage space ranges from 10 MB for Earobics to 500 MB for Sound and Beyond. CD ROM drive speed could be as low as 2× to run Earobics or as high as 8× to run Otto's World of Sound. One consideration mentioned previously is whether or not the program will operate independently of a CD ROM. This provides greater flexibility for the user to not be dependent on having the CD ROM in place during training. The final column in Table 6–4 indicates whether the program is CD ROM dependent, meaning, that a program CD ROM must be in the computer's CD ROM drive to run the program.

As noted in Table 6–4, software has been developed for a variety of audiences. The primary groups that have been targeted for training include those with language impairments and those with hearing loss. Much software also has been developed to treat children with reading difficulties. Many programs include some activities directed at phonemic awareness including discrimination of speech sounds and sound symbol association (see Table 6–1). As suggested by Gillam et al. (2005), the critical factors contributing to success through auditory training may not be the specific program content, but rather the intensiveness of training.

With the possibility for significant overlap in applications of these programs, the selection of an appropriate program may be difficult. For example, there are several programs designed to enhance language skills. It could be very time consuming to review all these programs to select one for a particular child; therefore, it is suggested that age be the first criterion for program selection. Within that age category, one may determine from a more limited set of programs which ones have appropriate levels for training.

Table 6–4. Summary of (C)APD Programs

Software	Author	Publisher	Date	Web Address	Age	Intended Audience	CD ROM
Brain Train	Joseph A. Sanford, Ann Turner	Brain Train, Inc.	1989	http://www.braintrain.com/soundsmart/soundsmart_home.htm	Preschool to Adult	Cognitive impaired	Yes
Conversation Made Easy	Nancy Tye-Murray	Central Institute for the Deaf	2002	http://www.cid.wustl.edu/deafhome/PUBLICATIONS/books.htm	Upper Elementary to Adult	Hearing impaired	Yes
Earobics	Jan Wasowicz	Cognitive Concepts	1996	http://www.earobics.com/	Preschool to Adult	Language impaired, Dyslexic, Auditory processing	Yes
Fast ForWord	Paula Tallal, Michael Merzenich	Scientific Learning	1997	http://www.scilearn.com/	Preschool to Adult	Language impaired, Dyslexic, Pervasive developmental disorder	No
Foundations in Speech Perception	Cochlear Corp.	Cochlear Corp.	2000	No longer marketed	Elementary	Hearing impaired	Yes
Laureate Learning Systems	Mary Sweig Wilson, Bernard J. Fox, Marion Blank, Eleanor Semel, Barbara Couse Adams	Laureate Learning Systems	1982	http://www.llsys.com/professionals602/products/descriptions/mldesc.html	Elementary to Adults	Language impaired, Developmental disabilities, Physical impairments, Visual impairments, Hearing impairments, Autism, ESL students	Yes

Software	Author	Publisher	Date	Web Address	Age	Intended Audience	CD ROM
Learning Fundamentals	Marna Scarry-Larkin	LocuTour Multimedia	1994	http://www.locutour.com/products/product.php?id=40	Preschool to Teens	Language impaired, Dyslexic, Attention problems	No
Listening and Communication Enhancement (LACE)	Robert Sweetow	NeuroTone, Inc.	2004	http://www.neurotone.com/index.html	Adult	Hearing impaired	No
Otto's World of Sounds	Oticon Corporation	Oticon Corporation	2005	http://otikids.oticon.nl/eprise/main/Oticon/com/SEC_AboutHearing/Learn AboutHearing/Products/SEC_OtiKids/Parents/Helping/OWS/_Index	Elementary	Hearing impaired	Yes
Sound and Beyond	Cochlear Corp.	Cochlear Corp.	2005	www.cochlearamericas.com/support/169.asp	Adult	Hearing impaired	No

For example, for a 10-year-old child with auditory processing difficulties with no associated language delays, CBAT software that includes activities focused on memory, attention, and speech recognition in degraded acoustic conditions such as Captain's Log of Brain Train may be more useful than software focusing on language concepts, such as MicroLads of Laureate programs. Although a complete analysis of all the components of each of these programs is beyond the scope of this chapter, a brief synopsis of the software listed in Table 6–4 is provided below to guide one to appropriate exploration in greater detail.

Brain Train

Brain Train is a series of programs using natural speech designed to improve attention, memory, self-control, problem-solving, and listening skills designed for those with brain injury, learning disabilities, attention deficit hyperactivity disorder (ADHD), or other cognitive impairments. Unlike other CBAT, Brain Train includes activities to develop mental math skills and help reduce impulsivity. The software uses natural speech to encourage, praise, and challenge users to perform.

Conversation Made Easy

This series of programs is designed for persons with hearing loss to learn skills to improve conversation skills and therefore increase self-confidence. There are three instruction modules: (1) speechreading enhancement, (2) repair strategies, and (3) facilitative strategies to optimize the environment. Separate programs are available for adults and teenagers, children with low-level language skill, and children with advanced language skills. For each age, there are three CD ROM-based programs covering sounds, sentences, and everyday situations. The actual movies and photos of real-world scenes help to maintain attention. Because of these graphic requirements, however, some computers require changes to the display settings to allow the scenes to be seen.

Earobics

Earobics is a comprehensive, phonologic awareness and auditory-language processing training software designed for those with difficulties in reading and language processing. Programs are grouped for application in the school, clinic, or home. The school version consists of a package of games designed to strengthen language development, phonemic awareness, alphabetic knowledge, decoding and spelling, beginning reading, and beginning writing. The clinic version has three levels (i.e., steps) for prekindergarten, school-age, and adolescents/adults. The activities focus on the following:

Step 1: sound awareness, discrimination of sound in noise and quiet, sequencing sound, and associating sound with letters;

Step 2: complex directions with and without background noise, memory for sounds and words;

Step 3: activities to strengthen reading, spelling, and comprehension.

The home version is similar to the three steps, but designed to be used by only two participants and a guest. Earobics is known for its reasonable cost and accessibility for home use. The graphics are entertaining and activities maintain interest for the respective age level.

Fast ForWord

Fast ForWord training is based on the premise that language and reading difficulties stem from poor temporal processing (Merzenich et al., 1996). Activities are designed to increase temporal resolution and stimuli may be nonspeech tones or acoustically modified speech with lengthened features (i.e., formant transitions) compared to natural speech. Based on the user's success, the stimuli progress from longer to shorter, toward the acoustics of formant transitions found in natural speech. Fast ForWord has many levels for all age levels. In general, programs are designed for young children to develop basic skills necessary for language and reading development; for school-aged children to strengthen fundamental cognitive skills of memory, attention, processing, and sequencing with a focus on phonologic awareness and language structures; and for older students to focus on processing skills similar to the previous level and strengthen reading through sound-letter comprehension, phonologic awareness, beginning word recognition, and English language conventions.

Foundations in Speech Perception

This program is designed to teach listening skills to children, ages 3 to 12 years, with moderate to severe hearing loss, including those with cochlear implants. Lessons start at the basic level of matching words to pictures and progress to complex tasks such as identifying words or phrases without visual cues. Using recorded natural speech, the activities are adaptive to the child's performance level. Each activity begins with a training task to familiarize the participant with the lesson prior to being scored. There is a hierarchy of training ranging from basic (matching words with pictures) to advanced (distinguishing between similar sounding words) to complex (identifying words or phrases without visual cues). When a skill is achieved, the program automatically moves the user to the next level. The child can also record his or her speech and replay it to compare to the computer model. Reinforcement is provided by a computer painting activity at the conclusion of a lesson. The screen layout may be confusing at first because there are blocks to correspond to speech segments that are discovered through frequent exploration with the computer mouse.

Laureate Learning Systems

Laureate Learning Systems includes over 80 programs that address a wide array of auditory-language processing skills. The programs are designed for those functioning from preverbal level up to adult language levels. They are conveniently organized by category and by linguistic level. The categories include games designed for early instructional, early vocabulary, expressive language, early categorization training, syntax training, auditory discrimination, vocabulary and concept development, functional language training, advanced categorization training, and finally reading and spelling. The software also may be selected based on linguistic stages, which include interpreted communication, intentional communication, single words, word combinations, early syntax, syntax mastery, and complete generative grammar. The Laureate Web site includes descriptions of these stages along with training goals and the recommended software.

Learning Fundamentals

This set of programs is designed for use by parents, clinicians, and teachers and includes four main areas: speech, language, literacy, and attention. Each area has several programs with skill levels that vary from beginning to advanced. For example, in the area of memory the tasks begin with simple sustained attention and move to alternating and divided attention with response delays and auditory distractors. The programs include bright photographs on simple screens designed to allow those with attention difficulties to focus on the concept with minimal distractions. In addition to listening to quality audio recordings of natural speech, speech may be recorded and compared to the speaker's productions. Four programs also are offered that train phonology, vocabulary, and syntax in Spanish.

Listening and Communication Enhancement (LACE)

The purpose of LACE is to provide interactive, computerized training to improve listening and communication. It is designed for adult hearing-aid users to train at home. It is recommended that training be done for 30 minutes a day, 5 days a week, for 4 weeks. The interactive and adaptive tasks are divided into three

main categories: degraded speech, cognitive skills, and communication strategies. These activities also train auditory memory, speed of processing, and auditory-verbal closure, which are believed to be important skills for understanding language in noisy or otherwise challenging environments. The results of the training session are plotted for the adult as well as sent to a Web site so that the audiologist can monitor progress. Although the opportunity to train at home is attractive, the vocabulary may be challenging for some clients with limited urban experience. The response accuracy is based on the honor system because the program will provide the correct answer in print and listeners are to respond yes or no to indicate whether they had perceived the stimulus correctly.

Otto's World of Sounds

Otto's World of Sounds, designed for children with hearing loss, focuses on basic auditory skills of sound detection, discrimination, and identification. It is intended for home use and as a supplement to a traditional auditory training program. Through the use of 10 different auditory environments, the child encounters sounds analogous to those in their daily listening experiences. The activities within each environment increase in complexity as more sounds are added as the basis for training discovery, memory, and recognition. This program is based on Otto, a prairie dog, which may be most attractive to younger children. The program is distributed free of charge.

Sound and Beyond™

Sound and Beyond is designed for adults with cochlear implants or those with hearing aids who have severe to profound hearing loss. The eight modules include auditory discrimination of pure tones, discrimination and identification of environmental sounds, male/female voice identification, vowel recognition, consonant recognition, word recognition, everyday sentences, and music appreciation. The modules can be completed at home with no specific recommended schedule.

Treatment Outcomes, Efficacy, and Effectiveness

The recent technical report issued by experts in the field of (C)APD and published by the American Speech-Language-Hearing Association (ASHA) recognized the potential benefits of CBAT (ASHA, 2005). They reported that intervention for (C)APD consists of three concurrent approaches, including direct skills remediation, compensatory strategies, and environmental modifications. Despite their recognition that computer-mediated software has several advantages of "multisensory stimulation in an engaging format that provides generous feedback and reinforcement and facilitates intensive training," (p. 11), they admonish that "additional data are needed to demonstrate the effectiveness and efficacy of these approaches" (p. 11).

Table 6–5 includes a summary of auditory training research that specifically included computer-based techniques. Many of the studies evaluating CBAT methods reported positive treatment outcomes (Gillam, 1999; Merzenich et al., 1996; Tallal et al., 1996). However, demonstrating efficacy and effectiveness is more involved, because of the need for control groups, counterbalanced designs, and real-world conditions. On average, most studies show improved scores on some outcome measure following auditory training in children with language impairments (Friel-Patti et al., 2001; Loeb, Stoke, & Fey, 2001; Merzenich et al., 1996; Tallal et al., 1996), hearing loss (Schopmeyer, Mellon, Dobaj, Grant, & Niparko, 1998; Zwolan et al., 2000), and reading difficulties (Rouse & Krueger, 2004; Tallal et al., 1996; Troia & Whitney, 2003). Only one of the studies summarized in Table 6–5 involved a randomly assigned control group that received no CBAT (Rouse & Krueger, 2004).

Efficacy is demonstrated when results show that the treatment is capable of working in the best-case scenario, that is, when appropriate listeners participate and the treatment protocol is followed (Robey & Schultz, 1998). Effectiveness, however, is demonstrated when the program is shown to be effective in real-life situations where there may be fewer controls (Robey & Schultz, 1998). In the few studies properly designed to demonstrate efficacy of CBAT (e.g., included control groups that did not receive CBAT), support was not seen for a specific CBAT; however, these studies did reveal gains derived from intensive treatment with CBAT (Cohen, Hodson, O'Hare, Boyle, Durani, McCartney, et al., 2005; Gillam, et al., 2005; Pokorni, Worthington, & Jamison, 2004; Rouse & Krueger, 2004; Troia & Whitney, 2003). One study conducted by Gillam et al. (2005) designed to separate intensiveness of treatment from treatment mode found that the improvements in language skills by children who received intensive intervention from a speech-language pathologist were equivalent to those achieved by children who received intervention for the same time period via CBAT.

Table 6–5. Summary of CBAT Research

Study			Subjects				Procedures	Results
Author	Year	Title	Journal	Exper N	Control N	Ages	Diagnosis	CBAT	Effect
Merzenich, Jenkins, Johnston, Schreiner, Miller, & Tallal	1996	Temporal Processing Deficits of Language-learning Impaired Children Ameliorated by Training	*Science*	11	11	5;4 to 10;0	Language impaired	Group 1: Modified Speech in FFW games Group 2: Video Games and training with natural speech	Positive treatment for both groups; Greater gains on Receptive Tasks for Group 1
Tallal, Miller, Bedi, Byma, Wang, Nagarajan, Schreiner, Jenkins, & Merzenich	1996	Language Comprehension in Language-learning Impaired Children Improved with Acoustically Modified Speech	*Science*	7	None	5:0 to 9;0	Language impaired and Poor readers	Portions of FFW	Positive treatment effect
Schopmeyer, Mellon, Dobaj, Grant, & Niparko	1998	Use of Fast ForWord to Enhance Language Development in Children with Cochlear Implants	7th Symposium on Cochlear Implants in Children	11	None	4;10 to 11;5	Hearing Impaired using cochlear implant	FFW	Positive treatment effect

	Study				Subjects				Procedures	Results
Author	Year	Title	Journal	Exper N	Control N	Ages	Diagnosis	CBAT	Effect
Zwolan, McDonald-Connor, & Kileny	2000	Evaluation of the Foundations in Speech Perception Software as a Hearing Rehabilitation Tool for Use at Home	*Journal of the American Academy of Audiology*	7	7	5;0 to 12;0	Hearing impaired using cochlear implant	Group 1: FSP Group 2: No Treatment	Positive treatment effect
Friel-Patti, DesBarres, & Thibodeau	2001	Case Studies of Children Using Fast ForWord	*American Journal of Speech-Language Pathology*	5	None	5;10 to 9;2	Language learning disability	FFW	Positive treatment effect for some students
Loeb, Stoke, & Fey	2001	Language Changes Associated with Fast ForWord	*American Journal of Speech-Language Pathology*	4	None	5;6 to 8;1	Language impaired	FFW in Homes	Positive treatment effect for some students
Gillam, Crofford, Gale, & Hoffman	2001	Language Change Following Computer-Assisted Language Instruction with Fast ForWord or Laureate Learning Systems Software	*American Journal of Speech-Language Pathology*	2	2	6;11 to 7;5	Language impaired	Group 1: FFW Group 2: CBAT-Tones	Positive treatment effect for some students

continues

195

Table 6–5. *continued*

Study			Subjects				Procedures		Results
Author	Year	Title	Journal	Exper N	Control N	Ages	Diagnosis	CBAT	Effect
Marler, Champlin, & Gillam	2001	Backward and Simultaneous Masking Measured in Children with Language-Learning Impairments Who Received Intervention with Fast ForWord or Laureate Learning Systems Software	*American Journal of Speech-Language Pathology*	2	2	6;10 to 9;3	Language impaired	Group 1: FFW Group 2: CBAT-Lang	No treatment effect
Thibodeau, Friel-Patti, & Britt	2001	Psychoacoustic Performance in Children Completing Fast ForWord Training	*American Journal of Speech-Language Pathology*	5	5	5;10 to 9;1	Language impaired and Normal language	Group 1: CBAT-Tones Group 2: CBAT-Tones	No treatment effect
Troia & Whitney	2003	A Close Look at the Efficacy of Fast ForWord Language for Children with Academic Weaknesses	*Contemporary Educational Psychology*	25	12	Grades 1–6	Academic weakness	Group 1: FFW Group 2: No Treatment	Limited treatment effect

Study			Subjects				Procedures		Results
Author	Year	Title	Journal	Exper N	Control N	Ages	Diagnosis	CBAT	Effect
Hayes, Warrier, Nicol, Zecker, & Kraus	2003	Neural Plasticity following Auditory Training in Children with Learning Problems	*Clinical Neuro-physiology*	27	15	8;0 to 12;0	Learning impaired	Group 1: Earobics Group 2: No Treatment	Positive treatment effect on some measures
Segers & Verhoeven	2003	Effects of Vocabulary Training by Computer in Kindergarten	*Journal of Computer Assisted Learning*	67	97	4;0 to 6;0	Normal language	Group 1: CBAT-Lang Group 2: No Treatment	Positive treatment effect
Temple, Deutsch, Poldrack, Miller, Tallal, Merzenich, & Gabrieli	2003	Neural Deficits in Children with Dyslexia Ameliorated by Behavioral Remediation: Evidence from Functional MRI	*Proceedings of the National Academy of Sciences*	20	None	8;0 to 12;0	Poor readers	FFW	Positive treatment effect
Pokorni, Worthington, & Jamison	2004	Phonological Awareness Intervention: Comparison of Fast ForWord, Earobics, and LiPS	*Journal of Educational Research*	36	16	7;6 to 9;0	Poor readers	Group 1: FFW Group 2: Earobics Group 3: Non CBAT	No treatment effect

continues

Table 6–5. *continued*

	Study			Subjects				Procedures	Results
Author	**Year**	**Title**	**Journal**	**Exper N**	**Control N**	**Ages**	**Diagnosis**	**CBAT**	**Effect**
Rouse & Krueger	2004	Putting Computerized Instruction to the Test: A Randomized Evaluation of a "Scientifically Based" Reading Program	*Economics of Education Review*	272	240	5;0 to 7;9	Poor readers	Group 1: FFW Group 2: No Treatment	Limited treatment effect
Troia	2004	Migrant Students with Limited English Proficiency: Can Fast ForWord Language Make a Difference in Their Language Skills and Academic Achievement?	*Remedial and Special Education*	99	92	Grades 1–6	Normal verbal IQ, Native Spanish speaker	Group 1: FFW Group 2: Trad Tx	Limited treatment effect
Warrier, Johnson, Hayes, Nicol, & Kraus	2004	Learning Impaired Children Exhibit Timing Deficits and Training-related Improvements in Auditory Cortical Responses to Speech in Noise	*Experimental Brain Research*	13	11	8;0 to 13;0	Learning problems	Group 1: Earobics Group 2: No Treatment	Positive treatment effect

Study				Subjects				Procedures		Results
Author	Year	Title	Journal	Exper N	Control N	Ages	Diagnosis	CBAT		Effect
Segers & Verhoeven	2004	Computer-supported Phonological Awareness Intervention for Kindergarten Children with Specific Language Impairment	*Language, Speech, and Hearing Services in the Schools*	24	12		Language impaired	Group 1: CBAT-Phon Awareness Group 2: CBAT-Syn Sp Group 3: CBAT-Vocab		Positive treatment effect but not for synthetic speech
Cohen, Hodson, O'Hare, Boyle, Durani, McCartney, et al.	2005	Computer-Based Intervention Through Acoustically Modified Speech (Fast ForWord) in Severe Mixed Receptive-Expressive Language Impairment: Outcomes from a Randomized Controlled Trial	*Journal of Speech, Language, and Hearing Research*	50	27	6;0 to 10;0	Receptive Specific language impairment	Group 1: FFW Group 2: CBAT-Lang Group 3: No Treatment		No treatment effect

continues

Table 6–5. *continued*

	Study			Subjects				Procedures	Results
Author	Year	Title	Journal	Exper N	Control N	Ages	Diagnosis	CBAT	Effect
Gillam, Loeb, Friel-Patti, Hoffman, Brandel, Champlin, et al.	2005	Comparing Language Intervention Outcomes	Paper Presented at ASHA	216	N/A	6;0 to 8;11	Language impaired	Group 1: FFW Group 2: CBAT-Lang Group 3: Trad Tx Group 4: CBAE	No treatment effect
Russo, Nicol, Zecker, Hayes, & Kraus	2005	Auditory Training Improves Neural Timing in the Human Brainstem	*Behavioural Brain Research*	9	10	8;0 to 12;0	Learning impaired	Group 1: Earobics Group 2: No Treatment	Positive treatment effect on some measures

Note: Exper = Experimental, CBAT = Computer-Based Auditory Training, FFW = Fast ForWord, CBAT-Lang = Computer-Based Auditory Training with Language Focus, CBAT-Tones = Computer-Based Auditory Training with Tone Stimuli, CBAT-Vocab = Computer-Based Auditory Training with focus on Vocabulary Training, CBAT-Syn Sp = Computer-Based Auditory Training with Synthetic Speech Stimuli, Trad Tx = Traditional Therapy, FSP = Foundations of Speech Perception, Non CBAT = Auditory Training that was not computer based, CBAE = Computer-Based Academic Enrichment

Sweetow and Palmer (2005) reviewed the limited published research regarding the efficacy of auditory training with individuals with hearing loss. They provided many insights into the quality of research needed for CBAT with children with (C)APD. Of the 213 articles they reviewed concerning adults with hearing loss, 42 were identified as studies with potential results related to effectiveness of auditory training. Of these, only six met inclusion criteria that required sufficient detail to allow evaluation of the quality of the research and a study design that involved a randomized controlled trial. These six studies did support, in fact, the efficacy of auditory training, particularly for the treatments that involved training with meaningful, sentence materials (synthetic approach), rather than noncontextual speech syllable drills (analytic approach). Sweetow and Palmer (2005) provide a framework for evaluation of research with CBAT.

Table 6–6, adapted from Sweetow and Palmer (2005) includes the criteria upon which CBAT research can be evaluated. The lack of a control group is perhaps the most important variable limiting many CBAT studies. Interestingly, several studies have demonstrated that the benefits of Fast ForWord or Earobics are no greater than the gains seen following the same intense computer experience but with academic enrichment games (Cohen et al., 2005; Gillam, 1999; Pokorni et al., 2004). This finding suggests that the gains that were made were not the result of specific training activities in the software, but perhaps the result of more generalized training of attending to auditory patterns and the strengthening of possible auditory representation used in perception.

In addition to comparing different types of CBAT, it is also interesting to compare a single CBAT treatment with a no-treatment control group. At least three studies have examined the benefits of Earobics compared to a control group that received no treatment (Hayes, Warrier, Nicol, Zecker, & Kraus, 2003; Russo et al., 2005; Warrier, Johnson, Hayes, Nicol, & Kraus, 2004). Results of each study confirmed significant benefits received

Table 6–6. Criteria for Evaluation of CBAT Research

1. Randomized assignment to treatment groups

2. Inclusion of a control group

3. Power analysis supports the number of subjects included

4. Experimenters and/or subjects blinded to the treatment

5. Psychometrically sound outcome measures related to communication disorders and/or treatment

6. Feedback employed in the training paradigms

7. Assessment of long-term benefits following dismissal from treatment

8. Generalization to other treatment settings

Source: Adapted from Sweetow and Palmer (2005).

by the experimental (treatment) group relative to the control group. These studies demonstrate the benefits of CBAT and, when considered in conjunction with the studies reviewed above that demonstrated absence of significant differences in treatment outcomes across different types of CBAT, it seems apparent that the intensity and frequency of treatment are perhaps the most important variables influencing treatment outcome.

Summary

CBAT can be an effective training tool for children with (C)APD and associated disorders. Three important elements influence the benefit derived from training: meaningfulness of stimuli, engagement of active or focused attention, and intensive training. Although research has supported the use of CBAT for children with language impairments (many of whose clinical profiles included reference to auditory or listening difficulties), there have been no studies specifically designed to determine the efficacy of CBAT for children diagnosed with (C)APD. It is important to note, however, that many of these same studies measured abnormal auditory evoked potential activity in their subjects with language impairment and learning impairment prior to treatment, suggesting the presence of central auditory deficits in these subjects (Jirsa, 1992; Russo et al., 2005; Tremblay, Kraus, McGee, Ponton, & Otis, 2001; Warrier et al., 2004)]. CBAT seems ideally suited to strengthen auditory perception skills through repetitive tasks that can be presented in an engaging format with reinforcement that allows intensive training necessary for maximum benefit.

Currently there are several programs available that range in price, sophistication, and ease of use. Selection of software is expedited by first selecting the age category followed by training area. Additional research involving individuals diagnosed with (C)APD in well-designed studies incorporating randomly assigned control groups are needed to determine the efficacy of CBAT, including the most important program features underlying treatment success. Further research is needed to determine the most appropriate stimuli, hierarchy of tasks, and training format (home vs. school vs. clinic) to use with children with (C)APD.

References

American Speech-Language-Hearing Association. (1996). Central auditory processing: Current status of research and implications for clinical practice. *American Journal of Audiology, 5*(2), 41–54.

American Speech-Language-Hearing Association. (2005). (Central) Auditory Processing Disorders. Available at http://www.asha.org/members/deskref-journals/deskref/default.

Borden, G. J., Harris, K. S., & Raphael, L. J. (2003). *Speech science primer* (4th ed.). Baltimore: Lippincott Williams & Wilkins.

Carhart, R. (1960). Auditory training. In S. R. S. Hallowell Davis (Ed.), *Hearing and deafness* (pp. 368–386). New York: Holt, Rinehart and Winston.

Chermak, G., & Musiek, F. (1997). *Central auditory processing disorders: New perspectives.* San Diego: Singular.

Chermak, G., & Musiek, F. (2002). Auditory training: Principles and approaches for remediating and managing auditory processing disorders. *Seminars in Hearing, 23*(4), 297–308.

Cohen, W., Hodson, A., O'Hare, A., Boyle, J., Durani, T., McCartney, E., et al. (2005). Effects of computer-based intervention through acoustically modified speech (Fast ForWord) in severe mixed receptive-expressive language impairment: Outcomes from a randomized controlled trial. *Journal of Speech, Language, and Hearing Research, 48*, 715-729.

Cox, R. M., & Alexander, G. C. (1992). Maturation of hearing aid benefit: Objective and subjective measurements. *Ear and Hearing, 13*(3), 131-141.

Dawson, M. M., Hallahan, D. P., Reeve, R. E., & Ball, D. W. (1980). The effect of reinforcement and verbal rehearsal on selective attention in learning-disabled children. *Journal of Abnormal Child Psychology, 8*(1), 133-144.

De Csipkes, R. A., Smouse, A. D., & Hudson, B. A. (1975). Influence of reinforcement on the paired-associate learning of retarded and nonretarded children. *American Journal of Mental Deficiency, 80*(3), 357-359.

Eggermont, J. J., & Komiya, H. (2000). Moderate noise trauma in juvenile cats results in profound cortical topographic map changes in adulthood. *Hearing Research, 142*(1-2), 89-101.

Friel-Patti, S., DesBarres, K., & Thibodeau, L. (2001). Case studies of children using Fast ForWord. *American Journal of Speech-Language Pathology, 10*, 203-215.

Galvan, V. V., & Weinberger, N. M. (2002). Long-term consolidation and retention of learning-induced tuning plasticity in the auditory cortex of the guinea pig. *Neurobiology of Learning and Memory, 77*(1), 78-108.

Garstecki, D. C. (1982). Rehabilitation of hearing-handicapped elderly adults. *Ear and Hearing, 3*(3), 167-172.

Gatehouse, S. (1992). The time course and magnitude of perceptual acclimatization to frequency responses: evidence from monaural fitting of hearing aids. *Journal of the Acoustical Society of America, 92*(3), 1258-1268.

Gatehouse, S. (1993). Role of perceptual acclimatization in the selection of frequency responses for hearing aids. *Journal of the American Academy of Audiology, 4*(5), 296-306.

Gillam, R. (1999). Computer-assisted language intervention using Fast ForWord: Theoretical and empirical considerations for clinical decision-making. *Language, Speech, and Hearing Services in Schools, 30*, 363-370.

Gillam, R., Crofford, J., Gale, M., & Hoffman, L. (2001). Language change following computer-assisted language instruction with Fast ForWord or Laureate Systems software. *American Journal of Speech-Language Pathology, 10*, 231-247.

Gillam, R., Loeb, D., Friel-Patti, S., Hoffman, L., Brandel, J., Champlin, C., et al. (2005, November). *Comparing language intervention outcomes.* Paper presented at the American Speech, Language and Hearing Association, San Diego, CA.

Goldstein, M. A. (1939). *The acoustic method for the training of the deaf and hard-of-hearing child.* St. Louis, MO: The Laryngoscope Press.

Hayes, E. A., Warrier, C. M., Nicol, T. G., Zecker, S. G., & Kraus, N. (2003). Neural plasticity following auditory training in children with learning problems. *Clinical Neurophysiology, 114*(4), 673-684.

Horwitz, A. R., & Turner, C. W. (1997). The time course of hearing aid benefit. *Ear and Hearing, 18*(1), 1-11.

Irvine, D. R. (2000). Injury- and use-related plasticity in the adult auditory system. *Journal of Communication Disorders, 33*(4), 293-311.

Jirsa, R. E. (1992). The clinical utility of the P3 AERP in children with auditory processing disorders. *Journal of Speech and Hearing Research, 35*(4), 903-912.

Jusczyk, P. W., & Luce, P. A. (2002). Speech perception and spoken word recognition: Past and present. *Ear and Hearing, 23*, 2-40.

Kent, R. D., & Read, C. (2002). *The acoustic analysis of speech* (2nd ed.). Clifton Park, NY: Delmar Thomson Learning.

Kilgard, M. P., & Merzenich, M. M. (1998a). Cortical map reorganization enabled by nucleus basalis activity. *Science, 279*(5357), 1714-1718.

Kilgard, M. P., & Merzenich, M. M. (1998b). Plasticity of temporal information processing in the primary auditory cortex. *Nature Neuroscience, 1*(8), 727-731.

Kraus, N., McGee, T., Carrell, T., King, C., Tremblay, K., & Nicol, T. (1995). Central auditory system plasticity associated with speech discrimination training. *Journal of Cognitive Neuroscience, 7*(1), 25-32.

Kuhl, P. K., & Meltzoff, A. N. (1996). Infant vocalizations in response to speech: Vocal imitation and developmental change. *Journal of the Acoustical Society of America, 100*(4 Pt. 1), 2425-2438.

Levitt, H. (1978). Adaptive testing in audiology. *Scandinavian Audiology* (Suppl. 6), 241-291.

Loeb, D., Stoke, C., & Fey, M. (2001). Language changes associated with Fast ForWord—language: Evidence from case studies. *American Journal of Speech-Language Pathology, 10*, 216-230.

Marler, J. A., Champlin, C., & Gillam, R., (2001). Backward and simultaneous masking measured in children with language-learning impairments who received intervention with Fast ForWord or Laureate Learning Systems software. *American Journal of Speech-Language Pathology, 10*, 258-269.

Merzenich, M. M., Jenkins, W. M., Johnston, P., Schreiner, C., Miller, S. L., & Tallal, P. (1996). Temporal processing deficits of language-learning impaired children ameliorated by training. *Science, 271*(5245), 77-81.

Montgomery, A. A., Walden, B. E., Schwartz, D. M., & Prosek, R. A. (1984). Training auditory-visual speech reception in adults with moderate sensorineural hearing loss. *Ear and Hearing, 5*(1), 30-36.

Musiek, F. E., Baran, J. A. & Shinn, J. (2004). Assessment and remediation of an auditory processing disorder associated with head trauma. *Journal of the American Academy of Audiology, 15*(2), 117-132.

Pokorni, J., Worthington, C., & Jamison, P. (2004). Phonological awareness intervention: Comparison of Fast ForWord, Earobics, and LiPS. *The Journal of Educational Research, 97*(3), 147-157.

Prensky, M. (2001). *Digital game-based learning*. New York: McGraw-Hill.

Recanzone, G. H., Schreiner, C. E., & Merzenich, M. M. (1993). Plasticity in the frequency representation of primary auditory cortex following discrimination training in adult owl monkeys. *Journal of Neuroscience, 13*(1), 87-103.

Rideout, V., Vandewater, E., & Wartella, E. (2003). *Zero to six: Electronic media in the lives of infants, toddlers, and preschoolers* (No. 3378). Menlo Park, CA: Henry J. Kaiser Family Foundation.

Robertson, D., & Irvine, D. R. (1989). Plasticity of frequency organization in auditory cortex of guinea pigs with partial unilateral deafness. *Journal of Comparative Neurology, 282*(3), 456-471.

Robey, R., & Schultz, M. (1998). A model for conducting clinical/outcome research: An adaptation of the standard protocol for use is aphasiology. *Aphasiology, 12*, 787-810.

Rouse, C., & Krueger, A. (2004). Putting computerized instruction to the test: A randomized evaluation of a "scientifically based" reading program. *Economics of Education Review, 23*, 323-338.

Russo, N. M., Nicol, T. G., Zecker, S. G., Hayes, E. A., & Kraus, N. (2005). Auditory training improves neural timing in the human brainstem. *Behavioral Brain Research, 156*(1), 95-103.

Schopmeyer, B., Mellon, N., Dobaj, H., Grant, G., & Niparko, J. (1998, June). *Use of Fast ForWord™ to enhance language development in children with cochlear implants.* Paper presented at the Seventh Symposium on Cochlear Implants in Children, Iowa City, IA.

Scott, J., & Thibodeau, L. (2006, April). *The effects of auditory training on hearing aid acclimatization.* Paper presented at the annual meeting of the American Academy of Audiology, Minneapolis, MN.

Scott, L. (1992). Attention and perseverance behaviors of preschool children enrolled in Suzuki violin lessons and other activities. *Journal of Research in Music Education, 40,* 225-235.

Segers, E., & Verhoeven, L. (2003). Effects of vocabulary training by computer in kindergarten. *Journal of Computer Assisted Learning 19,* 557-566.

Segers, E., & Verhoeven, L. (2004). Computer-supported phonological awareness intervention for kindergarten children with specific language impairment. *Language, Speech, and Hearing Services in the Schools, 35*(3), 229-239.

Suzuki, S. (1981). *Ability development from age zero.* Miami, FL: Warner Brothers Publications.

Suzuki, S. (1983). *Nurtured by love: The classic approach to talent education.* Miami, FL: Warner Brothers Publications.

Sweetow, R., & Palmer, C. V. (2005). Efficacy of individual auditory training in adults: A systematic review of the evidence. *Journal of the American Academy of Audiology, 16,* 494-504.

Tallal, P., Miller, S. L., Bedi, G., Byma, G., Wang, X., Nagarajan, S. S., et al. (1996). Language comprehension in language-learning impaired children improved with acoustically modified speech. *Science, 271*(5245), 81-84.

Temple, E., Deutsch, G. K., Poldrack, R. A., Miller, S. L., Tallal, P., Merzenich, M. M., et al. (2003). Neural deficits in children with dyslexia ameliorated by behavioral remediation: evidence from functional MRI. *Proceedings of the National Academy of Sciences of the United States of America, 100*(5), 2860-2865.

Thibodeau, L., Friel-Patti, S., & Britt, L. (2001) Psychoacoustic performance in children completing Fast ForWord™ training. *American Journal of Speech-Language Pathology, 10,* 248-257.

Tremblay, K., & Kraus, N. (2002). Auditory training induces asymmetrical changes in cortical neural activity. *Journal of Speech, Language, and Hearing Research, 45,* 564-572.

Tremblay, K., Kraus, N., Carrell, T. D., & McGee, T. (1997). Central auditory system plasticity: Generalization to novel stimuli following listening training. *Journal of the Acoustical Society of America, 102*(6), 3762-3773.

Tremblay, K., Kraus, N., & McGee, T. (1998). The time course of auditory perceptual learning: Neurophysiological changes during speech-sound training. *NeuroReport, 9*(16), 3557-3560.

Tremblay, K., Kraus, N., McGee, T., Ponton, C., & Otis, B. (2001). Central auditory plasticity: Changes in the N1-P2 complex after speech-sound training. *Ear and Hearing, 22*(2), 79-90.

Troia, G. (2004). Migrant students with limited English proficiency. *Remedial and Special Education, 25*(6), 353-366.

Troia, G., & Whitney, S. (2003). A close look at the efficacy of Fast ForWord language for children with academic weaknesses: Can Fast Forword Language make a difference in their language skills and achievement? *Contemporary Educational Psychology, 28,* 465-494.

Tyler, R. S., & Summerfield, A. Q. (1996). Cochlear implantation: relationships with research on auditory deprivation and acclimatization. *Ear and Hearing, 17*(3 Suppl.), 38S-50S.

Walden, B. E., Erdman, S. A., Montgomery, A. A., Schwartz, D. M., & Prosek, R. A. (1981). Some effects of training on speech recognition by hearing-impaired adults. *Journal of Speech and Hearing Research, 24*(2), 207-216.

Warrier, C. M., Johnson, K. L., Hayes, E. A., Nicol, T., & Kraus, N. (2004). Learning impaired children exhibit timing deficits and training-related improvements in auditory cortical responses to speech in noise.

Experimental Brain Research, *157*(4), 431–441.

Wedenberg, E. (1951). Auditory training of deaf and hard of hearing children. *Acta Oto-laryngologica Supplement, 94,* 1–129.

Willott, J. F. (1996). Physiological plasticity in the auditory system and its possible relevance to hearing aid use, deprivation effects, and acclimatization. *Ear and Hearing, 17*(3 Suppl.), 66S–77S.

Zwolan, T., McDonald Connor, C., & Kileny, P. (2000). Evaluation of the foundations in speech perception software as a hearing rehabilitation tool for use at home. *Journal of the Academy of Rehabilitative Audiology, 33,* 39–51.

CHAPTER 7

SIGNAL ENHANCEMENT
Personal FM and Sound Field Technology

CAROL FLEXER

Management for children with central auditory processing disorder ([C]APD) typically includes three events: direct therapeutic remediation, compensatory strategies, and environmental modifications. This chapter focuses on the environmental modifications piece by exploring the functional use of personal FM and sound field FM and IR (infrared) technology as a partial treatment for (C)APD. While functioning to improve the signal-to-noise ratio, this technology may not solve all of a child's (C)APD issues; other treatments discussed in this Handbook also are likely to be necessary.

One of the most challenging learning domains for all children and especially those with (C)APD is the classroom. Youngsters spend much of their time in noisy classroom environments where teachers demand constant, detailed listen-ing to critical, often fast-paced instruction that is spoken far from them. The major factors that affect auditory learning in the classroom include the hearing and attention capabilities of the child and the actual classroom environment. Additional variables include the speech of the teacher and of pupils, and their relative positions in the room.

A child with (C)APD has the same neurologic, linguistic, and psychosocial limitations experienced by all children, plus extra auditory baggage. Children with (C)APD and attention deficit hyperactivity disorder (ADHD) typically have normal hearing sensitivity at the time of diagnosis (note: they may have had otitis media-caused fluctuating hearing loss during infancy or preschool years) but are very distractible and have a great deal of difficulty paying attention for prolonged periods of time. They often are annoyed, confused and even agitated by typical classroom noise levels with subsequent difficulty focusing on their teacher's voice.

Let us begin by exploring the listening limitations common to all children, including those with (C)APD.

How Children Hear

We "hear" with the brain. The ears are just a way in. The problem with hearing loss and with poor auditory environments is that accurate sound repesentation does not reach the brain. The purpose of having favorable listening environments and amplification technologies is to enhance acoustic saliency by channeling complete words efficiently and effectively to the brain (Flexer, 1999).

To begin at the beginning, studies in brain development show that stimulation of the auditory centers of the brain is critical (Berlin & Weyand, 2003; Boothroyd, 1997; Chermak & Musiek, 1997; Sharma, Dorman, & Spahr, 2002; Sloutsky & Napolitano, 2003). Sensory stimulation influences the actual growth and organization of auditory brain pathways (Bhatnagar, 2002; Sharma, Dorman, & Spahr, 2002; Sloutsky & Napolitano, 2003; Tallal, 2005). Therefore, anything that can be done to access, grow, and "program" those important and powerful auditory centers of the brain with acoustic detail expands children's opportunities for enhancement of life function. Poor acoustic environments or a child's hearing loss, no matter how minimal, can be roadblocks to sufficient sounds getting to the brain unless amplification technologies are used. Signal enhancement, such as that provided by personal FM or sound field technology, is really about brain stimulation with subsequent development of auditory-neural pathways.

It is important to recognize that children are not small adults. They are not able to listen like adults listen. Indeed, children bring different listening capabilities to a communicative and learning situation than do adults in two main ways. First, human auditory brain structure is not fully mature until about age 15 years; thus, a child does not bring a complete neurologic system to a listening situation (Bhatnagar, 2002; Boothroyd, 1997). Second, children do not have the years of language and life experience that enable adults to fill in the gaps of missed or inferred information (such filling in of gaps is called auditory/cognitive closure). Therefore, because children require more complete, detailed auditory information than adults, all children need a quieter room and a louder signal (Anderson, 2001). The goal is to *develop* the brains of children, unlike adults where sound enters a *developed* brain.

Typical mainstream classrooms are auditory-verbal environments; instruction is presented through the teacher's spoken communication (Berg, 1993). The underlying assumption is that children can hear clearly, attend to, and focus on the teacher's speech. Thus, children in a mainstream classroom, whether or not they have hearing problems, must be able to hear the teacher for learning to occur. If children cannot consistently and clearly hear and focus on the teacher, the major premise of the educational system is undermined. The point is, all children and especially those with (C)APD, require a favorable signal-to-noise ratio.

Signal-to-Noise Ratio

The signal-to-noise ratio (S/N ratio) is the intensity relationship between a primary signal, such as the teacher's speech, and background noise. Noise is anything and everything that conflicts with the auditory signal of choice and may include other talkers, heating or cooling systems, classroom or hall noise, playground sounds, computer noise, and wind, among others. The quieter the room and the more favorable the S/N ratio, the clearer the auditory signal will be for the brain. The farther the listener is from the desired sound source and the noisier the environment, the poorer the S/N ratio and the more garbled the signal will be for the brain. The dominant source of noise in a room is the children in the room and the number of acoustic events that are co-occurring. As mentioned earlier, all children—especially those with (C)APD—need a quieter environment and a louder signal than adults do in order to learn (Anderson, 2004).

Adults with normal hearing and intact listening skills require a consistent S/N ratio of approximately +6 dB for the reception of intelligible speech (Bess & Humes, 2003). Children need a much more favorable S/N ratio because their neurologic immaturity and lack of life and language experiences reduce their ability to perform auditory/cognitive closure. It has long been known that all children require the signal to be about 10 times louder than competing sounds (Nábêlek & Nábêlek, 1985). Due to noise, reverberation, and variations in teacher position, the S/N ratio in a typical classroom is unstable and averages out to only about +4 dB and may be 0 dB, often less

than ideal even for adults with normal hearing and normal auditory processing capabilities (Crandell & Smaldino, 2002).

A key concept regarding the value of enhancing the S/N ratio is acoustic saliency. Language challenges typically coexist with (C)APD. Tallal (2005) found that children with language impairment make more errors on acoustically nonsalient, as compared to acoustically salient, grammatical morphemes. To explain, in a sentence context, acoustically nonsalient morphemes are shorter in duration and softer than louder phonemes in adjacent portions of the utterance (Tallal, 2005). Thus, the environmental management of enhancing the S/N ratio of spoken instruction has the added benefit of increasing acoustic saliency of more difficult to hear speech sounds.

Signal-to-Noise Ratio Enhancing Technology

It has long been recognized that a remote microphone improves the S/N ratio for a listener. That is, a microphone worn by a talker that uses radio or light waves to send the talker's voice to the listener who wears a receiver makes the desired signal louder and clearer by overcoming distance, background noise, and to some extent excessive reverberation, especially in the personal FM configuration (Berg, 1993). Numerous studies show that academics, literacy, attention, and behavior improve when children have better access to the desired signal (Crandell, Smaldino, & Flexer, 2005.). The question remains, will children with (C)APD show similar benefits of FM use? That is, can personal and/or sound field technology be considered a viable treatment for children with (C)APD? Given that children in general benefit from an enhanced S/N ratio, will children with (C)APD benefit more? Will the use of such technology reduce the necessity of additional treatments for some children? How can we determine if S/N ratio enhancing technology is effective for a particular student? The following sections explore these issues.

Necessary Versus Sufficient Distinctions

A discussion of environmental modifications must be preceded by a discussion of "necessary versus sufficient" benefit. There is general agreement that acoustic accessibility is a necessary prerequisite for academic success. However, acoustic accessibility and enhanced signal saliency in the absence of additional treatments may not be sufficient for children with (C)APD (Chermak & Musiek, 1997).

An analogy in the visual realm might involve a child who has difficulty drawing geometric figures. A necessary first step in addressing this problem would be ensuring clear lighting that enhances visual saliency of the drawing field. The lighting alone might be insufficient to correct a child's drawing of geometric designs; additional treatments may be necessary. One does not remove the lights if they did not solve the entire problem. One keeps the lighting as a necessary first step and then adds additional instruction and accommodations. In a similar vein, one does not remove FM systems if they do not solve the entire problem. One adds other treatments discussed in this Handbook to achieve sufficiency.

Personal FM Technology

Personal FM systems are like individual, private radio stations where the talker (typically the teacher) wears the wireless microphone transmitter, and the child wears the receiver coupled to his or her ears via headphones, ear buds, or through personal hearing aids. The purpose of a personal FM system is to improve the S/N ratio by effectively overcoming the typical classroom acoustic problems of distance and noise (Crandell, Kreisman, Smaldino, & Kreisman, 2004).

Personal FM systems, typically designed for children with hearing loss, have been too powerful for children with normal hearing sensitivity. As children with (C)APD tend to have normal hearing sensitivity at the time of diagnosis, typical FM systems may result in overamplification that could cause hearing loss through noise exposure. In addition, personal FM styles using body-worn receivers or headphones may be perceived as undesirable by parents and pupils with (C)APD. If personal FM systems are selected as an environmental treatment option, they must have low-power output and minimum gain to avoid overamplification.

The EduLink by Phonak (see Figure 7-1) was designed specifically for listeners with normal hearing sensitivity. The EduLink is a miniaturized FM receiver that can be used with a variety of FM transmitters. The discreet, ear-level receiver is easily fit by an audiologist. Its primary purpose is to improve listening and attention skills and perhaps the academic abilities of children with ADHD and (C)APD by improving the S/N ratio and enhancing signal saliency.

A study by Updike (2005) asked if personal FM systems, specifically the EduLink, actually improved the attention

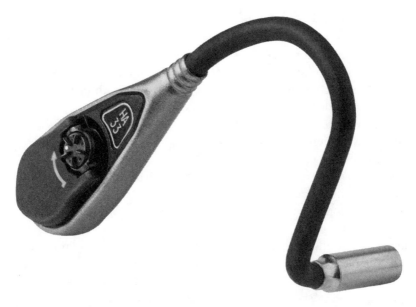

Figure 7–1. The EduLink, a miniaturized FM receiver, was designed for listeners with normal hearing sensitivity and can be used with a variety of FM transmitters. (Photo Courtesy of Phonak Hearing Systems.)

and achievement of children with ADHD and (C)APD. Specifically, Updike wanted to know if the EduLink could be used as a tool to enhance the speech discrimination skills, classroom behavior, and academic performance of children with ADHD and (C)APD. As subjects, she had 12, 8- to 10-year-old children; six with diagnosed (C)APD and six with diagnosed ADHD. All were given the following tests: hearing screening, tympanometry, acoustic reflex thresholds (screening), word recognition testing, and the SCAN Subtest 3—competing words. The results of the study clearly illustrated that with the use of the personal FM system: the students with (C)APD and ADHD's word recognition for phonetically balanced kindergarten word lists (PBK) performance improved significantly in quiet and in noisy classrooms using a +5 dB signal-to-noise ratio; (C)APD and ADHD students' attending and classroom behaviors improved significantly using attention surveys and classroom observations; (C)APD students' academic scores improved significantly in all subject areas in both fall and spring semesters; ADHD students' academic scores improved significantly in some subject areas; and both teachers and students highly approved of the EduLink personal FM system.

Another long-term field trial of the EduLink is being conducted in Switzerland in a school for children with learning disabilities (Phonak, 2004). In total, 28 children diagnosed with performance deficits related to (C)APD participated in the trial. Half the children were equipped with EduLink personal ear-level FM systems (treatment group A), and half the children comprised the matched control group B. It is important to note that FM system use added onto and did not replace any other therapies that the children were receiving, such as speech-language or occupational therapy. Speech intelligibility in noise was assessed using the Basler Sentence Test; a test designed to adaptively determine the speech-to-noise ratio where 50% speech intelligibility was reached. Results to date show that the EduLink improved clarity and the S/N ratio received by the children in school environments. Speech understanding in noise was improved. The teachers reported that the children could understand them better when wearing their personal FM systems and the pupils confirmed that report. In addition, the children and their peers accepted the EduLink. Acceptance is of great practical importance and is a prerequisite for successful use of personal FM systems (Phonak, 2004).

A study by Friederichs and Friederichs (2005) investigated whether changes in electrophysiologic late event potential patterns could be used to reflect clinical changes that occurred from using the EduLink personal FM system with children with (C)APD. They found that, indeed, auditory event-related potentials are sensitive to changes in clinical development of children with (C)APD who have received the treatment of an EduLink personal FM system. Specifically, they found that in the case of infrequent tone responses, development of the classical P2/P3 distribution pattern with an increase in P2 amplitude was observed in the experimental group after both 6 months and 1 year of FM use; this maturation was not observed in the control group. The EduLink did not replace other intervention measures such as speech-language therapy, but rather augmented them.

To summarize, the few studies that have been conducted to date support the use of personal FM systems for children with (C)APD. Certainly additional research is needed; however, these initial studies strongly suggest that personal FM systems be considered as a viable treatment option, with or without additional accommodations.

Sound Field Systems— FM or Infrared?

This section provides general information about sound field technology and its use in the classroom for all children, and particularly for those with (C)APD. Sound field technology is an exciting educational tool that allows control of the acoustic environment in a classroom, thereby facilitating acoustic accessibility of teacher instruction for all children in the room (Crandell, Smaldino & Flexer, 2005; Flexer, 2004a). A sound field system looks like a wireless public address system, but it is designed specifically to ensure that the entire speech signal, including the weak high-frequency consonants, reaches every child in the room. By using this technology, an entire classroom can be amplified through the use of one, two, three, or four wall- or ceiling-mounted loudspeakers.

The teacher wears a wireless microphone transmitter, just like the one worn for a personal FM unit, and his or her voice is sent via radio waves (FM), or light waves (infrared) to an amplifier that is connected to the loudspeakers (Figure 7–2). There are no wires connecting the teacher with the equipment. The radio or light wave link allows the teacher to move about freely, unrestricted by wires. To avoid FM interference when every classroom is amplified with two microphones, infrared transmission is recommended.

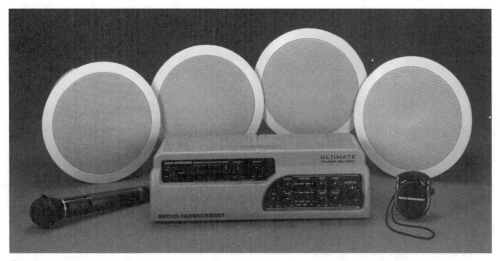

A.

Figure 7–2. Sound field technology functions by having the teacher wear a wireless microphone transmitter, which transmits the teacher's speech via light waves—infrared (**A**), or radio waves—FM (**B**) to an amplifier and loudspeakers. (A provided courtesy of Audio Enhancement; B provided courtesy of FrontRow.)

B.

Sound Field Distribution Systems: A More Descriptive Term

The term sound field distribution system is more descriptive of sound field function. To explain, some teachers, parents, and acoustical engineers interpret the labels "sound field amplification" or "classroom amplification" to mean that all sounds in the classroom are made louder. This misunderstanding may give the impression that sound is blasted into a room causing rising noise levels, interfering with instruction in adjacent rooms, and provoking anxiety in pupils. In actuality, when the equipment is installed and used appropriately, the reverse is true. The amplified teacher's voice can sound soothing as it is evenly distributed throughout the room easily reaching every child. The room quiets as students attend to spoken instruction. In fact, the listener is aware of the sound distribution and ease of listening only when the equipment is turned off. The overall purpose of the equipment is to improve *acoustic saliency* by having the details of spoken instruction continually reach the brains of all pupils.

Children Who Might Benefit from Sound Field Distribution Systems

It could be argued that virtually all children could benefit from sound field distribution systems because the improved S/N ratio creates a more favorable learning environment. If children could hear better, clearer, and more consistently,

they would have an opportunity to learn more efficiently (Rosenberg et al., 1999). Some school systems have as a goal the use of sound distribution systems in every classroom in their district (Knittel, Myott, & McClain, 2002).

No one disputes the necessity of creating a favorable visual field in a classroom. A school building never would be constructed without lights in every classroom. However, because hearing is invisible and more difficult to understand, the necessity of creating a favorable auditory field may be questioned by school personnel. Nevertheless, studies continue to show that sound distribution systems facilitate opportunities for improved academic performance (Crandell, Smaldino, & Flexer, 2005; Flexer, 2004a).

The populations that seem to be especially in need of S/N ratio-enhancing technology include children with: fluctuating conductive hearing impairments; unilateral hearing impairments; "minimal" permanent hearing impairments; cochlear implants; cognitive disorders; learning disabilities; attention problems; articulation disorders; and behavior problems (Rosenberg et al., 1999). Children with (C)APD are in particular need of this equipment as a first line of treatment because, by definition, their auditory neural brain centers are impaired (Friederichs & Friederichs, 2005).

Teachers who use sound field technology report that they also benefit (Rosenberg et al., 1999). Many state that they need to use less energy projecting their voices; they have less vocal abuse, and are less tired by the end of the school day. Teachers also report that the unit increases their efficiency as teachers, requiring fewer repetitions, thus allowing for more actual teaching time.

With more and more schools incorporating principles of inclusion where children who would have been in self-contained placements are in the mainstream classroom, sound field distribution systems offer a way of enhancing the classroom learning environment for the benefit of all children. It is a win-win situation.

Selection, Installation, and Monitoring of Sound Field Systems

Multiple issues need to be considered for the effective selection and installation of sound field distribution systems, the first being the number and positioning of loudspeakers (Boothroyd, 2004). How many loudspeakers and where to place them are probably the most frequently asked questions when considering a sound field distribution system. More data-based studies are needed to investigate these questions because many geometric and acoustic variables are present in each classroom environment. Classroom variables include size, shape, construction materials, and seating arrangements. Learning styles also vary considerably; whole group instruction, individual learning, small group interactive learning, learning centers, independent learning, self-contained classes, and open-concept classrooms. Teaching style is another important variable and includes single-teacher lecture, team teaching, or multiple teaching occurring simultaneously at several learning centers throughout the room. The students themselves add yet additional variables according to their ages, numbers in a class, compliance, and any additional disabling conditions.

A pragmatic approach is useful for ordering and installing sound field equipment. This pragmatic approach considers the individual classroom, the individual teacher and teaching style(s) used in it, and the pupils who learn in that particular classroom. A simulation approach is another strategy that holds great promise of resolving many of the unknowns in loudspeaker placement (Boothroyd, 2000, 2004).

A typical design goal for a sound field system is to increase the signal intensity by about 10 dB uniformly throughout the classroom (Crandell et al., 2004). To accomplish this goal, one must know something about the room and also about the loudspeakers used in the sound field system. Interestingly, reverberation can either help or hinder speech perception. Late room reflections interfere with the speech signal and are considered noise (Crandell & Smaldino, 2002). However, earlier reflections add to the original speech signal and actually increase the intensity of the original signal in a positive way (Boothroyd, 2002). By seating the student close to a loudspeaker, two goals are accomplished: the intensity of the signal is increased by amplification, and the addition of noise by late reverberation is avoided because the student receives only early reflections (Crandell & Smaldino, 2002).

Desktop or totable sound field systems have been introduced to provide ideal sound field conditions for individual students. Figure 7–3 depicts a small loudspeaker placed on a student's desk. Usually students with exceptional listening needs such as cochlear implant students or students with more severe auditory processing problems use this form of sound field amplification. Obviously, not all students

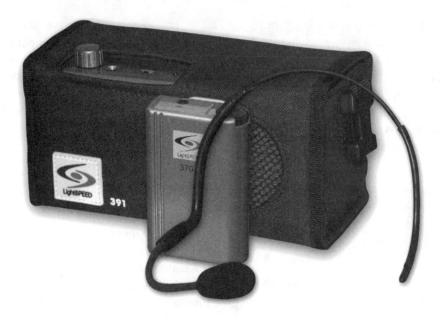

Figure 7–3. A small loudspeaker (personal sound field system) placed on a pupil's desk can increase the loudness of the teacher's speech for a particular student. (Photograph courtesy of LightSPEED Technologies.)

in the room benefit from this kind of system because it does not provide uniform amplification throughout the classroom.

Adequate acoustic dispersion of the teacher's voice throughout the classroom is a function of many factors including the wattage of the sound field amplifier, the directionality of the loudspeakers, and the location and number of the loudspeakers in the room. It has been common practice to use multiple loudspeakers to accomplish adequate dispersion, although there is little research to base this decision on other than intuition and what sounds good to the installer. It is well recognized that carelessly installed, multiple loudspeakers can alter the acoustic spectrum of the talker's signal and increase the negative effects of reverberation (Siebein, 2004). On the other hand, single, point loudspeakers may not allow for an even distribution of sound throughout the room (Boothroyd, 2000).

There is some evidence that four or more loudspeakers installed and distributed in the ceiling provide the best dispersion of sound to all students in the room (Boothroyd, 2000). Some different loudspeaker designs such as bending wave flat panel, and high directivity loudspeakers may provide more placement options (Prendergast, 2001). Ongoing research is needed in this area to ascertain the best way to accomplish adequate dispersion of speech energy in classrooms.

Obviously, the goal is for all students in the learning field to have access to an even, consistent, and favorable S/N ratio at a 10-dB improvement over unamplified speech (Crandell et al., 2004). Thus, if group learning is the mode of teaching, the entire classroom needs to be amplified evenly; all the pupils need to be able to hear the teacher at all times. The larger the classroom, typically the greater number of loudspeakers (three or four) that need to be used so that each child is closer to a loudspeaker than he or she could be to the teacher (Boothroyd, 2002). Close proximity avoids loss of critical speech elements as the sound signal is transmitted across a physical space.

If the classroom has learning centers, a loudspeaker can be positioned close to each learning center for maximum effective amplification at the critical locations (Crandell, Smaldino, & Flexer, 2005). If only one learning center is used at a time, then the other loudspeakers should be turned off.

If a small resource classroom is used, two loudspeakers could provide an even and consistent S/N ratio throughout the area. In fact, if the room is quite small, and there are only a few students who can be seated close to the teacher, even a single loudspeaker might be effective (Crandell, Smaldino, & Flexer, 2005).

If the classroom and class size are small with only one teacher-instructed learning center in use at any given time, then the teacher can carry a single battery-powered loudspeaker to each teaching location to amplify that specific environment. This single, portable loudspeaker arrangement has worked very effectively in some preschool settings.

Understanding Sound Field Technology from a Universal Design Rather Than from a Treatment Perspective

Historically, amplification technologies such as hearing aids, personal FM systems, and now cochlear implants have been recommended as treatments for hearing loss. Because there certainly are populations for whom an enhanced signal-to-noise ratio can mean the difference between passing and failing in school, sound field technologies came to be recommended as treatments for hearing problems. If viewed as a treatment, sound field technology is recommended for a particular child and managed through the special education system. When recommended for a specific child with (C)APD, sound field fits in the treatment category.

However, with the recognition that all children require an enhanced signal-to-noise ratio comes the necessity of moving beyond thinking of sound field technology as a treatment. Sound field distribution systems need to be integrated into the general education arena. The concept of universal design can be useful in this regard.

The concept of universal design originated in the architectural domain with the common examples of curb cuts, ramps, and automatic doors. After years of use, it was found that the modifications that were originally believed to be relevant for only a few people turned out to be useful and beneficial for a large percentage of the population.

In terms of learning, universal design means that the assistive technology is not specially designed for an individual student but rather for a wide range of students. Universally designed approaches are implemented by general education teachers rather than by special education teachers (Research Connections, 1999). It is critical to note that implementation of sound field technologies is shifting from the special education to the general education arena (Flexer, 2004b). Universal design is good news for children with (C)APD because it means that they will be going into classrooms that are automatically equipped with the signal-to-noise ratio enhancing equipment necessary to address their limitations.

Teacher In-Service Education: A Necessity for Effective Equipment Use

Difficulties with sound field technology can result from two primary categories: lack of teacher and administrator information about the rationale and use of the technology, and inappropriate setup and function of the equipment itself (Boothroyd, 2002).

Initial in-service workshops for teachers and administrators need to emphasize the "brain development" purpose of acoustic accessibility (Flexer, 2004a). The relationship of hearing to literacy needs to be targeted, as does the fact that children listen differently than adults do. The concept of signal-to-noise ratio needs to be explained. Microphone techniques need to be demonstrated to teachers so that they can learn how to use the equipment to teach incidental listening strategies. Teachers can use a much softer and more interesting voice because the sound field distribution system provides the vocal projection. Problems can result when teachers place limitations on their teaching, or when they teach the same way with the technology as without it. A second microphone in the classroom —a pass-around microphone for the students—can greatly enhance teacher effectiveness. The pass-around microphone also allows children to hear each other, thereby increasing incidental learning and creating an auditory feedback loop through enhanced auditory self-monitoring of speech.

One point to emphasize when advocating for S/N ratio-enhancing technology for all children, and especially for a child with (C)APD, is that acoustic accessibility is not a luxury—it is a necessity. Hearing is a first-order event for children in mainstreamed classrooms. If children cannot clearly and consistently hear classroom instruction, the entire premise of the educational system is undermined. Few families or schools have money for devices that are perceived as frills. However, when hearing takes its proper place at the head of the line relative to academic opportunities, then recommendations for S/N ratio-enhancing technologies are taken seriously.

Collectively, results of sound field amplification research suggest significant benefits for students in the areas of literacy and academic achievement, speech recognition enhancement in quiet and noise, and on-task behavior related to attentional skills and learning behaviors (Mendel, Roberts, & Walton, 2003). Students, teachers, parents, and school administrators have indicated positive approval for the use of sound field technology in classrooms (Crandell, Smaldino, & Flexer, 2005).

Legal Issues

Section 504 of the Rehabilitation Act of 1973

In most states, children with (C)APD do not qualify for special education services through IDEA unless they also have other documented/covered disabilities. Unlike special education legislation, Section 504 is not based on failure; rather, it is predicated on accessibility (Rehabilitation Act of 1973). The law is a civil rights act that prohibits recipients of federal funds (such as agencies and organizations) from discriminating against "qualified individuals with disabilities in the United States." Specifically, a recipient of federal funds that operates a public elementary or secondary education program shall provide a free, appropriate public education (FAPE) to each qualified person with a disability who is in the recipient's jurisdiction, regardless of the nature or severity of the person's disability. The emphasis in Section 504 is equal opportunity or equal access. Section 504 does not link the child's disability to his or her need for special education services, but rather to the existence of limitations on a major life activity (Rehabilitation Act Amendments of 1992). Therefore, Section 504 is financed by general education and not by special education funds. On the other hand, Public Law 94-142 (now called IDEA), also known as the Education for All Handicapped Children Act of 1975, requires that a child's disability be linked directly to the need for special education services in order to benefit from the educational process (U.S. Dept. HEW, 1977).

The 504 plan can outline access support with accommodations. However, 504's regulations are not as clearly defined nor as financially supported as IDEA's. Any student who qualifies for an IEP automatically qualifies for a 504 Plan, but the reverse is not true. In order to qualify for a 504 Plan, some documentation must be provided showing that equal access cannot be obtained without it.

Show the Need for Technology

The key to securing technology from the school system is to obtain data documenting need (Ackerhalt & Wright, 2003). A Multifactored Evaluation (MFE), which is a thorough evaluation by a multidisciplinary team, is necessary to document the need for a child to receive special services. The last category on most MFE forms is "Assistive Technology Needs." In order for assistive technology to be recommended within any legislative framework, some type of evaluation must be conducted. That is, can we document that the child in question cannot obtain an appropriate education unless personal FM or sound field amplification is utilized? Can the child's failure in the regular education system be linked to hearing difficulties in the classroom?

Efficacy Measures for S/N Ratio Enhancing Technology

Efficacy can be defined as the extrinsic and intrinsic value of a treatment (Crandell, Smaldino, & Flexer, 2005). Even though an environmental modification might have general value, some measurement needs to be made to show that the individual student in question is obtaining some benefit. Benefit may be measured through educational performance, behavioral speech perception tests, direct measures of changes in brain development, or through functional assessments. Functional assessments are the most common and easily administered efficacy measure.

Functional Assessments as a Measure of Efficacy for a Child with (C)APD

Functional assessments as a measure of efficacy are typically accomplished by having the teacher, student, or parent complete a questionnaire before and after use of the personal FM or sound field system.

Several functional assessment measures are available commercially; The Screening Instrument for Targeting Education Risk (SIFTER), Listening Inventories for Education (LIFE), and Children's Auditory Performance Scale (CHAPS). Several of the most commonly used tools, are described below.

SIFTER—Screening Instrument for Targeting Educational Risk

The SIFTER is a one-page form that is easily filled out by the teacher or teachers at multiple intervals during a school year (Anderson, 1989). The form allows the teacher to observe and rate the student's performance as compared to typical students in the class according to the five content areas of academics, attention, communication, class participation, and school behavior. The total score in each area is recorded as pass, marginal, or fail. Even though the SIFTER was originally developed to identify students at risk for listening problems, it has proven to be useful in establishing efficacy of intervention in the classroom. When used in a pretest, post-test paradigm, any change in the child's classroom performance as a result of the FM intervention can be noted and documented.

LIFE—Listening Inventories for Education

The LIFE is an extension of the SIFTER (Anderson & Smaldino, 1998). The LIFE also uses a teacher self-report questionnaire, but it adds a self-report questionnaire that is filled out by the student. The addition of students' input about their personal classroom listening difficulties improves the overall validity of this subjective approach to efficacy.

CHAPS—Children's Auditory Performance Scale

This questionnaire, appropriate for children age seven and older, consists of six subsections that were selected to represent the most often reported auditory difficulties experienced by children diagnosed as having (C)APD (Smoski, Brunt, & Tannahill, 1998). The 36-item scale concerns six listening conditions: quiet, ideal, multiple inputs, noise, auditory memory/sequencing, and auditory attention span. Parents or teachers are asked to judge the amount of listening difficulty experienced by the child in question as compared to the listening difficulty of a typical child of similar background and age.

Summary

The key issue explored in this chapter concerns the role of technology in the overall program for children with (C)APD. To summarize, the first issue or perhaps question is, what outcome/results are we expecting the technology to provide? There are potentially both short- and long-term results demonstrated by studies summarized in this chapter. Short-term results could include better auditory focus, increased attention span, longer time on task, and fewer disruptive behaviors. Of course, measuring these results can be tricky and may involve videotaping, or at the least, multiple pre-FM use and post-FM classroom observations and functional assessments. In addition, the child with (C)APD may have spent many years "practicing" his or her diffuse focus and disruptive behaviors, so these unwanted behaviors may not disappear overnight. Long-term results are based on learning and practicing new skills and strategies. New skills can take many months to show up as improved learning and performance because we are growing new neural connections in the brain and creating new "data files" of life and language experience. Measurement of new skills could include improved grades, accurate class participation, and higher marks on standardized tests. In addition, functional tools such as the SIFTER, LIFE, and CHAPS could be useful.

The second issue concerns expectations. Are we expecting the equipment to solve all of the student's problems, to.be the magic bullet? Or have we targeted a few, critical behaviors that we are expecting the equipment to address. That is, extensive research has demonstrated that signal-to-noise ratio enhancing technology is a *necessary* first step toward creating a viable classroom learning environment for students. However, that technology may not be *sufficient* to address all the challenges experienced by a child with (C)APD; additional accommodations and therapies may be required.

An evaluation strategy could begin by identifying short- and long-term desired outcomes of FM use and the tools needed to measure those outcomes. Next, one ought to identify if the equipment is expected to occur with additional accommodations, instead of any additional accommodations or therapies, or prior to additional accommodations. What is realistic?

In summary, environmental modifications in the form of personal FM systems or sound field technology likely are viable first steps toward enhancing signal saliency and auditory focus for the child with (C)APD. Numerous studies suggest that every classroom ought to have a well-installed and used sound field

system as a *necessary* learning condition for all children. The universal use of sound field technology reduces the need for special education referrals; the technology nips many potential problems in the bud before they have a chance to blossom, including (C)APD problems (Flexer & Long, 2004).

References

Ackerhalt, A. H., & Wright, E. R. (2003). Do you know your child's special education rights? *Volta Voices, 10*(3), 4-6.

Anderson, K. (1989). *Screening instrument for targeting educational risk (SIFTER)*. Tampa, FL: Educational Audiology Association.

Anderson, K. L. (2001, April). Voicing concern about noisy classrooms. *Educational Leadership*, 77-79.

Anderson, K. (2004). The problem of classroom acoustics: The typical classroom soundscape is a barrier to learning. *Seminars in Hearing, 25*(2), 117-129.

Anderson, K., & Smaldino, J. (1998). *The listening inventory for education (LIFE)*. Tampa, FL: Educational Audiology Association.

Berg, F. S. (1993). *Acoustics and sound systems in schools*. San Diego, CA: Singular Publishing Group.

Berlin, C. I., & Weyand, T. G. (2003). *The brain and sensory plasticity: Language acquisition and hearing*. Clifton Park, NY: Thompson Delmar Learning.

Bess, F. H., & Humes, L. E. (2003). *Audiology: The fundamentals* (3rd ed.). Philadelphia: Lippincott Williams & Wilkins.

Bhatnagar, S. C. (2002). *Neuroscience for the study of communicative disorders* (2nd ed.). Philadelphia: Lippincott Williams & Wilkins.

Boothroyd, A. (1997). Auditory development of the hearing child. *Scandinavian Audiology, 26*(Suppl. 46), 9-16.

Boothroyd, A, (2000). *The sound field wizard*. Phonic Ear Web site. Available at www.phonicear.com.

Boothroyd, A. (2002, March). *Optimizing FM and sound-field amplification in the classroom*. Paper presented at the American Academy of Audiology National Convention, Philadelphia.

Boothroyd, A. (2004). Room acoustics and speech perception. *Seminars in Hearing, 25*(2), 155-166.

Chermak, G. D., & Musiek, F. E. (1997). *Central auditory processing disorders: New perspectives*. San Diego, CA: Singular Publishing Group.

Crandell, C. C., Kreisman, B. M., Smaldino, J. J., & Kreisman, N. V. (2004). Room acoustics intervention efficacy measures. *Seminars in Hearing, 25*(2), 201-206.

Crandell, C., & Smaldino, J. (2002, March). *Classroom acoustics*. Paper presented at the American Academy of Audiology National Convention, Philadelphia.

Crandell, C. C., Smaldino, J. J., & Flexer, C. (2005). *Sound-field amplification: Applications to speech perception and classroom acoustics* (2nd ed.). Clifton Park, NY: Thomson Delmar Learning

Flexer, C. (1999). *Facilitating hearing and listening in young children* (2nd ed.). San Diego, CA: Singular Publishing Group.

Flexer, C. (2004a). The impact of classroom acoustics: Listening, learning, and literacy. *Seminars in Hearing, 25*(2), 131-140.

Flexer, C. (2004b). *Classroom amplification and the brain*. (Videotape). Layton, UT: Info-Link Video Bulletin.

Flexer, C., & Long, S. (2004). Sound-field amplification: Preliminary information regarding special education referrals. *Communication Disorders Quarterly, 25*(1), 29-34.

Friederichs, E., & Friederichs, P. (2005). Electrophysiologic and psycho-acoustic findings following one-year application of a personal ear-level FM device in children with attention deficit and suspected central auditory processing disorder. *Journal of Educational Audiology, 12*, 29-34.

Knittel, M. A. L., Myott, B., & McClain, H. (2002). Update from Oakland schools sound field team: IR vs FM. *Educational Audiology Review, 19*(2), 10-11.

Kreisman, B., & Crandell, C.C. (2002). Behind-the-ear FM systems: Effects of speech perception in noise. *Journal of Educational Audiology 10*, 21-25.

Mendel, L. L., Roberts, R. A., & Walton, J. H. (2003). Speech perception benefits from sound field FM amplification. *American Journal of Audiology, 12*, 114-124.

Nábêlek, A., & Nábêlek, I. (1985). Room acoustics and speech perception. In J. Katz (Ed.), *Handbook of clinical audiology* (3rd ed.). Baltimore: Williams & Wilkins.

Phonak Hearing Systems. (2004, May). Edu-Link: Improves speech understanding in noisy classrooms. *Field News*, pp. 1-2.

Prendergast, S. (2001). A comparison of the performance of classroom amplification with traditional and bending wave speakers. *Journal of Educational Audiology, 9*, 1-6.

Rehabilitation Act Amendments of 1992, P.L. 102-569. (1992, October 29). *United States Statutes at Large, 106*, 4344-4488.

Rehabilitation Act of 1973, P.L. 93-112. (1973, September 26). *United States Statutes at Large, 87*, 355-394.

Research Connections in Special Education. (1999, Fall). Universal design: Ensuring access to the general education curriculum. *5*, 1-2. Available at http://ericec.org/osep/recon5/rc5cov.html

Rosenberg, G. G., Blake-Rahter, P., Heavner, J., Allen, L., Redmond, B. M., Phillips, J., & Stigers, K. (1999). Improving classroom acoustics (ICA): A three-year FM sound field classroom amplification study. *Journal of Educational Audiology, 7*, 8-28.

Sharma, A., Dorman, M. F., & Spahr, A. J. (2002). A sensitive period for the development of the central auditory system in children with cochlear implants: Implications for age of implantation. *Ear and Hearing, 23*(6), 532-539.

Siebein, G. W. (2004). Understanding classroom acoustic solutions. *Seminars in Hearing, 25*(2), 141–154.

Sloutsky, V. M., & Napolitano, A. (2003). Is a picture worth a thousand words? Preference for the auditory modality in young children. *Child Development,* 74, 822–833.

Smoski, W. J., Brunt, M. A., & Tannahill, J. C. (1998*). Children's auditory performance scale (CHAPS).* Tampa, FL: Educational Audiology Association.

Tallal, P. (2005). Improving language and literacy is a matter of *time.* Paper presented at Speech, Language and Learning Center Beth Israel Medical Center, New York City.

Updike, C. (2005, July). Children with ADD and APD: *Do personal FM systems improve their attention and achievement?* Paper presented at the Educational Audiology Association Conference; Myrtle Beach, South Carolina

U.S. Department of Health, Education, and Welfare. (August 23, 1977). Rules and regulations for the administration of the education of all handicapped children act. *Federal Register* (Part IV), *42,* 163.

CHAPTER 8

CLASSROOM MANAGEMENT

Collaboration with Families, Teachers, and Other Professionals

JEANANE M. FERRE

Central auditory processing disorder ([C]APD) refers to a deficit in the perceptual processing of auditory stimuli and the neurobiologic activity underlying that processing (ASHA, 2005b). (C)APD is not the result of higher order language, cognitive, or related disorders, but may be associated with difficulties in higher-order language, learning, and communication function. That is to say that (C)APD may coexist with, but is not the result of, dysfunction in other modalities (ASHA, 2005b). In the diagnostic process, the audiologist administers well controlled tests designed to determine the presence or absence of the disorder and to identify the specific perceptual processes that are impaired. In assessment, related professionals use formal and informal procedures to obtain evidence of the extent to which there exist difficulties in other sensory processing or higher-order cognitive, language, or learning skills, as well as evidence of the functional strengths and weaknesses of the listener (ASHA, 2005b). This evaluation process leads to the differential diagnosis of (C)APD from neurocognitive and other related disorders and to the determination of the impact the disorder is likely to have on a listener's academic success, communication skills, and psychosocial well-being. The evaluation process is followed logically by intervention; the comprehensive, therapeutic treatment and management of the disorder designed to reduce or resolve specific impairments and to minimize the adverse impact of the disorder on the listener's life functions.

Intervention— A Balancing Act

For intervention to be effective, it is necessary to "balance" treatment and management components (see Figure 8–1). In remediation or treatment, deficit-specific procedures designed to improve deficient skills are implemented. In management, efforts are directed toward minimizing the impact of the disorder on the listener's everyday life settings. The reader will find detailed discussions of treatment and management strategies and techniques in Chapters 4 and 5 of this volume. In this chapter, environmental modifications and compensatory strategies commonly employed to minimize the adverse effects of (C)APD on school-aged children are described. Case studies are used to illustrate the importance and role of collaboration among professionals, students, and their families in the management of specific profiles of (C)APD.

The Management Team

Although most would agree that the audiologist's role in the diagnostic process is both essential and obvious, there is less agreement when it comes to intervention. Too often, the refrain is heard, "audiologists *diagnose*, speech-language pathologists or others *treat*." Presence of a (C)APD can exacerbate and be exacerbated by other sensory and neurocognitive disorders. Because (C)APD manifests with a variety of clinical profiles, case management should, like the assessment process, be multidisciplinary in nature (see Figure 8–2). Results from a compre-

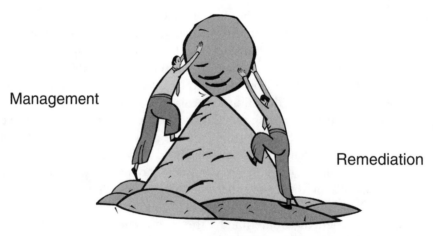

Effective Intervention

Management

Remediation

Knowledge and Principles

Figure 8–1. Intervention—The balanced efforts in management and remediation based on sound principles and accumulated neuroscientific knowledge.

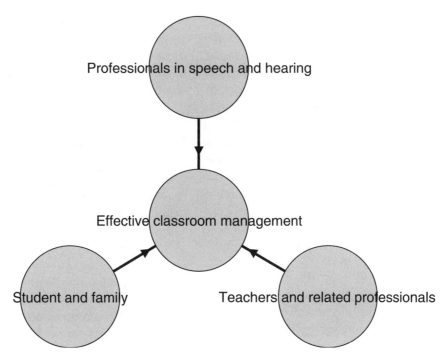

Figure 8–2. The management team.

hensive evaluation of auditory and language function should be included when discussing the overall academic, communicative, and psychosocial needs of the listener.

As a member of the assessment and intervention team, the audiologist offers insight regarding possible impact of (C)APD as it relates to other life skills. The audiologist works with other team members to develop specific, meaningful, and realistic treatment and management strategies designed to improve auditory and related skills, as well as to minimize the day-to-day impact of the disorder on the listener's academic success, communication abilities, and/or well-being. The audiologist applies neuroscientific principles to assist in developing deficit-specific treatment and management goals and strategies, to gauge the success of those strategies, and to extend interven-

tion principles to all environments to maximize benefit.

In most cases, input from related professional disciplines, including, but not limited to, neuropsychology/psychology, special education, speech-language pathology, occupational therapy (OT), and physical therapy (PT)—is incorporated in the intervention process. This input may include diagnosis of comorbid conditions and identification of specific communication or academic difficulties to which the (C)APD is a contributing or exacerbating factor. Parents, families, and other caregivers can offer important information regarding the disorder's impact on the student's day-to-day listening and well-being and, therefore, these individuals also should be considered integral to the intervention team. In addition to understanding treatment goals, parents, teachers, and others need to know how to manage the (C)APD on a daily basis. This aspect of intervention extends beyond individualized pull-out/push-in sessions with the speech-language pathologist or educational specialist, by complementing the efforts of specialists throughout the day, at school, and at home. These additional strategies encourage parents and teachers to modify the way they talk to and with children with (C)APD, help them choose games/activities to enhance listening skills, and modify a classroom or home environment to enable all children to meet their potential.

Interactive Intervention Approach

The goal of intervention for (C)APD should be to maximize the listener's access to and use of incoming auditory information. To that end, one must iden-

tify the components of a communication event. For any communication event, the three key components are the listening environment, the message, and the listener (see Figure 8–3).

Focus on the Environment

It is estimated that up to 60% of classroom activities involve students listening to and participating in spoken communication with teachers or other students (ANSI, 2002). Thus, it is essential that classrooms be free of acoustical barriers. When assessing the listening environment, consideration should be given to both acoustic and nonacoustic variables that can affect speech perception. Acoustic variables include presence, nature, and level of background noise, reverberation time, and distance between speaker and listener (Crandell & Smaldino, 2002). Nonacoustic factors include

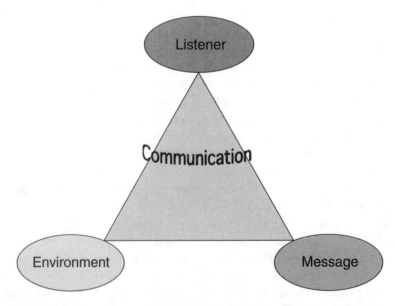

Figure 8–3. The communication triangle. The environment, message, and listener as the key elements in communication.

Background Noise

Background noise refers to any auditory disturbance in a room that interferes with listening (Crandell & Smaldino, 2002). Noise within a room can come from internal sources (in the building but outside the room), external sources (outside the building), and in-room sources. Background noise can adversely affect speech perception by masking the acoustic and linguistic cues of a message and by distracting the listener from the communication event (Crandell & Smaldino, 2002).

The audiologist can use a sound level meter to measure the intensity of noise, as well as its spectral and temporal aspects which also contribute to the degree to which the noise interferes with listening (Nábêlek & Nábêlek, 1994). Speech spectrum noise, multitalker babble and "real-life" in-room noise appear to affect more adversely the speech recognition skills of young children, college-age students, and adults with academic difficulties than does pink or non-speech-like noise (Chermak, Vonhof, & Bendel, 1989; Jamieson, Kranjc, Yu, & Hodgett, 2004; Papso & Blood, 1989).

Signal-to-noise ratio (SNR) refers to the intensity of the signal relative to the background noise. Holding other factors constant, as the SNR becomes less favorable, speech recognition becomes poorer for all listeners (Cooper & Cutts, 1971). For listeners with normal hearing, speech recognition is not severely reduced until the SNR reaches 0 dB (Crandell & Smaldino, 2002). For very young listeners and those with hearing impairment, speech-language disorders, limited English proficiency, academic disabilities, or (C)APD, SNRs that are at least 2 to 15 dB more favorable than those needed by normal hearing listeners are required (Bronzaft, 1982; Crandell & Smaldino, 1996, 2002; Evans & Maxwell, 1997; Finitzo-Heiber & Tillman, 1978; Maxwell & Evans, 2000; Plomp & Mimpen, 1979).

Reverberation

Reverberation, or echo, refers to the persistence of a sound in an enclosed space due to the multiple reflections of sound waves off hard surfaces. A room's reverberation may be expressed in terms of its reverberation time (RT), or the amount of time required for the sound to significantly decay (i.e., decrease by 60 dB) after the signal source has stopped. Reverberation affects speech recognition by masking direct sound (Nábêlek & Nábêlek, 1994). Although all rooms have some reverberation, large and irregularly shaped rooms tend to have longer RTs than smaller rooms or those with greater amounts of absorptive material. For normal hearing adults, recognition is not adversely affected until the RT exceeds 1.0 second (Finitzo-Hieber & Tillman, 1978); however, for children with disordered hearing, language, or processing skills, speech perception may be compromised at RTs as low as 0.4 seconds (Crandell, Smaldino, & Flexer, 1995).

Classroom Noise Abatement

Classroom noise abatement programs should seek to maintain an SNR of at least +15 with reverberation time of 0.4 seconds or less (ASHA, 1995; 2005a). Reverberation times can be somewhat longer (i.e., 0.6 seconds) in small and midsize classrooms, and up to 0.7 seconds in larger classrooms, without degrading speech intelligibility for normal hearing listeners, provided an SNR of +15 or better is maintained (ANSI, 2002).

Classroom noise abatement techniques ranging from relatively simple to rather extensive, can be implemented to achieve these SNR and RT goals. Extensive, and often expensive, solutions for improving classroom acoustics include: reduction or elimination of open classrooms; relocation of teaching spaces away from playgrounds, gymnasiums, or cafeterias; building infrastructure changes such as double-paned windows, noise control devices on heating, air conditioning, and ventilation systems; use of smaller and less irregularly shaped classrooms; changes in lighting fixture type (i.e., from fluorescent to incandescent) and location; and lowered ceiling levels. Simpler and less expensive classroom noise abatement can be accomplished by: closing windows; carpeting rooms; using curtains, drapes and/or acoustic ceiling tiles; placing baffles within the listening space; and damping highly reflective surfaces. Placing bookcases perpendicular to each other or creating a 6- to 8-inch space between side-by-side bookcases can create baffles and minimize noise. Cork bulletin boards and the use of fabric to cover hard surfaces increases sound absorption and dampens reflective surfaces. Felt pads or rubber caps on the bottoms of chair and table legs minimize furniture-to-floor noise. For more detailed information on specific acoustical modifications in the classroom the reader is referred to Sillman (2000), Crandell and Smaldino (2001), and Crandell and Smaldino (2004).

In the home, parents and caregivers should be reminded about simple ways to reduce noise and minimize acoustic barriers to listening such as closing doors and windows; reducing radio, stereo, and television volume; using carpet and drapes; rearranging furniture and changing lighting; and minimizing the number of speakers talking at the same time.

Distance from Source

Distance between the speaker and listener also can affect speech recognition. Generally, sound intensity decreases with increasing distance from the source (Ostergaard, 2000). Sound in a room may be direct or reverberant. Direct sound is the sound reaching the listener without obstruction. Reverberant sound is sound energy comprised of reflected waves within the space. As distance from the speaker increases, the amount of reverberant sound tends to increase and dominate the signal. Boothroyd (2004) noted that for students seated near the back of a classroom the signal was composed almost entirely of reverberant sound while listeners near the front of the room received almost all direct sound. He suggested that a distance of 3 to 6 feet from the source would create optimal audibility, with speech recognition decreasing beyond that critical distance.

Nonacoustic Factors

When assessing the physical space, attention also should be given to nonacoustic factors such as lighting, presence of visual cues, and presence of visual and physical distractions. Room lighting can affect ability to use visual cues and maintain attention on task. Replacing fluorescent lighting with incandescent lighting not only eliminates the hum often produced by these lights, it also improves access to visual cues by reducing harshness and glare. Speakers should avoid being *backlit*, that is, standing with the light coming from behind the speaker rather than on the speaker's face. Teachers should be reminded to speak *after* looking down at their notes or writing on a board rather than *while* writing or reading. The importance of maintaining eye contact and using visual cueing to assist and gauge understanding should be discussed with teachers, specialists, and parents.

Preferential classroom seating can be used to counteract the adverse effects of distance and poor lighting and enhance the listener's ability to use available relevant visual cues. In preferential seating, an effort is made to maximize both the acoustic and visual aspects of the signal based on the summative benefits of bimodal processing (Erber, 1969; Sanders & Goodrich, 1971). The listener's speech perception is enhanced when seated nearer the speaker. The student with (C)APD should be encouraged to *look and listen* to maximize speech-reading opportunities. Schow and Nerbonne (1996) noted that speech-reading is optimal at a distance of 5 feet from the speaker, decreasing significantly as distance from the speaker increases. By placing the listener near and facing the speaker at no more than a 45-degree angle and away from distracting noise, both signal audibility and accessibility of speech-reading cues are optimized (Ferre, 1997). Depending upon the type of auditory processing deficit that has been identified, it may be necessary to move students to a different listening, study or testing environment. Study/work carrels can be used to minimize visual distrac-

tions at school and in the home. Consultation with the OT/PT may result in changes in seating ergonomics (e.g., chair type or design) to minimize physical distractions that can interfere with listening or studying.

Summary

It has been established that by improving classroom acoustics, the listening and learning skills of all children can be enhanced (ANSI, 2002; Crandell & Smaldino, 2002). Before implementing environmental modifications, the audiologist should verify with other team members the specific needs of the student with (C)APD in the classroom and at home. In addition, the specific profile of processing deficits should be identified clearly, as not all modifications outlined above may be beneficial for all profiles of (C)APD, as illustrated in the case histories at the end of this chapter. Considerations when assessing the listening environment are included in Appendix 8A.

Focus on the Message

In addition to enhancing the environment, attention should be given to management strategies that enhance the acoustic, linguistic, and related instructional-language aspects of the signal or message. Acoustic signal enhancement can be accomplished through assistive listening technology and by using "clear speech" techniques. Linguistic modifications include rephrasing information and adding nonauditory sensory cues. Instructional modifications include using preview material, adjusting length and type of message, and modifying response time and response mode.

Assistive Listening Technology

Technology (i.e., assistive listening devices [ALD]) may be recommended to enhance the signal. The ALD is designed to improve the SNR reaching the listener's ear. Unlike traditional amplification where both the speech signal and the ambient noise are both amplified, the physical configuration of the personal ALD selectively amplifies the signal and has the effect of pulling the target signal away from the noise via mild gain amplification, thereby pushing the noise further into the perceptual background. This results in a significantly more favorable SNR and, in turn, improved speech reception. Sound field FM (i.e., frequency modulated) systems enhance the target signal for groups of listeners. When used with proper diagnosis and monitoring, assistive listening technology can lead to improved auditory attention, short-term memory, auditory discrimination, and speech perception (Blake, Field, Foster, Plott, & Wertz, 1991; Crandell & Smaldino, 2002; Rosenberg, 1998; Shapiro & Mistal, 1985; 1986; Stach, Loiselle, Jerger, Mintz, & Taylor, 1987). Direct signal enhancement via personal and soundfield technology is discussed in detail by Flexer in Chapter 7 of this volume.

Clear Speech

In the direct signal enhancement discussed above, speech recognition *of the listener* is enhanced. In "clear speech" the focus is on improving speech recognition by modifying the speech *of the talker*. Schum (1997) noted that in typical conversational speech it is not uncommon for speakers to articulate quickly, fail to project the voice, omit unnecessary or redundant sounds, and to run words and sounds together. These behaviors can adversely affect speech recognition not only for normal hearing listeners (Helfer, 1997), but also for those with hearing loss and auditory-based learning disabilities (Bradlow, Kraus, & Hayes, 2003; Payton, Uchanski, & Braida, 1994; Schum, 1996).

A common complaint among students with (C)APD is mishearing parts or all of a message. In clear speech, the speaker is trained to speak at a slightly reduced rate and to use a slightly increased volume (Picheny, Durlach, & Braida, 1985, 1986). In so doing, spectral boundaries and characteristics are enhanced, signal timing and prosody improves, and relative consonant-to-vowel intensities increase (Picheny et. al. 1986; Bradlow et. al., 2003; Ferguson & Kewley-Port, 2002; Krause & Braida, 2004).

With a minimal amount of instruction and practice, most talkers can be trained to produce clear speech (Schum, 1996; Caissie, Campbell, Frenette, Scott, Howell & Roy, 2005). With additional training, clear speech can be achieved without necessarily reducing overall speaking rate (Krause & Braida, 2002, 2004). By coupling clear speech with an auditory-visual presentation, speech recognition is enhanced further (Helfer, 1997). Both the audiologist and the speech-pathologist are in unique positions to assist classroom teachers, related professionals, and parents in learning to use clear speech to improve day-to-day communication.

Linguistic Modifications

Other beneficial changes in the message involve alterations to the nonacoustic and nonverbal aspects of the signal. By rephrasing a "misheard" signal, the speaker presents the listener with a more linguistically familiar and less ambiguous target, thereby fostering improved comprehension. For example, the ambiguous "Stop that!" can be replaced with the more explicit "Stop tapping your pencil (feet, desk)." Similarly, to gauge a listener's comprehension, use "Tell me what you think I said" rather than "Do you understand?" That is, ask the listener to paraphrase the message to assess understanding. Adding complementary visual cues, examples, demonstrations, and manipulatives can improve understanding, particularly for unfamiliar or abstract information. Limiting the overall amount of information given at one time, breaking long messages down into shorter (5-6 word) sequences, and adding or emphasizing "tag" words (e.g., *first, last, before, after, if, then*, etc.) enhances message salience and understanding. When listening in class, some students with (C)APD will require a tape recorder or scribe to assist them with note-taking and improve their ability to "get the message" (Ferre, 2006).

Instructional Modifications

Preteaching or previewing material is designed to enhance familiarity, and thereby scaffold the listener's overall comprehension challenge. In general, the more familiar one is with the target, the easier the processing becomes. Books on tape, copies of teachers' notes/texts, Cliffs Notes™,[1] seeing movies, and reading aloud to children can enhance their familiarity with the subject, task demands, main ideas, key elements, and vocabulary. For children with (C)APD, knowledge of the rules, structure, and task demands *up front* can minimize overload. It is important to note that for many

of these children this knowledge is not acquired through mere exposure, but through explicit instruction, repeated practice, and review across a variety of contexts and settings (Ferre, 2006). When the message is in the form of a test, those that have closed-set questions (i.e., multiple choice or fill-in) rather than more open-ended questions (e.g., essays) are preferred for students with (C)APD. Some students may need test questions read to them to ensure understanding.

Many children with (C)APD report experiencing excessive auditory fatigue. Scheduling "listening breaks" in which auditory message demands are limited, can minimize this reported auditory overload. For example, do not schedule a spelling lesson right after a reading class. Intersperse lecture classes with activities that are more hands-on or less academically challenging (e.g., physical education). Do not schedule homework or therapy immediately after school. Instead schedule some minutes of *down time* following school (Ferre, 2002).

Sometimes the listening challenge simply exceeds the capability of the student with (C)APD such that course substitutions or waivers may be required. For example, consideration may be given to a nonverbal alternative to meet foreign language requirements. Many states not only recognize American Sign Language as a foreign language, but also accept it for credit at the high school and collegiate levels (NICD, 2001). Some students may require a waiver or substitution (e.g., a culture course) for a foreign language requirement based on the nature of their auditory processing difficulties. A highly structured and well-ordered language such as Hebrew or Latin may meet

---

[1]*Cliffs Notes* is a registered trademark of Hungry Minds, Inc.

the second language needs of some children with (C)APD.

Finally, how students are asked to respond to the message may require modification. For some students with (C)APD, it may be necessary to allow extended time, dictated responses on written exams, reduced use of wholly oral exams, and answers to be written in a test booklet rather than transferred to a score sheet, especially for standardized testing. As with modifications to the environment, any modification to the type, quality, or length of the message or comparable adjustments to the required response to the message should be made only after clearly defining the specific profile of the (C)APD and establishing the specific needs of the individual student. Appendix 8B provides a checklist for aspects of the message that may be modified to enhance instructional success.

Focus on the Listener

As illustrated in Figure 8–3, the listener plays an important role in the communication event. Students with (C)APD need to understand and be able to respond to the question, "How can *I* change the environment, the message, or myself to improve the listening situation?" Students can be taught and encouraged to use (or ask others for) many of the modifications discussed in this chapter.

One way to encourage this self-reflection and proactivity is by encouraging students to use *rules for good communication* (Ferre, 1997). These 10 simple "rules" can help students learn to monitor the listening environment, message quality, and their own listening behavior to manage the impact of the (C)APD. In

addition, top-down compensatory strategies or central resource training can teach the student to use specific compensatory strategies to improve access to and understanding of auditorily presented information. Compensatory strategies or central resource training is discussed in depth by Chermak in Chapter 5 of this volume.

As a member of the management team, the audiologist can facilitate the student's use of compensatory strategies. Both the student and team members need a clear understanding of the client's specific listening needs. Audiologists should work with parents and teachers to understand instructional styles and curricular demands to ensure that appropriate modifications are implemented. As the expert in (C)APD, the audiologist provides resources for materials, products, and activities that can be used, often informally, at home and school to improve understanding of the disorder, enhance the use of compensatory strategies, and to develop students' self-advocacy skills. Finally, the audiologist can facilitate access to appropriate related professionals and support groups as needed. A checklist of self-advocacy tips that can be shared with students, teachers, and families is presented in Appendix 8C.

Communicating the Results

As a member of the intervention team, the audiologist should convey diagnostic test results, impressions, and recommendations both in writing and through participation at the student's case conference or team meeting. Both formats provide the opportunity to educate the student, parents, teachers, and related professionals about (C)APD, in general, as well as the specific auditory processing and related listening/learning needs of the particular student.

A clearly written diagnostic report is key to this communication. The statement of problem, reason for referral, and relevant case history information should be included, followed by a reporting of test results in which vocabulary, professional terms, and acronyms have been clarified. Although results from individual tests are important, a summary of the cumulative audiologic test battery findings may be more appreciated by parents and related professionals with whom the student works. The audiologic characteristics and nature of the specific profile (i.e., deficient skill areas) should be explained clearly and concisely followed by a discussion of the possible impact on communication, academics, and day-to-day listening skills. Recommendations should be based on sound principles of intervention, include deficit-specific rationale, take into account recognized educational philosophies and practices, and include descriptions of desired changes and prognosis. Audiologists should be familiar with educational options in their geographic area, as well as state and local service eligibility criteria.

Finally, both oral and written reports should include recommendations and time lines for measuring outcomes, both subjectively and objectively. Effectiveness of classroom management strategies may be reflected, formally, in improved grades and improved function as reflected on listening performance checklists such as the CHAPS (Children's Auditory Performance Scale) (Smoski, Brunt, & Tannahill, 1998). Less formal evidence may include observation of increased use of

self-advocacy techniques by the student, decreased fatigue, reports of less frequent need for repetition and reinstruction, and students' self-reports of improved "hearing" in the classroom.

Case Studies of Specific (C)APD Profiles

To summarize and conclude this chapter, three cases illustrate the application of an interactive, collaborative approach to (C)APD intervention in an educational setting. The students described were diagnosed with (C)APD using the Bellis-Ferre model (1999) for characterizing specific profiles. This model delineates five profiles of (C)APD based on key central auditory test findings, and describes typical behavioral manifestations associated with each deficit. The model consists of three primary profiles of (C)APD, characterized by the presumed underlying site of central nervous system dysfunction, and two secondary profiles that, while yielding unique patterns of results on central auditory tests, may be more appropriately described as manifestations of supramodal or cognitive-linguistic disorders. For a detailed discussion of these profiles, the reader is referred to Bellis (2003). Brief descriptions of the three primary (C)APD profiles precede the case illustrations.

Auditory Decoding Profile

The auditory decoding profile is characterized by poor discrimination of fine acoustic differences in speech with behavioral characteristics similar to those observed among children with peripheral hearing loss. This profile is presumed to reflect left hemisphere dysfunction. Auditory decoding deficit can create secondary difficulties in communication (e.g., vocabulary, syntax, semantics, and second language acquisition) and academic skills (e.g., reading decoding, spelling, note-taking, and following directions). The listener with poor decoding typically exhibits difficulty recognizing speech in noisy or highly reverberant backgrounds, when visual and contextual cues are limited, and when unfamiliar with concepts or vocabulary. Children with auditory decoding deficit benefit from modifications and compensations that focus on improving the quality of and access to the acoustic signal (e.g., repetition, clear speech, preferential seating, noise abatement, and use of ALD or tape recorder).

Integration Profile

The integration deficit profile likely is due to inefficient interhemispheric communication and is characterized by deficiency in the ability to perform tasks that require intersensory and/or multisensory communication. The child does not synthesize information well, may complain that there is too much information, and has difficulty intuiting task demands, starting complex tasks, transitioning from task to task, or completing tasks in a timely fashion. Impact on communication is variable, and academic difficulties in reading, spelling, writing, and other integrative tasks are typically observed. Children with integration deficit who do not synthesize information as quickly and efficiently as other children benefit from modifications and compensations that adjust the quantity and structure of

the signal (e.g., repetition with related cues, manipulatives, shortened and simplified instructions, preteaching, extended time, closed set tests, and highly structured second-language learning).

Prosodic Profile

The prosodic deficit profile is characterized by deficiency in using prosodic features of a target, a predominantly right hemisphere function. The child displays difficulty in auditory pattern recognition, important for perceiving running speech, and may have difficulty recognizing and using other sensory patterns (e.g., visual, tactile). Difficulties are observed in pragmatic language (e.g., reading facial expressions, body language, and gestures; recognizing or using sarcasm or heteronyms), rhythm perception, music, and nonverbal learning. Children with prosodic deficits have difficulty recognizing and attaching meaning to auditory patterns and benefit from modifications that improve both the structure and meaning of the signal (e.g., repetition with emphasis, clear speech, knowledge of rules, untimed activities, highly structured second language learning).

Case Profiles

DB, age 9 years, 8 months, was referred for evaluation by the school speech-language pathologist as part of a multidisciplinary case study. Speech-language evaluation indicated poor sound blending, vocabulary, and word memory skills. Parents reported that DB had an embolism in the left hemisphere that was reportedly stable; however, MRI data was not available at the time of testing.

DB was enrolled in a dual curriculum (English-Hebrew) regular education environment. Academic achievement was at expected levels for English-language curriculum but significantly below grade level in Hebrew-language classes. Results of central auditory evaluation revealed normal peripheral auditory function and impaired auditory closure and related discrimination skills as evidenced by abnormal performance on low-redundancy speech tasks (e.g., low-pass filtered speech, time-compressed speech, with and without reverberation, and listening in noise). Performance on tasks of binaural integration, binaural separation, and temporal patterning were within normal limits for age, suggesting no specific deficits in these areas. Overall pattern of performance provided evidence of Auditory Decoding profile, suggesting dysfunction in the primary auditory cortex and consistent with reported presence of left hemisphere embolism. At the student's case conference, additional pull-out therapy time was added to allow the speech-language pathologist to include auditory rehabilitation (e.g., discrimination training, speech-reading, compensatory strategies training, and self-advocacy training). Recommended management strategies for this student included: preferential classroom seating; additional noise abatement at school and home with draperies added to classroom; direct signal enhancement via personal FM system and use of a tape recorder for use in Hebrew classes only; repetition of information as needed; use of clear speech by parents and teachers; adjusted class schedule to minimize auditory fatigue (e.g., Hebrew classes moved to mornings); preteaching new information, especially vocabulary; multisensory instruction (e.g., verbal information supplemented

with written and graphic materials); and informal checklist developed collaboratively by the speech-language pathologist and the audiologist to gauge strategy effectiveness.

RB, age 10 years, 6 months, was referred for testing as part of a triennial evaluation to clarify auditory needs. RB is in a self-contained classroom for students with learning disabilities with reports of limited improvement. Central auditory evaluation indicated normal peripheral auditory function and evidence of specific deficit in auditory pattern recognition (i.e., prosodic) skills, characterized by excessive left ear suppression on dichotic listening tests and inability to mimic or label temporal patterns. Overall test results indicated a prosodic profile, suggesting right hemisphere dysfunction. In addition to speech-language therapy currently in place to improve social and pragmatic language skills, therapy was recommended to improve temporal patterning skills, recognition and use of prosody, self-advocacy and compensatory skills, and speech-reading ability. The small classroom size and nature of RB's learning environment precluded the need for specific recommendations for noise abatement, preferential seating, or a multisensory learning environment that would be offered for other children with this profile. The following management strategies were recommended: repetition of targets emphasizing key items and components of the message; use of clear speech by teacher and classroom aide; teacher encouraged to use more "animated" instructional style; preteaching and use of concrete manipulatives for instruction of abstract concepts; tape recording of lectures, provision of copies of teachers' notes; extended time for tests and assignments; and classroom aide to track improvement/progress via observation checklist.

CF, age 8 years, 9 months, was seen for testing at the parents' request. CF received private occupational therapy (OT) for reported sensory integration disorder and special education services in reading and written language. Parents reported that CF had two febrile seizures during early childhood. Annual electro-encephalography (EEG) testing to monitor brain activity reportedly indicated generally immature responses but no specific abnormalities. Central auditory evaluation indicated normal peripheral auditory function, normal performance on degraded speech tests, good ability to mimic tonal patterns but poor ability to label patterns, and excessive left ear suppression on dichotic listening tests. Evaluation results indicated an integration profile, suggesting deficient interhemispheric communication, consistent with report of generalized neurologic immaturity. Activities to improve auditory-visual integration skills were recommended for inclusion in CF's therapy plan, to be implemented by both the OT and the special education resource teacher. In addition, the following management strategies were recommended: use of manipulatives for instruction of abstract concepts; teacher encouraged to use sequential, rather than simultaneous, presentation of directions (e.g., students told to "look" at and copy written instructions from board first, then teacher presented instructions verbally); teacher encouraged to present information with demonstration and modeling and to repeat rather than rephrase instructions; opportunities for previewing of new material; provision of books on tape; extended time for tests; for computer-scored tests, CF allowed to write answers

in test booklet rather than transfer to computer-scored answer sheet; integration skills to be tracked at three-month intervals by OT and audiologist.

Summary

The three preceding case presentations illustrate the importance of collaboration and teaming to best develop individualized intervention programs for students with (C)APD. Shared responsibility by professionals, families, and students is most likely to achieve intervention goals and lead to effective treatment outcomes.

References

American National Standards Institute. (2002). *ANSI S12.60-2002. Acoustical performance criteria, design requirements and guidelines for schools.* Melville, NY: Author.

American Speech Language Hearing Association. (1995). *Guidelines for acoustics in educational settings.* Rockville, MD: Author.

American Speech Language Hearing Association. (2005a). *Guidelines for addressing acoustics in educational settings.* Rockville, MD: Author.

American Speech Language Hearing Association. (2005b). *Technical report: (Central) auditory processing disorders.* Rockville, MD: Author.

Bellis, T. (2003). *Assessment and management of central auditory processing disorders in the educational setting* (2nd ed.). Clifton Park, NY: Thomson Delmar Learning.

Bellis, T., & Ferre, J. (1999). Multidimensional approach to differential diagnosis of central auditory processing disorders in children. *Journal of the American Academy of Audiology, 10,* 319–328.

Blake, R., Field, B., Foster, C., Plott, F., & Wertz, P. (1991). Effect of FM auditory trainers on attending behaviors of learning-disabled children. *Language-Speech-Hearing Services in the Schools, 22*, 111-114.

Boothroyd, A. (2004). Room acoustics and speech perception. *Seminars in Hearing, 25*, 155-166.

Bradlow, A., Kraus, N., & Hayes, E. (2003). Speaking clearly for children with learning disabilities: Sentence perception in noise. *Journal of Speech Language Hearing Research, 46*, 80-97.

Bronzaft, A. L. (1982). The effect of a noise abatement program on reading ability. *Journal of Environmental Psychology, 1*, 215-222.

Caissie, R., Campbell, M., Frenette, W., Scott, L., Howell, I., & Roy, A. (2005). Clear speech for adults with a hearing loss: Does intervention with communication partners make a difference? *Journal of the American Academy of Audiology, 15*, 157-171.

Chermak, G. D., Vonhoff, M. R., & Bendel, R. B. (1989). Word identification performance in the presence of competing speech and noise in learning disabled adults. *Ear and Hearing, 10*, 90-93.

Crandell, C., & Smaldino, J. (1996). Speech perception in noise by children for whom English is a second language. *American Journal of Audiology, 5*, 47-51.

Crandell, C., & Smaldino, J. (2001). Acoustical modifications for the classroom. In C. Crandell & J. Smaldino (Eds), Classroom acoustics: Understanding barriers to learning. *Volta Review, 101*(5), 33-46.

Crandell, C., & Smaldino J. (2002). Room acoustics and auditory rehabilitation technology. In J. Katz (Ed.), *Handbook of clinical audiology* (5th ed., pp. 607-630). Philadelphia: Lippincott Williams & Wilkins.

Crandell, C., & Smaldino, J. (Eds.). (2004). Classroom acoustics. *Seminars in Hearing, 25*(2), 189-200.

Crandell, C., Smaldino, J., & Flexer, C. (1995). *Soundfield FM amplification: Theory and practical applications.* San Diego, CA: Singular Publishing Group.

Cooper, J., & Cutts, B. (1971). Speech discrimination in noise. *Journal of Speech and Hearing Research, 14*, 332-337.

Erber, N. (1969). An interaction of audition and vision in recognition of oral speech stimuli. *Journal of Speech and Hearing Research, 12*, 423-425.

Evans, G. W., & Maxwell, L. (1997). Chronic noise exposure and reading deficits: The mediating effects of language acquisition. *Environment and Behavior, 29*, 638-656.

Ferguson, S., & Kewley-Port, D. (2002). Vowel intelligibility in clear and conversational speech for normal-hearing and hearing-impaired listeners. *Journal of the Acoustical Society of America, 112*, 259-271.

Ferre, J. (1997). *Processing power: A guide to CAPD assessment and management.* San Antonio, TX: The Psychological Corporation.

Ferre, J. (2002). Managing children's auditory processing deficits in the real world: What teachers and parents want to know. *Seminars in Hearing, 23*, 319-326.

Ferre, J. (2006). Management strategies for APD. In T. K. Parthasarathy (Ed.), *An introduction to auditory processing disorders in children.* Mahwah, NJ: Lawrence Erlbaum Associates.

Finitzo-Heiber, T., & Tillman, T. (1978). Room acoustical effects on monosyllabic word discrimination ability for normal and hearing impaired children. *Journal of Speech and Hearing Research, 21*, 440-448.

Helfer, K. (1997). Auditory and auditory-visual perception of clear and conversational speech. *Journal of Speech Language and Hearing Research, 40*, 432-443.

Jamieson, D. G., Kranjc, G., Yu, K., & Hodgett, W. E. (2004). Speech intelligibility of young school-aged children in the presence of real-life classroom noise. *Journal of the American Academy of Audiology, 15*, 508-517.

Krause, J., & Braida, L. (2002). Investigating alternative forms of clear speech: The effects of speaking rate and speaking mode on intelligibility. *Journal of the Acoustical Society of America, 112,* 2165-2172.

Krause, J., & Braida, L. (2004). Acoustic properties of naturally produced clear speech at normal speaking rates. *Journal of the Acoustical Society of America, 115,* 362-378.

Maxwell, L., & Evans, G. (2000). The effects of noise on pre-school children's pre-reading skills. *Environmental Psychology, 20,* 91-98.

Nébêlek, A., & Nébêlek, I. (1994). Room acoustics and speech perception. In J. Katz (Ed.), *Handbook of clinical audiology* (4th ed., pp. 624-637). Baltimore: Williams & Wilkins.

NICD: National Information Center on Deafness. (2001). *States that recognize American Sign Language as a foreign language.* Washington, DC: Gallaudet University: Author.

Ostergaard. P. (2000). Physics of sound and vibration. In E. Berger, L. Royster, J. Royster, D. Driscoll, & M. Layne (Eds.) *The noise manual* (pp. 19-39). Fairfax, VA: American Industrial Hygiene Association.

Papso, C. F., & Blood, I. M. (1989). Word recognition skills of children and adults in background noise. *Ear and Hearing, 10,* 235-236.

Payton, K., Uchanski, R., & Braida, L. (1994). Intelligibility of conversational and clear speech in noise and reverberation for listeners with normal and impaired hearing. *Journal of the Acoustical Society of America, 95,* 1581-1592.

Picheny, M., Durlach, N., & Braida, L. (1985). Speaking clearly for the hard of hearing I: Intelligibility differences between clear and conversational speech. *Journal of Speech and Hearing Research, 28,* 96-103.

Picheny, M., Durlach, N., & Braida, L. (1986). Speaking clearly for the hard of hearing. II: Acoustic characteristics of clear and conversational speech. *Journal of Speech and Hearing Research, 29,* 434-446.

Plomp, R., & Mimpen, A. (1979). Speech-reception threshold for sentences as a function of age and noise level. *Journal of the Acoustical Society of America, 66,* 1333-1342.

Rosenberg, G. G. (1998). FM soundfield research identifies benefits for students and teachers. *Educational Audiology Review, 15,* 6-8.

Sanders, D., & Goodrich, S. (1971). Relative contribution of visual and auditory components of speech intelligibility as a function of three conditions of frequency distortion. *Journal of Speech and Hearing Research, 14,* 154-159.

Schow, R., & Nerbonne, M. (1996). *Introduction to audiologic rehabilitation* (3rd ed.). Boston: Allyn & Bacon.

Schum, D. (1996). Intelligibility of clear and conversational speech of young and elderly talkers. *Journal of the American Academy of Audiology, 7,* 212-218.

Schum, D. (1997). Beyond hearing aids: Clear speech training as an intervention strategy. *Hearing Journal, 50,* 36-39.

Shapiro, A., & Mistal, G. (1985). ITE-aid auditory training for reading and spelling-disabled children: Clinical case studies. *Hearing Journal, 38,* 14-16.

Shapiro, A., & Mistal, G. (1986). ITE-aid auditory training for reading and spelling-disabled children: A longitudinal study of matched groups. *Hearing Journal, 39,* 14-16.

Sillman, E. (Ed). (2000). Improving acoustics in American schools. *Language-Speech-Hearing Services in Schools, 31,* 4.

Smoski, W., Brunt, M., & Tannahill, C. (1998). *Children's Auditory Performance Scale.* Tampa, FL: Educational Audiology Association.

Stach, B., Loiselle, L., Jerger, J., Mintz, S., & Taylor, C. (1987). Clinical experience with personal FM assistive listening devices. *Hearing Journal, 40,* 24-30.

APPENDIX 8A. Checklist for Assessing the Listening Environment

*E*ducate the listener, family and teachers about environmental impact on listening.

*N*oise—check noise levels at school and home.

*V*erify suspected adverse effects with management team.

*I*ndividualize the plan—choose modifications that are deficit specific.

*R*everberation—minimize echo in classroom or at home.

*O*ptimize access to visual and related cues.

*N*ew technology—investigate assistive listening device options.

*M*inimize distance between speaker and listener.

*E*liminate acoustic barriers whenever possible.

*N*ote impact, both positive and negative, that environmental changes have on the listener.

*T*ell parents and teachers how to enhance school and home environments using least restrictive means.

APPENDIX 8B. Checklist for Message Modifications that Enhance Listening Comprehension

*M*ake sure you have the listener's attention.

*E*ye contact and visual cues help.

*S*peak clearly.

*S*ay what you mean.

*A*void ambiguity.

*G*ive listening breaks to minimize fatigue.

*E*xtend response time for both verbal and written messages.

APPENDIX 8C. Checklist for Self-Advocacy and Good Communication Rules

*S*it still—we keep our bodies still while listening.

*E*veryone makes mistakes—don't give up on yourself.

*L*isten to the message not just the words—listen for the meaning.

*F*igure it out—use all the clues and guess when you can.

*A*llow yourself time to put your thoughts together before answering.

*D*o ask your buddy, peer, or teacher for help.

*V*oice concerns or questions if you don't understand.

*O*kay to get ahead in your reading and learn new vocabulary words ahead of time.

*C*hoose a quiet place to study or try to move away from noise.

*A*sk for repetition, clarification, or an example if you didn't hear or understand information.

*C*hange your environment when you can to help you hear well.

*Y*ou can use your eyes to hear better—use visual cues.

CHAPTER 9

MANAGING (CENTRAL) AUDITORY PROCESSING DISORDERS IN ADOLESCENTS AND ADULTS

JANE A. BARAN

Introduction

The preceding eight chapters in this text provided detailed information on many of the intervention approaches that can be used to remediate or alleviate the functional deficits experienced by individuals with (central) auditory processing disorder ([C]APD). Although much of the focus in these chapters was on the application of these procedures with children, each of the approaches discussed can be incorporated into an efficacious management plan for the adolescent or adult with (C)APD. As is the case with children, management programs developed for adolescents or adults with (C)APD should be individualized to address the specific deficit areas that were uncovered during the diagnostic process (Baran, 1998, 2002; Chermak & Musiek, 1997). In addition, it is important that the presence of any comorbid conditions be considered as the behavioral manifestations associated with many comorbid conditions (e.g., peripheral hearing loss, attention deficit disorder, behavioral disorder, etc.) can impact the utility of a given management plan or approach for the child or the adult with (C)APD (Baran, 1998, 2002; Chermak & Musiek, 1997).

Older individuals with (C)APD often present unique challenges and circumstances that will affect the design and effectiveness of their rehabilitative programs. Brain plasticity, which is optimal during early childhood, slows as one ages (Musiek & Berge, 1998). As a result of this recognized change in brain plasticity with advancing age, there is likely to be less emphasis on auditory training approaches in the management programs used with adults and greater reliance on approaches that are designed to improve the quality of the signal or enhance the individual's cognitive and linguistic resources (Baran, 2002; Musiek, Shinn, & Hare, 2002). Also, as children mature into adolescents and adults, their lives are reconfigured in different and complex ways and they are called upon to function in many different contexts. Children are commonly viewed as existing or functioning in one context at a time (i.e., as learners in school or as family members outside of school). Adults, on the other hand, are not configured primarily within the context of a single setting, but rather within and across the context of a number of settings—many of which often overlap (e.g., home, family, work, community, recreational activities, etc.) (Baran, 2002; Kleinman & Bashir, 1996). Therefore, distinctively different behaviors and performance are expected of the adult. Children with (C)APD and other related disabilities are provided educational support services that focus on the specific disability; however, there are few support services available for adults with (C)APD, and the focus is typically not on the individual's disability, but rather on such things as job performance, community involvement, family relationships, and parental effectiveness—all of which can be negatively affected by the disorder. Moreover, the effects of the disorder often are not consistent across contexts or even within one context. An individual may experience little or no difficulty functioning in a given context, but then begin to experience difficulty at another time in the same setting or environment. Fatigue or changes in the listening environment (e.g., an air

conditioner being turned on) may be sufficient to create a situation where the individual's compensatory strategies or cognitive resources are taxed, and problems arise. Different contexts will present different listening demands due to such variables as room acoustics, degree of familiarity with the topic(s) of conversation, the number of participants in the conversation, and so forth. Finally, cultural and personal values, motivation, and the availability of support from family or friends can all have an impact on the development and success of a management program designed for the adolescent or adult with (C)APD.

It is essential, therefore, that each of these factors and influences (specific auditory deficits, comorbid disorders or disabilities, age, motivation, communication contexts, communication styles, personal roles and responsibilities, and cultural values) be taken into consideration when designing a management program for the adolescent or adult patient with (C)APD. Failure to do so is likely to result in the development of a rehabilitative program that will not meet with optimal success.

Nature of (C)APD in Adolescents and Adults

Patient Characteristics

Adolescents and adults with (C)APD present with a variety of etiologic bases and behavioral symptoms. Professionals who provide rehabilitative or intervention services for older individuals with (C)APD are likely to encounter four distinct groups of patients in their clinical practices. These groups include: (1) individuals with central auditory deficits associated with confirmed compromise of the central auditory nervous system (CANS), such as in cases of head injuries, cerebrovascular accidents, and degenerative neurologic or neurodegenerative diseases (e.g., multiple sclerosis, Alzheimer's disease), (2) individuals who are experiencing degenerative processes within the CANS that are related to "normal" aging processes, (3) individuals who were initially identified with (C)APD at an earlier age and who were likely to have received one or more of the interventions discussed in the previous chapters, and (4) individuals who present for the first time as adults with a diagnosis of (C)APD, often in the absence of other significant findings (Baran, 2002; Musiek, Baran, & Pinheiro, 1994). Many of the individuals who fall into this latter group were likely to have experienced auditory difficulties in the past that went undiagnosed. In these cases, the individuals either identified and adopted strategies on their own that helped them compensate for their auditory problems, or they received individualized attention from teachers and/or parents who helped them deal effectively with their auditory difficulties in the absence of a specific diagnosis and any type of formalized intervention program (Baran, 2002).

The preceding comments focused on individuals with auditory problems that are related to some type of compromise of the CANS; however, there are other patients who will present with auditory difficulties that will not be directly related to involvement of the CANS. Generally these patients (like many of the patients with [C]APD) will present with significant hearing difficulties in the absence of a peripheral hearing loss. In many of these patients, the functional deficits may initially appear to be auditory in nature (i.e., related to CANS dysfunction), but when more comprehensive testing is undertaken it may be determined that the deficits are related to some other type of underlying etiology or cause (Jerger & Musiek, 2000). Common etiologic bases for the auditory deficits in these individuals include psychological or emotional difficulties, language differences (e.g., communication contexts where one of the conversational partners is an individual for whom English as a second language and the other is a native speaker of English), or significant changes in the acoustic environment (Baran, 1996; Baran & Musiek; 1994; Saunders & Haggard, 1989). In other patients, the deficits reported may be related to some type of subclinical compromise of the auditory system that is not detected by routine peripheral hearing assessment (Baran, 1996; Baran & Musiek, 1994). For many of these individuals (e.g., those with psychological or emotional problems), referral to another professional for intervention is critical as the types of services that will be required are clearly outside the scopes of practice for either audiologists or speech-language pathologists.

Although it is possible to categorize patients with (C)APD into one of the four groups identified above, it is not possible to associate "specific" and "unique" auditory deficits with each of these four groups. (C)APD represents a complex and heterogeneous group of deficits and there is considerable overlap in the deficits experienced by individuals who fall into these four categories of patients. Table 9–1 presents a list of some of the commonly reported symptoms noted by individuals being seen for central auditory processing diagnostic workups. As can

Table 9–1. Common Presenting Symptomatology Associated with Auditory Processing Disorders and Related Disorders in Adolescents and Adults

Inordinate difficulty hearing in noisy or reverberant environments
Lack of music appreciation
Difficulty following conversations on the telephone
Difficulty following multistep directions/instructions
Difficulty taking notes during lectures
Difficulty following long conversations
Difficulty learning a foreign language
Difficulty learning technical or discipline-specific vocabulary where the language is largely unfamiliar or novel
Difficulty in directing, sustaining, or dividing attention
Auditory memory deficits
Spelling difficulties
Reading difficulties
Organizational problems
Behavioral, psychological, and/or social problems
Academic or vocational difficulties

Source: From M. Gay Masters, N. A. Steckers, & J. Katz in *Central Auditory Processing Disorders* (p. 199) © 1998. Published by Allyn and Bacon, Boston, MA. Copyright © 1998 by Pearson Education. Reprinted by permission of the publisher.

readily be seen as one considers this table, this is a rather extensive list of deficits; however, it should be noted that many, if not most, of the patients seen for (C)APD evaluations will not experience all of these deficits. Therefore, it is important when developing a plan for a given patient that the professional take into consideration any functional deficits that were reported by the patient during intake procedures, and the specific auditory deficits that were identified during the diagnostic process, as well as any additional information that may have been uncovered during the diagnostic process (e.g., the existence of comorbid conditions).

Comorbid Conditions

Many patients with (C)APD will also present with one or more comorbid conditions that can impact the management program that is being developed to address the individual's auditory deficits. These comorbid conditions can include speech and language disorders, learning disabilities, attention deficit disorders with or without hyperactivity, frank neurologic involvement of the CANS, peripheral hearing loss, psychological disorders, and emotional disorders (Baran & Musiek, 1999; Chermak & Musiek, 1997). There has been much interest in establishing potential cause and effect relationships between each of these disorders and (C)APD; however, these causal relationships have been difficult to establish, and they remain elusive for the most part at this time (Baran, 2002). What is generally appreciated by the professional and research community is that these relationships are complex, interconnected, and most likely not unidirectional. Also, it is important to understand that it is possible that in some individuals the two conditions (or in some cases more than two conditions) simply coexist and are not directly linked to one underlying cause or etiology. Take, for example, the case of a person who has a peripheral hearing loss and then acquires a (C)APD as a result of a neurologic insult. In this patient the two conditions are clearly not related to the same etiology and therefore exist as separate conditions. Regardless of the precise nature of these relationships (i.e., causal, related, or simply coexisting), it will be critical for the professional to take all presenting conditions into consideration when developing a management or intervention program for the patient with (C)APD and other comorbid conditions, as these other conditions can (and often will) affect the individual's ability to benefit from the interventions that are specifically designed to address the auditory deficits.

The behavioral symptoms (Table 9–1) often noted in adolescents and adults with (C)APD are not unique to (C)APD, with many, if not most, of these behavioral symptoms being associated with more than one of the other disorders mentioned above. It is important, therefore, that a comprehensive, and preferably multidisciplinary, assessment of the individual's auditory, linguistic, cognitive, academic, and vocational functioning be

undertaken before a (C)APD management plan is developed, especially if deficits or problems are anticipated in any of these other areas.

Overview of Management Approaches

Management approaches used to remediate or alleviate the auditory deficits associated with (C)APD can be categorized into three major categories based upon their goals and objectives. These goals and objectives are as follows: (1) to improve signal quality, (2) to improve the individual's auditory perceptual skills, and (3) to enhance the individual's language and cognitive skills (ASHA, 1996). Chermak and Musiek (1997) have proposed an alternative classification system that divides the procedures into two main categories based upon the nature of the mechanisms that underlie the processing requirements involved. In this classification system, the approaches are classified as either bottom-up (i.e., stimulus-driven) or top-down (i.e., concept-driven) (Chermak & Musiek, 1997) and are represented in Figure 9–1. Bottom-up procedures involve approaches specifically used to facilitate the individual's ability to receive and process acoustic signals, whereas top-down approaches encompass procedures that are specifically designed to facilitate the *interpretation* of auditory information according to linguistic rules and conventions, other available sensory information, and knowledge and experience. Although there is not necessarily a one-to-one conversion from one categorization scheme to the other, for the most part approaches that are designed to improve the signal quality or to improve

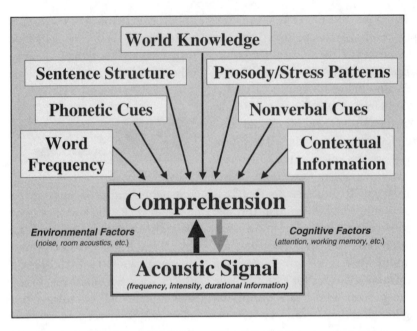

Figure 9–1. A schematic showing the relationship between bottom-up (i.e., stimulus-driven) and top-down (i.e., concept-driven) processes in the processing of verbal stimuli.

the individual's auditory perceptual skills would be classified as bottom-up or stimulus-driven procedures, whereas approaches that are used to enhance the individual's linguistic and cognitive skills would be classified as top-down or concept-driven procedures.

Many of the management options used with children can be used with adolescents and adults; however, as indicated earlier, adolescents and adults with (C)APD often present with unique challenges and special needs. Brain plasticity, which is optimal during childhood, is typically reduced in the older individual, with the amount of plasticity decreasing with increasing age (Musiek, Baran, & Schochat, 1999). Therefore, alterations or changes in the neural substrate of the CANS as a result of auditory training may be less likely to occur; they may require more time and training; and they may be

less extensive following auditory training than is typically seen in a younger person. However, even more mature brains do maintain some level of plasticity (Musiek et al., 1999). Therefore, auditory training techniques should not be summarily dismissed as an option for inclusion in a management plan for the adolescent or adult with (C)APD. Given the expectation of reduced brain plasticity for the older patient, it is likely that the management plan developed for an adult with (C)APD will focus less on formal and informal approaches specifically designed to improve the individual's auditory perceptual skills and more on the other management strategies which are designed to improve the signal quality and/or enhance the individual's compensatory cognitive and linguistic strategies and skills.

As the individual with a (C)APD matures from childhood through adolescence and then into his or her adult years, new academic, vocational, psychological, and emotional issues often surface and/or pre-existing issues become more consequential. Along with increasing age and maturity comes exposure to new and varied listening contexts (e.g., large college classrooms, technical or trade schools with noisy classrooms, civic or religious group meetings)—all of which can place increased demands on the individual's auditory processing skills. Previously successful individuals may now find that the same strategies that once served them well fail to provide the assistance they need to face the challenges they experience as adolescents and young adults in these new contexts. As a result, additional management options such as academic or vocational modifications, psychological counseling, career counseling, and transition planning must be considered when a management plan is being developed for the adolescent or adult with (C)APD. Some of these interventions may be provided most efficiently by the audiologist, whereas other services may be more appropriately provided by other professionals (e.g., speech-language pathologists, psychologists, special educators, vocational rehabilitation counselors, etc.). For these reasons, the value of a multidisciplinary approach to management of (C)APD cannot be underestimated.

Signal Enhancement Approaches

Signal enhancement procedures typically involve the use of specialized equipment, environmental modifications, and/or speaker training techniques that are specifically designed to improve the quality of the acoustic signal that reaches the auditory system of the individual with (C)APD. Commonly used approaches include the provision of either a personal FM (frequency-modulated) system or a classroom/group amplification system, the reduction of extraneous or competing environmental noise through the application of sound attenuating materials in the listening environment (e.g., classroom, workplace, etc.), the assignment or personal selection of preferential seating, the enhancement of the acoustic parameters of a spoken message through a variety of means, such as through the use of *clear speech* procedures (Picheny, Durlach, & Braida, 1985, 1986, 1989), and the use of specialized technology (e.g., telephone amplifiers). Although the use of a personal FM system would often be beneficial for the adolescent or adult student with (C)APD, this type of device is frequently rejected by older students, especially those in their teenage years, as these students are likely to be concerned about "appearances" and are often subjected to considerable peer pressure in this regard. In these instances, the professional will need to explore alternative methods of enhancing the quality of the acoustic signal (e.g., classroom amplification devices). Finally, it should be noted that all of the approaches listed above can be applied in a variety of contexts (e.g., home, school, or workplace, etc.) with appropriate modifications (Baran, 1998; Bellis, 2003; Chermak & Musiek, 1992; 1997; Masters, Stecker, & Katz, 1998; Musiek, 1999; Musiek et al., 1999; Musiek & Schochat, 1998; Ray, Sarff, & Glasford, 1984; Rosenberg, 2002; Stein, 1998). For additional discussion of personal FM systems, classroom modifications and group amplification systems, and other approaches to maximize the acoustics of the listening environment, the reader is referred to Chapters 3, 7, and 8.

Auditory Training

Auditory training approaches involve those intervention techniques that are specifically directed at improving the individual's auditory perceptual skills. As discussed earlier, these approaches tend to be more effective with younger patients than with older patients as neurophysiologic changes in the CANS are more likely to occur in younger patients due to the higher level of plasticity noted in these individuals. However, even more mature brains maintain some level of plasticity. Therefore, auditory training techniques should not be summarily dismissed as an option for inclusion in a management plan for the adolescent or adult with (C)APD. As would be the case for children, the selection of the specific type or types of auditory training should be made based upon the results of a comprehensive central auditory assessment through which the specific auditory deficit areas can be identified and then targeted for remediation. Musiek and his colleagues have identified a number of auditory processes that can be assessed using specific auditory tests and they have outlined specific management procedures that can be used to address each deficit area identified by these tests (Table 9–2) (Musiek, 1999; Musiek et al., 1999, Musiek & Schochat, 1998). Information on these procedures as well as a discussion of other issues and considera-

Table 9–2. Examples of Test-Related Auditory Processes and Suggested Auditory Training Procedures

Auditory Process	Tests That Assess Process	Habilitation Techniques
Auditory closure	Distorted speech tests (e.g., filtered speech, compressed speech, etc.)	Miller-Gildea vocabulary building
Auditory discrimination	Difference limens for intensity, frequency, duration	Discrimination training, auditory vigilance
Binaural interaction	Dichotic rhyme, localization, and lateralization tests	Signal detection in sound field with changing target positions
Binaural integration	Dichotic speech tests: divided attention	Intensity-altered dichotic listening, temporally altered dichotic listening, auditory vigilance tasks
Binaural separation	Dichotic speech tests: directed attention	Intensity-altered dichotic listening, temporally altered dichotic listening, auditory vigilance tasks
Temporal processing	Two element ordering, pattern perception tests, click fusion	Gap detection, sequencing tasks, prosody training

Source: Adapted with permission from Musiek, Baran, and Schochat (1999), p. 65.

tions in the selection of formal and informal auditory training procedures can be found in these resources, as well as in Bellis (2003), Musiek et al. (2002), and Chermak and Musiek (1997; 2002) and Chapter 4 of this Handbook.

Linguistic and Cognitive Interventions

As the individual with (C)APD matures into adolescence and then adulthood, the rehabilitative program designed for the individual is less likely to focus on specific skill acquisition (e.g., phonological awareness training, auditory discrimination training, etc.) and is more likely to focus on the development of metalinguistic and metacognitive skills and strategies (i.e., central resources training). Many well-conceived strategies have been developed and used with individuals with (C)APD. Specific information on these procedures can be found in a number of sources and will not be detailed here (Baran, 1998, 2002; Bellis, 2003; Chermak, 1998; Chermak & Musiek, 1992; 1997; Masters et al., 1998; Musiek, 1999; Musiek et al., 1999; Musiek & Schochat, 1998. The reader is also referred to Chapter 5 for in-depth discussion of metalinguistic and metacognitive approaches.

Although many of the strategies that have been described in these publications may appear to be obvious, and therefore should require little instructional effort or therapeutic intervention, this may not be the case (Baran, 2002). If the application of a given strategy was obvious to the individual with (C)APD, then it is likely that this individual would have adopted the use of the strategy without the need for any type of specific instruction. Moreover, even if an individual "self" identifies a strategy that works

well for a given situation or context, if that individual does not learn how to generalize the adopted strategy to new situations or contexts, the individual is likely to continue to experience communicative breakdowns or failures in new contexts. For these reasons, it is advisable that formalized, strategy instruction be considered as a potential component of the management plans that are being developed for adolescents or adults with (C)APD (Baran, 2002).

Although there have been a number of different approaches described for strategy instruction interventions, these procedures usually involve a number of common activities or steps. Most instructional approaches will include (1) some type of preassessment of strategy use and commitment to the use of newly acquired strategies, (2) the identification and description of the strategies, (3) the modeling of the strategies, (4) verbal rehearsal of the strategies, (5) controlled practice and feedback on the application of the strategies, and (6) generalization of the strategies to new contexts. The reader interested in additional information on the application of strategy instruction procedures is referred to the following resources (Baran, 1998, 2002; Bender, 2004; Deschler, Alley, Warner, & Schumaker, 1981; Deschler, Shumaker, Lenz, & Ellis, 1984; Hallahan, Lloyd, Kauffman, Weiss, & Martinez, 2005; Harris, Graham, & Pressley, 1991).

Ecological Perspectives

Auditory processing problems are complex and the manner in which they are manifested can vary with different contexts. Often persons with (C)APD will experience problems in one context, but they may fail to show evidence of their auditory difficulties in another context, as elaborated below. Even within a given context, it is not uncommon for an auditory deficit to be noted at times and not evident at other times. As mentioned earlier, older students and adults need to function in a number of different contexts with varying communicative demands. Children are typically viewed within two relatively distinct and separate contexts. During the day they are viewed as "learners" and function primarily within the context of school. Outside of school, they are viewed primarily as members of a family, even when they are engaged in school-related activities, such as completing homework assignments (Baran, 2002, Kleinman & Bashir, 1996). However, distinctively different behaviors and roles are expected of an adult. The lives of adolescents and adults are not so neatly compartmentalized, as they are expected to function in a number of different and often overlapping contexts (home, work, community and civic organizations, recreational settings) (Baran, 2002; Kleinman & Bashir, 1996).

At the same time, adults with (C)APD (as well as many adolescents, especially those who leave school prior to high school graduation) do not often enjoy the same level of support that is typically provided to a child with such a disability. For the postsecondary student or the adult, there may be no educational team, advocate, or parent to inform others of the difficulties that the individual is experiencing. For the adolescent who is moving into the upper grades (e.g., junior high and high school placements), new challenges are likely to arise—even for those students who may still be on an individualized education plan (IEP). The

student in the upper grades is expected to move from classroom to classroom to complete coursework with various teachers who have expertise in particular subject matters. With each different course comes a different teacher with his or her own unique teaching style and philosophy—some of which may be complementary to the individual's learning and communication style/needs, while others may prove to be at odds with the individual's learning style and needs. Not only will the teachers change throughout the course of the school day, but so will the environment within which the student must function. Differences in classroom acoustics, the location of the classrooms relative to noise sources both inside and outside the school building, and the size and composition of the various classes in which the student is enrolled will all function to provide the student with (C)APD with more or less favorable listening environments as he or she changes classes throughout the day.

These issues become even larger when the individual transitions from a secondary educational program to a postsecondary or technical school placement. In these latter contexts, classes are generally much larger, especially for freshmen enrolled in large postsecondary institutions as first year college students are typically enrolled in general education or "core" courses, which tend to be among the largest courses offered at an institution. As a result of the large number of students enrolled in these courses and the large classrooms that are needed to accommodate these large enrollments, classroom noise often becomes more of a problem and instructors often do not have the opportunity to get to know each student's individual learning style and needs (at least not in a timely manner). In addition, the instructors are less likely to be able to monitor students' faces for indications that they have understood or grasped the information being presented. Moreover, the postsecondary student is less likely to have an individual who can serve as an advocate on his or her behalf. Therefore, it is important that the older student with (C)APD assume responsibility for his or her own listening and academic success.

The postsecondary student needs not only to become an effective self-advocate, but also needs to become "strategic" to succeed. Strategies that worked well in elementary or high school may not provide the same assistance in the new and more advanced academic context. In order to succeed in a postsecondary program the older student must be able to assess each new listening situation, to identify the strategies that might help compensate for any processing difficulties that are anticipated in the novel listening environment, to select the strategy (or strategies) that appears to be the best alternative given the circumstances, and to find another, alternative strategy if the selected strategy fails to meet the individual's needs in the particular context. In other words, adolescents and adults with (C)APD need not only to know how to implement a strategy, but they also need to become *strategic*—knowing when or under which conditions to deploy a strategy (Baran, 1998; Chermak & Musiek, 1997). What worked in one environment or context may not prove to be useful in another environment or context—or possibly, even within the same environment or context if factors either intrinsic to the individual (e.g., increased fatigue) or extrinsic to the individual (e.g., increases in environmental noise levels) function to negate

the usefulness of a "proven" and commonly used strategy.

Although much of the previous discussion focused on the adolescent or the adult with (C)APD who is in a secondary or postsecondary educational placement, much of what was discussed would be important for the adolescent or adult with (C)APD regardless of whether the individual is a student, an employee, a community member, and so forth. Contexts or environments seldom remain constant. In fact, changes in the listening environment are more commonly the rule rather than the exception. It is important, therefore, that individuals with (C)APD learn to become *strategic,* as it is likely that the manifestations of their auditory deficits will change both within and across contexts (Baran, 2002).

Working with Multiculturally and Linguistically Diverse Clients and Families

It is likely that most professionals working with adolescents and adults with (C)APD will work with a culturally and linguistically diverse clientele, especially when one considers the changing demographics of the U.S. population. Recent demographic projections suggest that by 2050 the number of Americans racially classified as other than "White" will exceed the number of Americans who fall into the "White" classification (Day, 1996). These changing demographics underscore the need for professionals to be prepared to work with an increasing number of individuals who may not share the same racial/ethnic backgrounds or cultural values as the professional. To do so, the professional must gain an understanding and appreciation of the cultural differences that may mold an individual's (and his or her family's) needs and expectations and which may also influence or determine the individual's ability to access or benefit from professional services.

In some cultural groups, the parameters defining a communication disorder are influenced by the cultural values (Battle, 1997). Behaviors that are considered to be abnormal in one cultural group may well meet the norm for acceptable behavior in another cultural group. So what is perceived to be a disorder by members from the predominant cultural group(s) in the United States, may not be considered a disorder by other cultural groups. Also, in some cultural groups, seeking help for a communication disorder may not be considered as an option, even if the presence of the disorder is recognized. Different cultures assign different meanings to health, wellness, and disability (Battle, 1997). In some cultures, these definitions or meanings may impact access to rehabilitative or intervention services. For example, individuals from a Chinese culture are likely to believe that an individual with a disability or disorder is a curse that has been visited upon the family as a result of the sins or wrongdoings of one's ancestors. In other cultures, an individual with a disability is viewed as a gift from a higher being. In either case, it is unlikely that the individual or the family of the individual with a disorder will seek counseling and/or intervention services (Battle, 1997).

In Western cultures there is a commonly held assumption that individuals need to change to fit the system, but many cultural groups believe that the system can be altered to fit the individual (Battle, 1997). Also, there is an assumption among persons from Western cul-tures that individuals with disorders are helped by formal intervention services, whereas in many non-Western cultures there is a commonly held belief that the individual can be helped by the natural support of the family and the community. These differences in cultural values and beliefs will clearly influence an individual's willingness to seek out rehabilitative services (see Battle, 1997, 2002, for additional discussion of these topics).

An understanding of a cultural group's values and traditions can provide a framework for working with an individual from a cultural background that is different from that of the individual providing the services. It is essential, nonetheless, to consider each patient as an individual. Over time, individuals from a different cultural background may take on some of the values of the mainstream group as they are immersed in the Western culture. This process of internalizing some of the values of the new culture to which the individual is exposed is referred to as acculturation (Battle, 2002). As a result of this process, the individual's values may no longer overlap completely with those of the original culture and it will be important for the professional providing services to understand the individual's new (and often hybrid) values system.

In addition to cultural differences, there may be linguistic differences or communication style differences that may affect the rehabilitative process. Such linguistic differences are obvious when one is working with a non-English-speaking client and his or her family. However, some of these differences may not be as obvious when one is working with an individual for whom English is a second language. In many languages, there are differences in language use that may carry over into the second language, which if not recognized by the professional providing services may be misinterpreted as a language or auditory processing deficit. Take for example, the use of silence in conversions. For most Americans, silence in a conversation is interpreted as a hesitancy to speak or an inability to process or respond appropriately. However, in other cultural and linguistic groups, silence can indicate respect for elders (Japanese, Native American), agreement with the previous speaker's message or intent (Russian, Spanish, and French), or disagreement or inability to accept a speaker's attitude, opinions, or beliefs (Chinese) (Battle, 1997). There are many other examples of language use (both form and function) that can be culturally determined. The reader interested in a more in-depth discussion of these topics is referred to Battle (1997).

To summarize, it is essential that the provider who is offering services to individuals from different racial, cultural, or ethnic groups have an appreciation for and an understanding of the potential differences in behaviors, values, and/or beliefs that may be represented among the individuals with whom the professional is working. Such an understanding will assist the professional in designing a culturally appropriate intervention for each individual that then should meet with the greatest support and involvement from both the patient and his or her family.

Academic Modifications for Secondary and Postsecondary Students

Secondary and postsecondary programs often present new challenges for the individual with (C)APD. As the individual moves from the early grades through middle school, high school, and then on to college, class sizes often are larger, especially in postsecondary programs. Unfortunately, large classes pose unique challenges for the student with a (C)APD. As discussed above, faculty are not likely to get to know each student individually in large classes and there is likely to be more noise present in larger classrooms (e.g., college students often come late to class and some students will leave early, some students will shuffle papers, and others will converse with classmates, etc.). In addition, the postsecondary student is less likely to have an advocate or a case manager to help the student gain access to the support services and/or academic modification that are needed to ensure success.

At the postsecondary level, there is an increased reliance on independent learning and the student is expected to take responsibility for his or her own success or failure. Depending upon the nature of the services received as a student in previous school placements, the individual may enter a postsecondary educational placement ill-equipped to face these new challenges. Many students who have been on IEPs for several years have not had to function independently as there typically has been an individual or a team of professionals within the school assigned the responsibility of ensuring that the goals and the objectives of the individual's IEP are met. Although this type of service delivery may work well for younger students, it does little to prepare these students as they transition from secondary to postsecondary placements, that is, unless the IEP specifically addresses some of the new skills that the individual will need to acquire to be successful in college or in an alternative postsecondary placement (e.g., technical or vocational schools). As discussed below, if students are to be prepared to meet these new academic demands and expectations they should receive both self-advocacy training and counseling and guidance on how to transition effectively into the new educational program. Both of these services will be most beneficial if they are provided before the time that the student matriculates into the postsecondary placement.

Facing increasing numbers of students requiring individual academic planning and support (e.g., students with learning and/or cognitive disabilities) as well as a number of federal mandates (e.g., Section 504 of the Rehabilitation Act of 1973 and the Americans with Disabilities Act of 1990), universities and colleges have instituted academic support services for their students with disabilities (Baran, 2002). However, the range of services available across university campuses varies along a continuum from minimal support services to more comprehensive support programs. Even in the institutions with more extensive programs, the services available to students are not likely to be as extensive or as individualized as those that were afforded them as students in elementary or secondary educational programs (Baran, 2002).

Table 9–3 lists some of the more common academic modifications often recommended to assist adult learners with

Table 9–3. Examples of Academic Modifications for Students in Secondary and Postsecondary Academic Placements

Test administration in alternative environments (e.g., less noisy, fewer distractions)
Provision of note-taking services
Provision of tutoring services (may also include peer tutoring)
Reduced course loads
Waiver of a foreign language requirement or approval of a course substitution for a foreign language requirement (e.g., American Sign Language or a culture course)
Creative scheduling of classes to ensure that course requirements and task demands are equally distributed over the course of the academic program
Preferential seating (if seating is assigned)
Tape recordings of lectures and presentations
Video recordings of lectures and presentations
Assignment or selection of course section where instructor's teaching philosophy and style are consistent with student's needs
Provision of outlines, lecture notes, or reading assignments prior to class presentation so that student can review materials in advance
Other accommodations to address comorbid learning difficulties (e.g., untimed tests, alternative test formats)

Source: From M. Gay Masters, N. A. Steckers, & J. Katz in *Central Auditory Processing Disorders* (p. 207) © 1998. Published by Allyn and Bacon, Boston, MA. Copyright © 1998 by Pearson Education. Reprinted by permission of the publisher.

their learning challenges. Some of these recommendations are more appropriate for secondary students, whereas others are more realistic for postsecondary students. For example, it is common practice for faculty in postsecondary institutions to provide a syllabus at the beginning of each course, which outlines course objectives, topics to be covered in class, the sequencing and time of coverage of these topics, as well as specific readings and other assignments that are linked to each topic. Therefore, it is unlikely that a recommended modification/accommodation for the college student would include a request that faculty provide this information prior to each class. In secondary programs, however, it is less likely that students would be provided this type of information for the entire course—most of which are year-long courses. In these instances, a reasonable accommodation would be for the teacher to provide reading assignments prior to the day/time that a topic is to be covered in class. The student with (C)APD can then review this information prior to its coverage in the class, thus increasing the likelihood that the information will be processed, understood, and hopefully internalized when it is presented in class.

Preferential seating is a common accommodation that is often recommended for a student with (C)APD. In secondary programs where seating is often assigned, it may be reasonable to recommend to the teaching staff that a given individual be provided preferential seating (i.e., seating that provides the greatest auditory and visual access to the primary signal, typically the teacher) when seating assignments are made. Often such preferential seating involves providing a seat at the front of the classroom for the student with (C)APD; however, when classroom discussions are taking place, a more advantageous seating position is likely to be in the center of the classroom. In postsecondary settings, however, seating assignments rarely are made by the instructor. In these cases, although preferential seating would be beneficial, and therefore recommended, it would typically be the student's responsibility for ensuring that he or she has secured such seating. This may mean coming to class early so that the desired seating will still be available.

One of the major challenges for many postsecondary students is fulfilling a university's or college's foreign language requirement—a common requirement for graduation at many colleges and universities. Some universities will waive this requirement for the student with (C)APD with sufficient documentation of the disability; others will not waive the requirement, but rather will offer a course substitution (or substitutions) to satisfy this course requirement. The most common modification accepted at many colleges is the substitution of a course that will expose the student to the culture of a different country (Baran, 2002). Another modification of the foreign language requirement accepted by some universities is the substitution of a course in American Sign Language. This modification of the foreign language requirement is particularly attractive for many students with (C)APD as the reliance on auditory skills for acquisition of the language is significantly reduced when compared to the heavy auditory demands of learning a foreign language that is taught primarily through the auditory modality.

The preceding comments highlight the need to consider the unique circumstances that surround each student before recommending any of the accommodations listed in Table 9–3. What works for one student in one context will not necessarily work (or be appropriate) for another student in what may appear on the surface to be the same context.

Vocational Modifications

Although academic modifications recommended for individuals with (C)APD are more extensively discussed in the literature, equally important is the need for vocational modifications when young adults graduate from high school and enter the workforce. Unfortunately, this is an area where limited assistance is readily available for young adults with (C)APD who may be in need of (and eligible for) this type of support because there are few professionals who provide this type of intervention and support. Consultations with the employer can help the employer understand the deficits that the employee is experiencing as well as how these deficits or difficulties may interact with job demands. In addition, the work environment can be evaluated and recommendations for potential modifications that will improve the listening environment may be offered (e.g., the application of sound attenuating materials in the work area, the relocation of a work area away from a significant noise source, etc.). Such protections are afforded to employees with disabilities by federal mandates (e.g., the Americans with Disabilities Act of 1990) and should be more readily available to individuals with (C)APD and related disabilities. It is therefore essential that more professionals (i.e., audiologists) become involved in the provision of these types of intervention services. When equipped with professional advice and recommendations employers can implement workplace modifications that will help ensure that employees with disabilities can meet with job success and job satisfaction.

Career Counseling and Transition Planning

Career counseling and transition planning are often overlooked components of a management plan for the older student with (C)APD. Many adolescents and young adults with (C)APD have spent most of their time and energy throughout their educational programs learning how their auditory deficits affect their functioning as "learners." Often these individuals fail to develop an understanding of how these same auditory deficits may affect their performance in the workplace—where the listening demands and performance expectations may be very different from those that were encountered in the educational setting. This lack of understanding as to how their auditory deficits may potentially interact with new listening and performance demands may set the stage for frustration, possible job loss, and loss of self-esteem as these individuals enter the job market. Some of these undesirable outcomes may be avoided, or at least minimized, if students are provided guidance in this area before graduation through the use of appropriate counseling services. Students who can identify their strengths and weaknesses and who are prepared to explore a variety of career options will be more likely to choose a career where they can meet with reasonable success (Baran, 2002). In some cases, we have found that students may have chosen realistic career paths, but that parental or societal pressures are pushing these students toward careers for which they are ill equipped, uninterested, and unmotivated. Counseling may help these students learn how to become more self-assertive in dealing with these parental and societal pressures.

Even when a good "fit" exists between and among the individual's interests, strengths, and career, vocational, or educational choices, it is likely that the individual with (C)APD will encounter new and unanticipated challenges as he or she moves from one context to another (as discussed above). By working with a counselor, the individual may be able to begin to identify the potential difficulties that may be encountered in the new academic program or a job placement. Equipped with this knowledge, the individual can plan how he or she will react to these difficulties if they are encountered. Finally, an essential component of the management plan for individuals with (C)APD or related disorders is that of self-advocacy training. Although all of these interventions can be incorporated into the management program of a college student or the adult with (C)APD, they are likely to be most useful to the individual if they are provided, or at least introduced, during the junior/senior high school years.

not develop the skills and abilities needed to take on this advocacy role as the need arises and they may struggle in new and challenging situations rather than ask for assistance or accommodations. This is particularly true at the postsecondary level, where it is unlikely that the student will have an individual who advocates for the student. Without specific training in the development of self-advocacy skills, the postsecondary student may not be equipped to access the assistance and/or accommodations that will be needed in this new educational setting.

Although problems related to poor development of self-advocacy skills often surface in postsecondary environments, they also may be experienced in the workplace. Employees with (C)APD who are not able to advocate for their own needs may find themselves at risk for loss of employment or lack of advancement or promotion due to perceived employee ineffectiveness (Baran, 2002). These individuals also may find that they are not accepted by colleagues in the workplace, as they are perceived by coworkers as being disinterested, aloof, snobby, or antisocial as they may not readily participate in the conversations that often take place in the workplace because of their auditory deficits (Baran, 2002).

Self-Advocacy Training

Young students with disabilities in the educational mainstream typically have an IEP that specifies the various interventions and support services that will be received. They are also likely to have an advocate, case manager, or other professional who ensures that the child's educational needs are being met. As a consequence, many young students do

Management Considerations for Individuals with (C)APD and Peripheral Hearing Loss

There are many individuals who will experience both a peripheral hearing loss and a (C)APD. This particular comorbidity is more likely to affect adults as they age. In these individuals the (C)APD either coexists with, or is secondary to, the peripheral hearing loss. In either case, many of the interventions discussed in this chapter can be used to alleviate the auditory problems that these individuals may experience. However, this group of individuals can present unique challenges for the audiologist involved in the selection and fitting of hearing aids. Current preferred practice patterns in the field of audiology outline routine assessment procedures that should be used to evaluate the status of the auditory periphery prior to the fitting of amplification; however, at the present time the assessment of the integrity and function of the CANS in patients with peripheral loss who are being seen for fitting of amplification is currently not standard practice (ASHA, 1997; Musiek & Baran, 1996).

Today most patients with hearing loss are considered to be good candidates for amplification given the advances that have occurred in hearing aid technology over the past several years and binaural fittings have become the standard of care for patients with bilateral hearing losses as the benefits of binaural amplification have been well documented (Dillon, 2001). In spite of the documented benefits of binaural fittings for many patients with bilateral hearing losses, there is a subgroup of individuals with bilateral hearing losses for whom binaural amplification may be contraindicated. As clinicians and researchers learn more about the functioning of the CANS and the potential for less-than-optimal binaural processing of auditory information in some patients with CANS disorders, the customary practice of recommending binaural hearing aids for patients with bilateral hearing loss must be questioned.

Jerger and his colleagues (1993) found evidence of binaural interference using aided speech recognition measures and middle latency response (MLR) tests in four patients with symmetrical hearing losses. Aided speech recognition scores were obtained under three test conditions (aided right ear, aided left ear, and binaural fitting) for three of these subjects. In all three cases, sizable performance differences were noted between the scores obtained under the two monaural conditions in spite of the finding of symmetrical pure-tone hearing measures. More significant, however, was the observation that the binaural test condition resulted in reduced performance when the score obtained under this condition was compared to the aided speech recognition score of the better ear for each of the three subjects.

These same investigators also obtained MLRs for three of their four subjects under three conditions (monaural right, monaural left, and binaural presentation) and noted a similar pattern of results; that is, the waveforms derived under the binaural presentation condition for all three subjects were noticeably poorer than the waveforms derived from the better ear in each case (Jerger et al., 1993). For these subjects, the presentation of an auditory stimulus to the second or "poorer ear" somehow interfered with the processing of information presented to the "better ear." Although the exact mechanisms underlying this phenomenon have not been established, it is likely that some type of distortion is being introduced by the existing compromise of either the peripheral and/or the central system. Regardless of the exact mechanism(s) that may underlie this interference phenomenon, there remains an important implication of these findings, that is, that binaural processes within the auditory system must function appropriately if a patient is to make optimal use of binaural amplification.

Musiek and Baran (1996) outlined four other instances where binaural amplification may be contraindicated for patients with comorbid peripheral hearing loss and CANS dysfunction. They suggested that binaural amplification may be contraindicated under the following conditions: (1) if a symmetrical hearing loss is present, but the central auditory test performance of one ear is markedly poorer than that of the other ear; (2) if an asymmetrical hearing loss is present and the central auditory test performance of the *better ear* is significantly poorer than that of the poorer ear; (3) if a symmetrical hearing loss is present and abnormal middle and/or late potentials are noted over one hemisphere versus the other (i.e., a significant electrode effect); and (4) if a symmetrical hearing loss is present and an ear effect is noted on electrophysiologic testing (pp. 415–425). Case studies highlighting each of these four conditions or case profiles can be found in the reference cited above.

The cases presented by Jerger et al. (1993) and Musiek and Baran (1996) provide evidence of less-than-optimal binaural processing in at least a subgroup of patients with peripheral hearing loss. For an individual to take full advantage of binaural amplification, all of the binaural processes within the CANS must function at their optimum level. As the binaural processes of the CANS are not assessed by routine audiological testing, it is important that the audiologist consider the need to assess CANS function when working with patients with peripheral hearing loss, especially if a patient is considered to be at risk for (C)APD. (See Musiek and Baran, 1996, for discussion of alternative methods of incorporating such testing into the evaluation procedures used with patients who are being seen for hearing aid selection and fitting procedures.)

Professional Teaming

The effective management program for an adult or adolescent with (C)APD is likely to involve contributions from more than one professional. As noted above, it is frequently the case that the individual with (C)APD will also experience one or more comorbid conditions (e.g., speech and language disorders, attention deficit disorder with or without hyperactivity, psychological or emotional disorders, etc.). The coexistence of one or more of these disorders can significantly affect the effectiveness of any of the intervention programs or strategies that are specifically designed to address the individual's auditory processing deficits. It is therefore important that each of these areas be assessed by the professional with the appropriate training and credentials to conduct such evaluations, and that these professionals then collaborate on the development of an intervention plan for the individual.

Even in less typical cases where (C)APD appears to be the only deficit area, both the audiologist and the speech-language pathologist are likely to be involved in the development and delivery of a management plan or program. The audiologist will likely take responsibility for interventions designed to improve the quality of the signal (e.g., provision of a personal FM system, consultation with a school system to install a classroom amplification system) and to improve the listening environment (e.g., working with school personnel to improve classroom acoustics). In addition, the audiologist should be involved in the provision of auditory training activities, especially those training activities that can be provided most effectively with the use of sophisticated electronic instrumentation that permits the precise control of the stimulus parameters (e.g., the dichotic interaural intensity difference [DIID] procedure) (ASHA, 2005, Musiek et al., 2004). The speech-language pathologist's role in the management program is to work with the individual to enhance the individual's cognitive and linguistic resources (e.g., working with the individual to identify metacognitive and metalinguistic strategies that can improve his or her ability to follow conversations, communicate more effectively, etc.). In addition, speech-language pathologists are often involved in the delivery of auditory training programs, especially informal auditory training (e.g., auditory discrimination training) and computerized auditory-language training programs (see Chapter 6), as these are procedures that fall within their scope of practice and for which they are likely to receive reimbursement (ASHA, 2005; Chermak & Musiek, 2002).

When working with adolescents and many young adults with (C)APD, it is important to also include teachers, special educators, and guidance counselors in the "professional team." These professionals are in a position to help ensure that interventions designed by the audiologist, speech-pathologist, and/or other professional carry over to the school setting and that newly acquired skills and/or strategies generalize to other settings. In addition, these individuals can play important roles in career counseling, transition planning, and self-advocacy training.

Role of Paraprofessionals and Family Members

Paraprofessionals can play an important role in the provision of services to individuals with (C)APD. Aides in the classroom can assist students by ensuring that instructions, course content, and homework assignments are received and understood by the individual with (C)APD. They can provide additional explanation and clarification of concepts or topics that are not fully understood because the verbal message is not processed efficiently. They can also monitor the student's attention during class time, help the student refocus if lapses in attention occur, and provide other important support services in the classroom.

Speech-language pathology assistants can augment or reinforce the remedial services that are being provided by the school's speech-language pathologist or pathologists. In many schools, the speech-language pathologist's caseload is quite high, often limiting the amount and frequency of services that can be provided to the child with a disability. Speech-language pathology assistants can provide additional instruction and practice on the activities planned by the speech-language pathologist, which should lead to more timely attainment of therapy goals and objectives. These individuals can also play significant roles in implementing some of the strategy instruction techniques outlined above (e.g., they can be helpful in modeling behaviors for the student, listening to student's description of the strategies, etc.).

At the postsecondary level, tutors and note-takers can provide invaluable services to the college student with (C)APD. As noted above, postsecondary courses and programs often present new challenges for the student with (C)APD. Class sizes are often large, the acoustics of the classroom are frequently less than ideal, and new vocabulary items are likely to be introduced in advanced courses that may not be accurately perceived by the student with (C)APD. Each of these variables may hinder the reception and acquisition of course materials that are presented auditorily. Tutors and note-takers can help facilitate the acquisition of information and concepts that may be missed in the classroom due to the presence of (C)APD.

Finally, family members and friends can take on important roles in the rehabilitative program for adolescents and adults with (C)APD. They can, and will, play a significant role in the application of some recommended procedures (e.g., *clear speech*, which requires that the conversational partner with whom the person is communicating take responsibility for modifying his or her own speech according to the parameters specified in the approach). They also can take on the role of facilitator or monitor for many of the informal procedures that may be recommended for implementation at home, as many of these procedures will require a second person to provide feedback about the appropriateness of an individual's responses and/or to present the necessary auditory stimuli. (See Chapter 8 for elaboration of clear speech.)

Documenting Treatment Efficacy

It is important for professionals working with individuals with (C)APD to be able to document patient outcomes. As the health care industry works to control rising costs, it is demanding evidence of the effectiveness of treatment procedures. As noted by Musiek, Bellis, and Chermak (2005) "a solid base of evidence documents [should document] improved psychophysical performance, neurophysiologic representation of acoustic stimuli, and listening and related function in children and adults following targeted auditory training" (p. 2); Unfortunately, at this time, relatively few empirical studies have documented the efficacy of treatment approaches. This is largely because (C)APD is a relatively young area of clinical research, with the investigative energies in the field of (C)APD following a natural evolution. Following Bocca and his colleagues' findings (1954, 1955) that individuals with temporal lesions experience auditory deficits in spite of normal peripheral audiological findings, much of the clinical research that followed has involved the investigation of the nature of the auditory deficits in patients with confirmed lesions of the CANS as assessed by a number of auditory tasks/tests (Baran & Musiek, 1999). These investigations served to increase our understanding of normal and abnormal brain function and to link specific auditory processes with an area (or areas) of the brain. What then followed was research on the clinical application of these tests to the assessment of auditory processing abilities in children and the development of clinically feasible tests of central auditory function. More recently, research efforts have focused on the efficacy of (C)APD intervention programs. One of the first investigations in this area was a study conducted by Jirsa (1992), which was then followed by other studies that focused on the effects of intervention for (C)APD with children (e.g., Hayes, Warrier, Trent, Zecker, & Kraus, 2003; Schochat, Musiek, & Baran, 2005). However, additional studies are needed to produce the level of evidence (e.g., randomized controlled trials; meta-analyses of randomized controlled trials) that would be necessary to establish the efficacy of various CAPD interventions (Chermak, 2002).

Although no large scale studies have examined the efficacy of intervention approaches with adults, there have been some case studies that have shown changes in behavioral and electrophysiologic measures in adults with (C)APD following intervention (e.g., Musiek et al., 2004). In addition, there have been a number of studies with normal adults that have used various auditory evoked potential measures to see if neurophysiologic changes could be documented following training on novel auditory perceptual tasks (Kraus et al., 1995; Tremblay & Kraus, 2002; Tremblay, Kraus, Carrell, & McGee, 1997; Tremblay, Kraus, & McGee, 1998; Tremblay, Kraus, McGee, Ponton. & Otis, 2001). Each of these studies documented one or more electrophysiologic changes associated with the training, and as such, provide some evidence that behavioral interventions can result in physiologic changes in adults. Additional studies with adolescents and adults with (C)APD using similar methodologies (i.e., behavioral training approaches and electrophysiologic assessment measures) are likely to demonstrate similar findings—thus, supporting the efficacy of these approaches with adults despite the anticipated reduced plasticity of the mature brain.

Although much of the interest recently has been in using an objective measure (e.g., MLR, mismatched negativity, etc.) to document changes in neurophysiologic function associated with behavioral changes affected by auditory training, this is by no means the only approach to documenting treatment efficacy. Equally as important are ecological or functional measures that document changes in the individual's performance in a variety of contexts (e.g., school, home, work, and community). For these types of documentation, other measures would be needed. These could include various types of behavioral rating scales, communication effectiveness measures, and other performance measures that probe listening, communication, and academic achievement, and so forth.

Documenting Effectiveness for an Individual

Absent large scale investigations that document treatment efficacy for the various approaches that are being used in remediation and management of (C)APD with adolescents and adults, it is important for the professional to document on an individual basis the changes that are occurring, presumably as a result of intervention. Electrophysiologic measures as well as behavioral test measures can be used to document these changes; however, additional quantitative and qualitative measures should be included. Data collected should include measures that would document changes (or lack thereof) in a variety of contexts in which the individual would need to use the newly acquired processing skills and/or strategies. For adolescents in structured environments, these could include teacher questionnaires that probe for changes in auditory behaviors and academic performance. For the adult patient who is not in a structured environment, this could include a journal or a checklist where the individual indicates when a desired strategy or behavior was used. Additionally, the journal could include some type of evaluation or rating of the success of the strategy or behavior. The use of these latter techniques can also encourage self-monitoring and the use of executive processes, which can further enhance the treatment program (Chemak & Musiek, 1997). (See Chapter 2 for further discussion of evidence-based practice and treatment efficacy.)

Case Study

History

This case, which has been reported previously (Musiek, Baran, & Shinn, 2004), involves a 41-year-old female who sustained a traumatic head injury secondary to a horseback riding accident. The patient lost consciousness for a brief period of time at the time of the accident, but then recovered consciousness quickly and demonstrated few abnormal symptoms immediately following the accident. She was able to walk without major difficulty and showed no signs of amnesia, although she was slightly disoriented. She also experienced some disequilibrium and a tinnitus that was localized in her head following her accident. A neurologic exam conducted within a

few days of the incident, however, was essentially normal. Based upon these findings and the patient's initial post-trauma symptoms, it was the opinion of the attending physician that this patient had sustained a mild concussion.

A few days after the accident the patient began to experience some additional and/or worsening symptoms. She began to experience dizziness and her previously experienced disorientation became more of a problem. She also began sleeping excessively. In addition, she began experiencing difficulty understanding conversations and recalling information. The patient's physician indicated that these symptoms were not unusual following a concussion and he felt that these symptoms would resolve with time; however, there was little change in the patient's symptoms after a year had lapsed and other symptoms became apparent over this time frame. Listening became more of a challenge. The patient had difficulty maintaining attention, and she often needed "extended" time to process information. She also reported that the hearing in her left ear was poorer than in her right ear and that she experienced extreme difficulty with the comprehension of auditory directives, hearing in the presence of background noise or competing messages, and following the speech of speakers who spoke rapidly. Additional problems experienced by the patient included reading comprehension difficulties, memory, planning, and organizational problems (i.e., difficulties in executive function), and mathematical computation difficulties. At the time of her audiologic evaluation (13 months post-trauma), the patient noted that her tinnitus had resolved and that she had noted some "slight" improvements in her hearing abilities. Although somewhat improved, the patient's auditory problems continued to have a significant negative impact on her ability to function in normal everyday activities.

Audiological Evaluation

This patient was seen for an audiological evaluation at 13 months post-accident. Results of testing conducted at this time revealed normal peripheral auditory function; however, abnormal results were evident on four of five central auditory tests administered (i.e., dichotic digits, competing sentences, duration patterns, and compressed speech) (Figure 9–2). In addition, subtle electrophysiologic abnormalities were suggested by the MLR tests. These included smaller Na-Pa amplitudes for the right ear relative to the left ear, and poorer waveform morphology for right ear versus left ear recordings (Figure 9–3).

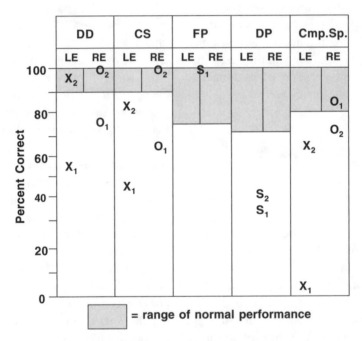

Figure 9–2. Central auditory test results for a 41-year-old female with a history of a mild head injury. Results are displayed for both pre- and postintervention assessments. Key: DD = dichotic digits, CS = competing sentences, FP = frequency patterns, DP = duration patterns, Cmp. Sp. = compressed speech, O_1, X_1, and S_1 = pretherapy test results for the right ear, left ear, and sound field, respectively; O_2, X_2, and S_2 = post-therapy test results for the right ear, left ear, and sound field, respectively. (Adapted from Musiek et al. [2004], with permission.)

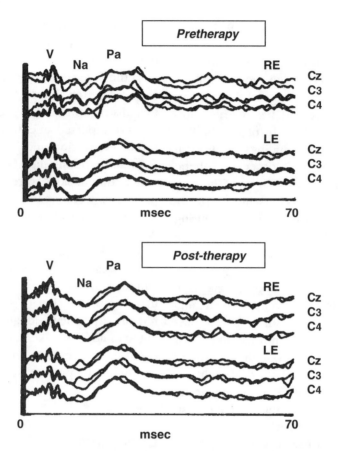

Figure 9-3. The middle latency responses (MLRs) from a 41-year-old female with a history of a mild head injury. Results are displayed for the right and left ears at three electrode sites (Cz, C3, C4) derived pre- and postintervention. (Adapted from Musiek et al. [2004], with permission.)

Rehabilitative Program

Because the patient lived some distance from our clinical facility, the decision was made to instruct her on a number of therapy approaches that she could work on daily with the assistance of her family. As the patient was highly motivated, we were confident that she would follow through on our recommendations. The specific therapy procedures recommended for her included clear speech, reauditorization strategies, a modified dichotic interaural intensity difference (DIID) procedure, a modified auditory memory enhancement procedure, temporal sequence training, auditory discrimination training, and the use of metacognitive strategies. The reader is referred to Musiek et al. (2004) for a detailed discussion of each of these procedures and how they were modified for this particular patient.

Postintervention Assessment

Postintervention testing was completed at approximately seven months following our initial assessment of this patient. A screening pure-tone test revealed normal test results. In light of this finding and the previous findings of normal peripheral function, other peripheral tests were not readministered. The four central auditory tests for which performance was found to be abnormal during the earlier testing session were readministered, as was the MLR procedure. As can be seen in Figures 9–2 and 9–3, comparisons of the pre- and postintervention results revealed improvements on a number of the test measures. Test scores improved to within normal limits for both ears on the dichotic digits test and to within normal limits for the right ear and close to normal performance for the left ear on the competing sentences test. Although test performance on the compressed speech test dropped slightly in the right ear, it improved significantly in the left ear. The MLR results showed better waveform morphology across all electrode sites for both ears and increased amplitudes for the Na-Pa wave across the three electrode sites when pre- and postintervention comparisons were made.

Postintervention Patient Status

The patient reported that she had noted a number of improvements in her auditory skills and cognitive functioning following her participation in the rehabilitative program. She reported that she could follow and participate in most conversations, although she did acknowledge

some continuing difficulty with people who speak rapidly. She also indicated that she could talk on the telephone with the receiver to her left ear and that she was better able to "tune out" auditory distractions and to attend to tasks. She also reported an enhanced ability to recall information and improved short-term and working memory. In addition, concentration skills were reportedly improved, as were organizational skills and speed of processing. She did, however, continue to experience some auditory and cognitive skills deficits. She reported that processing speed, although improved, had not improved to pre-accident levels, that comprehension of some messages remained problematic, and that attending to multiple speakers at the same time and following rapidly presented speech continued to present some difficulties for her.

Comments

This particular case was chosen for presentation because it highlights several important considerations and factors that are relevant to the management of the adult with (C)APD. These include the following: (1) that patient motivation is an important variable that will affect treatment outcomes, (2) that electrophysiologic measures can be useful in documenting neurophysiologic changes associated with improved behavioral measures, (3) that engagement of family members in the rehabilitative program can help facilitate the achievement of program goals and objectives, and (4) that auditory training can be used effectively with adults, even though the brain is known be less plastic as one ages.

Concluding Comments

(C)APD represents a complex and heterogeneous group of auditory deficits that can result from a variety of etiologic bases. For many individuals, the disorder will be a developmental disorder that persists from childhood into adulthood. For others, the disorder will be the result of some type of frank neurologic compromise of the CANS (i.e., an acquired disorder), whereas for others the disorder will be the result of normal aging processes. Although there are some clear differences in the etiologic bases of (C)APD, these differences do not seem to translate into distinct profiles of auditory deficits. It is important, therefore, that the specific auditory deficits that an individual is experiencing be identified before any management approaches are implemented so that the intervention program can target these specific deficits.

Ecological and context-specific perspectives provide a useful framework for understanding the nature and changing manifestations of (C)APD. These perspectives can be used to inform the development of a management plan. In addition, several other variables are important to consider as one prepares to work with a given individual. Variables, such as age, co-morbid conditions, communication styles, cultural values, and language differences, all can affect an individual's ability to access and benefit from an intervention program. Therefore, it is essential that each management program be individualized to meet the unique needs of each patient. In addition, it is important that each patient's intervention program be continually monitored and systematically evaluated to determine the need for program modification, which may be indicated if inadequate progress is being made or if the patient's needs change.

References

American with Disabilities Act of 1990. 49 U.S.C. §§12101 et seq.

American Speech-Language-Hearing Association. (1996). Central auditory processing: Current status of research and implications for practice. *American Journal of Audiology, 5*(2), 41–54.

American Speech-Language-Hearing Association. (1997). *Preferred practice patterns for the profession of audiology*. Rockville, MD: Author.

American Speech-Language-Hearing Association. (2005). (Central) auditory processing disorders. Available at http://www.asha.org/members/deskref-journals/deskref/default.

Baran, J. A. (1996). Audiologic evaluation and management of adults with auditory processing disorders. *Seminars in Hearing, 17*, 233–244.

Baran, J. A. (1998). Management of adolescents and adults with central auditory processing disorders. In G. A. Masters, N. A. Stecker, & J. Katz (Eds.), *Central auditory processing disorders: Mostly management* (pp. 195–214). Boston: Allyn & Bacon.

Baran, J. A. (2002). Managing auditory processing disorders in adolescents and adults. *Seminars in Hearing, 23*, 327–335.

Baran, J. A., & Musiek, F. E. (1994). Evaluation of the adult with hearing complaints and normal audiograms. *Audiology Today, 6*(5), 9–11.

Baran, J. A., & Musiek, F. E. (1999). Behavioral assessment of the central auditory nervous system. In F. E. Musiek & W. F. Rintelmann (Eds.), *Contemporary perspectives in hearing assessment* (pp. 375–413). Boston: Allyn & Bacon.

Baran, J. A., Shinn, J. B., & Musiek, F. E. (2006). New developments in the assessment and management of auditory processing disorders. *Audiological Medicine, 4,* 35–45.

Battle, D. E. (1997). Multicultural considerations in counseling communicatively disordered persons and their families. In T. A. Crowe (Ed.), *Applications of counseling in speech-language pathology and audiology* (pp. 118–141). Baltimore: Williams & Wilkins.

Battle, D. E. (2002). Communication disorders in a multicultural society. In D. E. Battle (Ed.), *Communication disorders in multicultural populations* (pp. 3–32). Boston: Butterworth-Heinemann.

Bellis, T. J. (2003). *Assessment and management of central auditory processing disorders in the educational setting: From science to practice* (2nd ed.). Clifton Park, NY: Thomson Learning, Inc.

Bender, W. A. (2004). *Learning disabilities: Characteristics, identification, and teaching strategies* (5th ed.). Boston: Allyn & Bacon.

Bocca, E., Calearo, C., & Cassinari, V. (1954). A new method for testing hearing in temporal lobe tumors. *Acta Otolaryngologica, 44,* 219-221.

Bocca, E., Calearo, C., Cassinari, V., & Migliavacca, F. (1955). Testing "cortical" hearing in temporal lobe tumors. *Acta Otolaryngologica, 45,* 289-304.

Chermak, G. D. (1998). Metacognitive approaches to managing central auditory processing disorders. In G. A. Masters, N. A. Stecker, & J. Katz (Eds.), *Central auditory processing disorders: Mostly management* (pp. 49-62). Boston: Allyn & Bacon.

Chermak, G. D. (2002). Deciphering auditory processing disorders in children. *Otolaryngology Clinics of North America, 35,* 733-749.

Chermak, G. D., & Musiek, F. E. (1992). Managing central auditory processing disorders in children and youth. *American Journal of Audiology, 1,* 62-65.

Chermak, G. D., & Musiek, F. E. (1997). *Central auditory processing disorders: New perspectives.* San Diego, CA: Singular Publishing Group.

Chermak, G. D., & Musiek, F. E. (2002). Auditory training: Principles and approaches for remediating and managing auditory processing disorders. *Seminars in Hearing, 23,* 297-308.

Day, J. C. (1996). *Population projections of the United States by age, sex, race, and Hispanic origin: 1995 to 2005* (U.S. Bureau of the Census, Current Population Reports, pp. 25-1130). Washington, DC: Government Printing Office.

Deschler, D. D., Alley, G. R., Warner, M. M., & Schumaker, J. B. (1981). Instructional practices for promoting skill acquisition and generalization in severely learning disabled adolescents. *Learning Disability Quarterly, 4,* 415-421.

Deschler, D. D., Schumaker, J. B., Lenz, B. K., & Ellis, E. S. (1984). Academic and cognitive interactions for LD adolescents. Part II. *Journal of Learning Disabilities, 17,* 170-187.

Dillon, H. (2001). *Hearing aids.* New York: Thieme Medical Publishers.

Hallahan, D. P., Lloyd, J. W., Kauffman, J. M., Weiss, M. P., & Martinez, E. A. (2005). *Learning disabilities: Foundations, characteristics, and effective teaching* (3rd ed.). Boston: Allyn & Bacon.

Harris, K. R., Graham, S., & Pressley, M. (1991). Cognitive-behavioral approaches in reading and written language: Developing self-regulated learners. In N. N. Singh & L. L. Beale (Eds.), *Learning disabilities: Nature, theory, and treatment* (pp. 415-541). New York: Springer-Verlag.

Hayes, E. A., Warrier, C. M., Trent, G., Zecker, S. G., & Kraus, N. (2003). Neural plasticity following auditory training in children with learning problems. *Clinical Neurophysiology, 114,* 673-684.

Jerger, J., & Musiek, F. E. (2000). Report of the consensus conference on the diagnosis of auditory processing disorders in school-aged children. *Journal of the American Academy of Audiology, 11,* 467-474.

Jerger, J., Silman, S., Lew, H. L., & Chmiel, R. (1993). Case studies in binaural interference: Converging evidence from behavioral and electrophysiologic measures. *Journal of the American Academy of Audiology, 4,* 122-131.

Jirsa, R. E. (1992). The clinical utility of the P3 AERP in children with auditory processing disorders. *Journal of Speech and Hearing Research, 35,* 903-912.

Kleinman, S. N., & Bashir, A. S. (1996). Adults with language-learning disabilities: New challenges and changing perspectives. *Seminars in Hearing, 17,* 201-216.

Kraus, N., McGee, T., Carrell, T., King, C., Tremblay, K., & Nichol, T. (1995). Central auditory system plasticity associated with speech discrimination training. *Journal of Cognitive Neuroscience, 7,* 25-32.

Masters, G. A., Stecker, N. A., & J. Katz (Eds.). (1998). *Central auditory processing disorders: Mostly management.* Boston: Allyn & Bacon.

Musiek, F. E. (1999). Habilitation and management of auditory processing disorders: Overview of selected procedures. *Journal of the American Academy of Audiology, 10,* 329-342.

Musiek, F. E., & Baran, J. A. (1996). Amplification and the central auditory nervous system. In M. Valente (Ed.), *Hearing aids: Standards, options, and limitations* (pp. 407-437). New York: Thieme Medical Publishers.

Musiek, F. E., Baran, J. A., & Pinheiro, M. L. (1994). *Neuroaudiology: Case studies.* San Diego, CA: Singular Publishing Group.

Musiek, F. E., Baran, J. A., & Schochat, E. (1999). Selected management approaches to central auditory processing disorders. *Scandinavian Audiology, 28*(Suppl. 51), 63-76.

Musiek, F. E., Baran, J. A., & Shinn, J. (2004). Assessment and remediation of an auditory processing disorder associated with head trauma. *Journal of the American Academy of Audiology, 15,* 117-132.

Musiek, F. E., Bellis, T. J., & Chermak, G. D. (2005). Nonmodularity of the CANS: Implications for (central) auditory processing disorder: A critique of Cacace and McFarland's "The importance of modality specificity in diagnosing central auditory processing disorder (CAPD)." *American Journal of Audiology, 14,* 128-138.

Musiek, F. E., & Berge, B. E. (1998). A neuroscience view of auditory training/stimulation and central auditory processing disorders. In G. A. Masters, N. A. Stecker, & J. Katz (Eds.), *Central auditory processing disorders: Mostly management* (pp. 15-32). Boston: Allyn & Bacon.

Musiek, F. E., & Schochat, E. (1998). Auditory training and central auditory processing disorders. *Seminars in Hearing, 19,* 357-365.

Musiek, F. E., Shinn, J., & Hare, C. (2002). Plasticity, auditory training and auditory processing disorders. *Seminars in Hearing, 23,* 263-276.

Picheny, M. A., Durlach, N. I., & Braida, L. D. (1985). Speaking clearly for the hard of hearing I. Intelligibility differences between clear and conversational speech. *Journal of Speech and Hearing Research, 28,* 96-103.

Picheny, M. A., Durlach, N. I., & Braida, L. D. (1986). Speaking clearly for the hard of hearing II. Acoustic characteristics of clear and conversational speech. *Journal of Speech and Hearing Research, 29,* 434-436.

Picheny, M. A., Durlach, N. I., & Braida, L. D. (1989). Speaking clearly for the hard of hearing III. Attempt to determine the contribution of speaking rate to differences in intelligibility between clear and conversational speech. *Journal of Speech and Hearing Research, 32,* 600-603.

Ray, H., Sarff, L. S., & Glassford, J. E. (1984, Summer/Fall). Sound field amplification: An innovative educational intervention for mainstreamed learning disabled students. *The Directive Teacher,* pp. 18-20.

Rosenberg, G. G. (2002). Classroom acoustics and personal FM technology in management of auditory processing disorder. *Seminars in Hearing, 23,* 309-318.

Saunders, G. H., & Haggard, M. P. (1989). The clinical assessment of obscure auditory dysfunction. *Ear and Hearing, 10,* 200-208.

Schochat, E., Musiek, F. E., & Baran, J. A. (2005, April). *Effects of auditory training on the MLR of children with APD.* Paper presented at the annual meeting of the American Academy of Audiology, Washington, DC.

Section 504 of the Rehabilitation Act of 1973, as amended, 29 U.S.C. §794.

Stein, R. (1998). Application of FM technology to management of central auditory processing disorders. In G. A. Masters, N. A. Stecker, & J. Katz (Eds.), *Central auditory processing disorders: Mostly management* (pp. 89–92). Boston: Allyn & Bacon.

Tremblay, K. L., & Kraus, N. (2002). Auditory training induces asymmetrical changes in cortical neural activity. *Journal of Speech, Language, and Hearing Research, 45,* 564–572.

Tremblay, K., Kraus, N., Carrell, T. D., & McGee, T. (1997). Central auditory system plasticity: Generalization to novel stimuli following listening training. *Journal of the Acoustical Society of America, 102,* 3762–3773.

Tremblay, K., Kraus, N., & McGee, T. (1998). The time course of auditory perceptual learning: Neurophysiological changes during speech-sound training. *NeuroReport, 9,* 3357–3560.

Tremblay, K., Kraus, N., McGee, T., Ponton, C., & Otis, B. (2001). Central auditory plasticity: Changes in the N1-P2 complex after speech-sound training. *Ear and Hearing, 22,* 79–90.

SECTION III

Multidisciplinary Perspectives Across the Spectrum of Related Disorders

CHAPTER 10

DIFFERENTIAL INTERVENTION FOR (C)APD, ADHD, AND LEARNING DISABILITY

JEANANE M. FERRE

The purpose of diagnosis is to determine the presence or absence of and describe the nature of a disorder. Once properly diagnosed, appropriate intervention can commence that is designed to treat directly the disorder and to manage the impact of the disorder on the client's day-to-day life. Resources to minimize the problem can be allocated effectively, but only after the nature of the problem has been diagnosed clearly.

Many disorders present behavioral characteristics similar to (central) auditory processing disorder (C)APD and can cause the listener to perform poorly on behavioral central auditory function tests. In addition, (C)APD may lead to or coexist with other disorders (ASHA, 2005). These include neurocognitive disorders (e.g., attention deficit hyperactivity disorder—ADHD, executive function

disorder), cognitive impairment (e.g., mental retardation), communication disorders (e.g., autistic spectrum disorder, Asperger's syndrome, language processing disorders), social-emotional disturbance (e.g., behavior disorders), learning disability, and other sensory processing impairments (e.g., sensory integration disorder) (ASHA, 2005; Bellis, 2006). Misdiagnosis of these disorders as (C)APD, or conversely, misdiagnosis of (C)APD as one of these disorders can lead to ineffective use of treatment resources, and thereby compromise intervention. To avoid misdiagnosis and subsequent ineffective intervention, *differential diagnosis* of (C)APD must be undertaken.

Differential diagnosis refers to the differentiation among two or more disorders that have similar symptoms and/or manifestations (ASHA, 2005; Bellis, 2006).

As Myklebust (1954) eloquently observed, "The practical importance of making a correct diagnosis is that children having different types of problems vary significantly in their needs and unless a differential diagnosis is made, their potentialities are lost" (p. 8).

The differential evaluation or diagnosis of (C)APD from other similar disorders requires input from a variety of disciplines, including, but not limited to, audiology, speech-language pathology, psychology/neuropsychology, occupational therapy (OT), physical therapy (PT), education, and other related professions. The audiologist administers well-controlled tests designed to demonstrate the presence and describe the nature of specific auditory deficits while other professionals contribute information regarding the extent to which there exist difficulties in other sensory processing skills or in higher-order cognitive, language, or learning skills that may confound auditory test results or which may be exacerbated by (C)APD. By examining intra- and intertest patterns within the (C)APD test battery and relating these findings to the functional, observed day-to-day difficulties experienced by the listener, the audiologist is able to identify the presence and nature of the (C)APD, describe the impact the disorder is likely to have on the listener's life, and determine the relative contribution of nonauditory factors to the listener's functioning (Bellis, 2006). This multidisciplinary approach to differential diagnosis leads logically to implementation of timely, deficit-specific intervention that mitigates lost potential, maximizes successful treatment outcomes, minimizes residual functional deficits, and utilizes resources efficiently (ASHA, 2005).

Because (C)APD can have varied manifestations, intervention should, like diagnosis, be multidisciplinary in nature. The audiologist works as part of a team of professionals to develop specific, meaningful, and realistic treatment and management strategies designed to improve auditory and related skills, as well as to minimize the day-to-day impact of the disorder on the listener's academic success, communication abilities, and well-being. The audiologist applies neuroscientific principles to assist in developing deficit-specific treatment and management goals, to gauge the success of those strategies, and to extend intervention principles to the variety of environments in which the client operates in order to maximize benefit. Detailed discussions of differential diagnosis of (C)APD can be found in Chapters 13 through 15 of Volume I of this Handbook.

This chapter describes the *differential intervention* of (C)APD and related disorders. Case studies are used to illustrate multidisciplinary collaboration, selection and development of deficit-specific intervention goals, and effectiveness and efficacy of the intervention plan.

Steps in Developing Customized Intervention Programs

Intervention for (C)APD involves the comprehensive, therapeutic treatment and management program designed to reduce or resolve specific impairments and to minimize the adverse impact of the disorder on the listener's life skills. In treatment, deficit-specific procedures designed to improve deficient skills are implemented. In management, efforts are directed toward minimizing the impact of the disorder on the listener's everyday life. The development of customized intervention programs for students with (C)APD involves four steps: (1) identification of the specific auditory deficit(s), (2) determination of functional impairments as they relate to the (C)APD, (3) selection of deficit-appropriate treatment and management strategies, and (4) evaluation of treatment effectiveness and management success (Bellis, 2002).

Identifying the Nature of the Auditory Disorder

The evaluation of (C)APD is accomplished through the administration of a battery of well-controlled, efficient tests designed to identify impairments in (central) auditory processing skills. These skills include: sound localization and lateralization; temporal processing, including temporal discrimination, ordering, integration, and masking; auditory performance in the presence of competing signals (including dichotic listening); auditory performance with degraded acoustic signals (including auditory closure); auditory discrimination; and auditory pattern recognition (ASHA, 1996, 2005; Bellis, 2003; Chermak & Musiek, 1997). By including tests designed to assess these skills, the audiologist not only determines the presence or absence of (C)APD, but also describes the auditory skill areas that are deficient.

Functional Impairments Related to (C)APD

Disorder refers to a disruption of, or interference with, normal functions or established systems (*Mosby Medical Dictionary*, 2002). Disability refers to a physical or mental impairment that substantially limits one or more of the major life activities of an individual (Americans with Disabilities Act, 1990). The term "child with a disability" means (1) a child with mental retardation, hearing impairments (including deafness), speech or language impairments, visual impairments (including blindness), serious emotional disturbance, orthopedic impairments, autism, traumatic brain injury, other health impairments, or specific learning disabilities; or (2) one who is experiencing developmental delays in physical development, cognitive development, communication development, social or emotional development, or adaptive development; and (3) one who needs special education and related services (Individuals with Disabilities in Education Act, 1997). The Americans with Disabilities Act (ADA) mandates safeguards afforded to and reasonable accommodations that must be provided for all citizens with disabilities; IDEA outlines these protections and services for children with respect to their educational experience. Because neither document specifies a federal category for (C)APD, in order to establish the presence of a disability, it is essential that the *impact* of (C)APD on the listener's life be described fully. It is not sufficient to identify only the presence of (C)APD. Diagnostic test results must be related to educational impact and everyday behaviors to qualify a child for services and for meaningful intervention to take place.

To this end, the Bellis-Ferre model (1999) describes five (C)APD profiles that identify the nature of the disorder based on key central auditory test findings and measures of cognition, communication, and/or learning, and associated behavioral manifestations. These manifestations include behavioral characteristics that also may be associated with other disorders. By identifying the nonauditory factors that may affect listening, as well as the auditory factors that may affect other life skills, the multidisciplinary team is able to diagnose differentially (C)APD from other related disorders in order to develop individualized intervention programs. The model describes three primary central auditory deficit profiles characterized by presumed underlying site of dysfunction. Two secondary profiles yield unique patterns of results on central auditory tests; however, they may be described more appropriately as manifestations of supramodal or cognitive-linguistic disorders. For a comprehensive discussion of these deficit profiles, the reader is referred to Bellis (2003, 2006) and Bellis and Ferre (1999). For the purposes of this discussion, they are described briefly here.

Processing Deficit Profiles

Auditory decoding profile is characterized primarily by a deficit in auditory closure representing dysfunction in the primary (usually left) auditory cortex. Auditory deficits are seen in the ability to discriminate fine acoustic differences in speech. On central auditory tests, this profile is characterized by poor performance on degraded speech tests and measures of temporal discrimination (e.g., temporal gap detection). Binaural and/or right ear deficits may be observed on dichotic listening tests. Listeners with Auditory decoding deficit exhibit behavioral listening difficulties similar to those observed among listeners with peripheral hearing loss, including auditory fatigue, and difficulty hearing in noisy or excessively reverberant backgrounds, when visual and/or contextual cues are limited, and when unfamiliar with vocabulary. Auditory decoding deficit can create secondary difficulties in communication skills (e.g., vocabulary, syntax, semantics, and second language acquisition) and academic skills (e.g., reading decoding, spelling, note-taking, and/or direction following) (Bellis & Ferre, 1999).

Integration profile is likely due to inefficient interhemispheric communication, characterized by deficiency in the ability to perform quickly and efficiently tasks that require intersensory and/or multisensory communication. On central auditory tests, integration deficit is characterized by deficits on dichotic listening tests, particularly for the left ear, combined with poor performance on temporal patterning tasks only when asked to label (i.e., verbally describe) the pattern. Behavioral difficulties include poor synthesis skills, complaints of "too much" information, and difficulty intuiting task demands, starting complex tasks, transitioning from task to task, and completing tasks in a timely fashion. Difficulty in sound-symbol association, visual-motor or auditory-visual integration, important for success in reading, spelling, and writing; may be present (Bellis & Ferre, 1999).

Prosodic profile is characterized by deficiency in using prosodic features of a target, a predominantly right hemisphere function. Diagnostically, the listener displays difficulty in auditory pattern recognition, regardless of response mode (verbal or mimicked), an important skill for perceiving running speech, as well as excessive left ear suppression on dichotic listening tasks. Difficulty recognizing and using other sensory patterns (e.g., visual, tactile) may be observed as well as difficulties with pragmatic language (e.g., reading facial expressions, body language, and gestures; and recognizing or using sarcasm or heteronyms), social language (e.g., perceiving message intent), affect and intonation, rhythm perception, nonspeech discrimination, and music perception (Bellis, 2006; Bellis & Ferre, 1999).

Associative profile is a secondary profile, characterized by significant auditory-language processing difficulties, believed to be related to dysfunction in the auditory association cortex (Wernicke's area). On central auditory tests, the listener with associative deficit typically presents with bilateral or right-ear deficits on dichotic listening tasks. Ability to attach linguistic labels to tonal patterns may be poor, whereas performance on degraded speech and temporal discrimination tasks is normal. Behavioral characteristics include impaired receptive language and language processing skills, inability to comprehend the content or meaning of a message, poor listening comprehension, and difficulties in working memory skills (Bellis, 2003, 2006; Bellis & Ferre, 1999; Ferre, 2006).

Output-organization profile is a secondary profile characterized by difficulty organizing a response to auditory information. Diagnostically, poor scores are observed on central auditory tests requiring the reporting of multiple or precisely sequenced targets, with normal performance seen on single target tasks. Behaviorally, the listener may exhibit difficulty hearing in noise, be disorganized, impulsive, or a poor planner, or experience difficulties in expressive speech and language skills, including word retrieval. Although no specific neurophysiologic region of dysfunction is implicated by test findings, the cohort of central auditory test results and behavioral manifestations implicate the frontal and prefrontal cor-

tices and efferent (i.e., motor) pathways as possible sites of dysfunction (Bellis, 2006; Bellis & Ferre, 1996; Ferre, 1997).

These profiles can occur singly or in combination, although one profile typically predominates. In this regard, it is important to note that if the listener exhibits deficits in all auditory processes assessed or test results suggest the presence of more than two of the five functional deficit profiles, consideration should be given to the likelihood of a more global, higher-order disorder rather than (C)APD as the primary condition creating the day-to-day listening, language, and learning difficulties.

Relationship of (C)APD to Other Disorders

As indicated previously, there is overlap among characteristics of (C)APD and the symptoms of other disorders. This is especially evident in the case of ADHD. The *Diagnostic and Statistical Manual IV* (DSM-IV) lists criteria for ADHD to include difficulty attending and sustaining attention, poor listening, inability to follow through on instructions and assignments, distractibility, forgetfulness, disorganization, hyperactivity, and impulsivity (APA, 2000). These symptoms also are associated with four of the five (C)APD profiles outlined above, including auditory decoding, integration, associative, and output-organization profiles. Similarly, executive functions are a complex set of behaviors reflecting metacognitive and control/organizational processes and include attention, working memory, strategy development, monitoring of strategies, and refinement of goals and strategies to meet needs (Hunter, 2005; Luria, 1973; Richard & Fahey, 2005). Deficits in these skills are among the behavioral characteristics of the output-organization and associative profiles. Also reflecting overlapping symptomatology, the diagnostic criteria for behavior disorders, such as oppositional defiant disorder, include symptoms of active defiance, noncompliance, and frequent arguing with adults (APA, 2000), characteristics that also may be observed among listeners who are unable to perceive message meaning or intent, such as those with prosodic or associative deficit profiles. Finally, Asperger's syndrome is characterized by impairments in social interaction including lack of social or emotional reciprocity (e.g., affect) and impaired use of multiple nonverbal cues, such as facial expressions and gestures (APA, 2000), characteristics that are shared by the prosodic deficit profile. The central auditory processing evaluation contributes to the clarification of the nature of the disorder underlying these shared symptoms leading to effective differential intervention of comorbid or coexisting conditions.

In addition to exhibiting shared symptomatology with other disorders, presence of poor (central) auditory processing may be among the criteria for diagnosing another disorder or disabling condition. Impairments of auditory processing are included in the checklist of symptoms associated with sensory integration disorder (Ayers, 1994). For many students, presence of poor speech sound discrimination, associated with the decoding profile, poor working memory skills, observed with the associative profile, or poor sound-symbol association and synthesis skills, noted for the integration profile are contributing factors when determining presence of speech-language impairment or specific learning disability (IDEA, 1997). Finally, difficulty recognizing and using prosodic cues are among

the characteristics of nonverbal learning disability (NVLD) (Palombo, 2001; Tanguay, 2001; Thompson, 1997). Inclusion of treatment and management of the (central) auditory processing component in the individual's overall intervention plan may minimize or resolve the associated disorder or disability.

Selecting Appropriate Intervention Strategies

Once differential diagnosis has been accomplished, appropriate intervention strategies can be selected. Treatment should be designed to reduce or resolve the auditory deficiency and compensatory strategies should be selected to minimize the impact of the disorder on the listener's daily functioning. Following a brief overview of treatment and management approaches for (C)APD, intervention programming customized for individuals presenting with (C)APD in conjunction with other sensory processing, neurocognitive, or language disorders is outlined. The reader is referred to Chapters 4, 5, and 7 for in-depth coverage of components of intervention for (C)APD.

Treatment Options

As noted previously, the inclusion of treatment in the intervention plan is designed to remediate deficient skills and teach compensatory strategies. When choosing a specific therapy, the clinician should consider the extent to which the therapy protocol is (a) based on sound neuroscientific principles (i.e., should it work?), (b) supported by treatment outcome data (i.e., does it work?), and (c) appropriate for the type of deficit and functional needs of the listener (i.e., does it fit?) (Ferre, 2006). Any treatment program chosen must adhere to currently accepted neuropsychological, neurophysiological, and/or neuroscience principles. Therapy programs that cannot be shown to be founded on these basic principles should not be considered in the intervention plan for the listener with (C)APD.

For any program under consideration, the clinician should attempt to locate reports of successful outcomes based on treatment efficacy data, treatment effectiveness data, and/or anecdotal evidence. Treatment efficacy refers to evidence of documented change for a specified population accrued under controlled conditions and provides the clinician with the highest quality evidence that the treatment program is likely to meet the listener's needs (Shapiro & Balthazar, 2004). Treatment effectiveness refers to evidence of positive outcomes for a specified population obtained in everyday conditions and is useful when efficacy data are not available (Shapiro & Balthazar, 2004). So-called anecdotal evidence, although having face validity, is not a reliable index of treatment effectiveness or efficacy. Programs supported only by anecdotal reports should not be among the treatment options under consideration for the listener with (C)APD. (See Chapter 2 for discussion of evidence-based practice and treatment efficacy.)

Because of the complexity of the central nervous system and the interactive and dynamic nature of the skills it subserves, it can be safely said that there is no "silver bullet" for treating (C)APD. A program that may be effective for one listener may be ineffective for another based on the specific auditory skills affected and the impact of the disorder on the listener's life. Before implement-

ing any treatment program, the audiologist should verify the specific needs of the listener with (C)APD in the classroom, workplace, and at home. In addition, the specific type of processing deficit should be identified clearly, as not all treatment programs may be beneficial for all types of (C)APD.

Regardless of type of deficit and functional sequelae, treatment goals for (C)APD should include both bottom-up therapy, designed to reduce the deficit, and top-down therapies designed to minimize the residual effects of the disorder (ASHA, 2005; Chermak & Musiek, 1997). The inclusion of bottom-up auditory training is based on neural plasticity/brain organization theory, referring to the brain's ability to reorganize itself in response to internal and/or external changes. An increasing body of work exists documenting the potential of bottom-up training to change auditory behavior (Kraus et al., 1995; Musiek, 2004; Tremblay & Kraus, 2002; Tremblay, Kraus, Carrell, & McGee, 1997; Tremblay, Kraus, McGee, Picton, & Otis, 2001). Bottom-up therapy for auditory and related skills may include, but is not limited to, auditory training, including binaural processing training, temporal patterning training, interhemispheric transfer training, speech recognition in noise training, and even speech-reading training (Bellis, 2003; Chermak & Musiek, 1997, 2002; Ferre, 1997, 2002a; Flowers, 1983; Kelly, 1995; Masters, 1998; Musiek, 2005; Sloan, 1995).

Although intensive bottom-up training exploits plasticity, top-down therapy is considered extensive treatment designed to complement bottom-up training efforts, maximize generalization of skills across settings, and minimize functional deficits. By strengthening higher order metalinguistic, metacognitive, and metamemory skills, day-to-day listening, language, and learning problems can be minimized (ASHA, 2005). Top-down therapies include auditory closure training, prosody training, metamemory skills training, metalinguistic skills training, and metacognitive strategies training (Bellis, 2003; Chermak, 1998).

Management Strategies

The goal of the management plan for the listener with (C)APD is to maximize the individual's ability to communicate effectively across a variety of settings (ASHA, 2005). To accomplish this goal, management strategies may include modifications to the environment, adjustments to auditory or academic demands at home, work, or school, or use of support services and/or technology. Environmental modifications include, but are not limited to, noise abatement in school, the workplace, or the home, preferential seating, physical and architectural changes to the listening environment, increased availability of visual cues, and instruction to talkers to speak more clearly (i.e., *clear speech*) in order to improve signal access. Adjustments to listening and learning demands may include preteaching and previewing new material, extended time or reduced workload, course substitutions or waivers, adjusted schedules, multisensory educational or work environment, repetition and rephrasing, and test-taking modifications. Finally, some listeners will require support for information access that takes the form of direct signal enhancement via assistive listening technology or supported learning via computer assistance, or the use of concrete manipulatives, organizers, tape recorder, note-taking service, or scribe.

Relationships Among Intervention Strategies for (C)APD and Other Disorders

Because (C)APD shares symptomatology with other disorders, it should not be surprising that intervention for (C)APD may be, in some cases, similar to the treatment and management strategies recommended for other disorders. Bottom-up therapy to improve speech recognition in noise, indicated for listeners with auditory decoding and, often, output-organization profiles (Ferre, 1997), also may be a useful addition to the behavioral treatment plan for the listener with ADHD. Temporal patterning training and its top-down extension, prosody training, are appropriate treatment options for listeners with the prosodic profile. Language therapy to improve use of prosodic elements (e.g., rhythm, stress, and intonation) is among the treatment recommendations for clients with Nonverbal Learning Disability (NVLD) (Tanguay, 2001; Thompson, 1997), as well as for students with phonologic processing disorders (Tyler, 1997). Interhemispheric transfer training, which often includes whole-body exercises, is an appropriate intervention not only for the listener with (C)APD-integration profile but also for students with sensory integration disorder (Ayers, 1994) and NVLD (Thompson, 1997). Finally, treatment options for listeners with ADHD, executive function disorder, NVLD, language processing disorders, and language-based learning disabilities include some of the same kinds of top-down therapies appropriate for (C)APD, including metamemory skills training, metalinguistic skills training, and metacognitive strategies training (Duesenberg, 2006; Gerber, 1993; Ingersoll & Goldstein, 1993; Johnson, 1983; Phillips-Keeley,

2003; Richard, 2001; Richard & Fahey, 2005; Thompson, 1997).

In the classroom, home, or workplace, listeners with auditory decoding deficit profile require modifications and compensations that improve the quality of and access to the *acoustic* signal and enhance access to nonauditory cues. For listeners with associative deficit profile, management strategies that transform the signal to improve *linguistic* comprehension are needed. Strategies that adjust the quantity and structure of the signal are indicated for the listener with the integration deficit profile, whereas listeners with the prosodic deficit profile require improvement to *both* the structure and the meaning of the signal. Finally, students presenting the output-organization deficit profile need enhanced signal salience and assistance in organization of a *response* to the signal (Ferre, 2002b). These same management strategies are among the environmental modifications and supports that are recommended for clients with ADHD (Duesenberg, 2006; Ingersoll & Goldstein, 1993), executive function disorder (Phillips-Keeley, 2003; Richard & Fahey, 2005), NVLD (Thompson, 1997), learning disability (e.g., dyslexia) (Horn & Horn, 2005), and language processing disorders (Richard, 2001). The degree of overlap among symptoms and intervention options for (C)APD and other disorders that can impair language, listening, and learning necessitates both the differential diagnosis and differential intervention of these disorders.

Gauging Success

Selection of appropriate treatment and management goals is incomplete without the inclusion of measurable outcomes to determine whether intervention goals and objectives have been achieved (ASHA, 2005). The multidisciplinary team has a variety of methods available to gauge the success of the intervention plan. To document treatment efficacy and/or effectiveness, one must establish that real change has occurred as a result of the treatment and not of some uncontrolled factor or, in the case of a child, maturation (Goldstein, 1990). For treatments designed to improve specific auditory skills, the clinician may rely on auditory test performance, measured pretreatment, at regular intervals during the course of the therapy, and again at a specified posttreatment interval to determine treatment effectiveness and/or efficacy. These data may include documentation from both behavioral and electrophysiologic measures (Ferre, 1998; Jirsa, 2002; Kraus et al., 1993; Putter-Katz et al., 2002; Seats, 1998).

Because (C)APD may lead to or be associated with other disorders, improved (central) auditory function may contribute to improvement in other skill areas. The overall goal of intervention, then, not only should be improved auditory performance but also improved language, learning, and listening skills. Outcome measures should not rely solely upon improvement in performance on tests of auditory function, but also include documented change in related functional skills at home and school (ASHA, 2005; Chermak & Musiek, 1997). Team members may find evidence of positive outcomes by examining changes in performance on academic and language tests following implementation of a customized intervention plan (Chermak, Curtis, & Seikel, 1996; Ferre, 1997; 1998; Shapiro & Mistal, 1985, 1986; Tallal & Merzenich, 1997). Improved values on listening performance checklists such as the CHAPS

(Children's Auditory Performance Scale) (Smoski, Brunt & Tannahill, 1998) or on self-assessment measures (Ferre, 1997; Kelly, 1995) provide outcome data concerning the extent to which overall communication skills across a variety of settings have improved.

Case Studies in Differential Diagnosis and Intervention

The following cases illustrate the application of differential diagnosis and intervention for (C)APD and related disorders. The students described here presented with a (C)APD profile diagnosed using the Bellis-Ferre model (1999), which also characterizes behaviors suggestive of comorbid disorders in other sensory, neurocognitive, and/or language skills. Multidisciplinary evaluations are needed to definitively determine the appropriate primary and secondary diagnoses.

Hannah—Management of Comorbid Sensory Processing Disorders

This 9-year-old student, with reported behavior disorder was referred for evaluation by the classroom teacher following observation of poor outcomes of a classroom behavior management program. The original management plan included verbal and visual cueing by the teacher and classroom aide (e.g., change in tone of voice, use of facial expressions) to assist the student in classroom listening, maintaining focus, remaining on-task, and following directions. Neuropsychologic evaluation had ruled out presence of

ADHD as a contributing factor. Central auditory evaluation was requested to examine (C)APD as a potential contributing factor. Central auditory test findings revealed excessive left ear suppression on dichotic listening tasks and inability to label or mimic auditory patterns, indicating prosodic deficit profile, a right-hemisphere-based processing deficit.

At the team meeting, the audiologist noted that inability to recognize and use prosodic features of speech might explain the student's inability to benefit from the verbal cueing and facial expressions incorporated in the original management plan. Recommendation was made for comprehensive evaluation by a developmental vision specialist who subsequently diagnosed deficits in visual tracking and visual pattern recognition. The use of verbal and visual cueing was temporarily suspended in favor of implementation of treatment to improve both auditory and visual pattern recognition skills.

This case highlights the importance of differential diagnosis and outcome measurement for effective intervention. This student had been misdiagnosed as having a behavior disorder with implementation of an intervention plan judged, by observation, to be ineffective. In this case, thorough diagnostic testing led to appropriate diagnosis of comorbid sensory processing disorders and effective differential intervention.

Seth—Management of (C)APD and Comorbid Language Disorder

This 14-year-old (8th grade) student was referred for central auditory testing by the speech-language pathologist to determine the extent to which apparent language processing difficulties might have resulted from (C)APD. Speech-language evaluation indicated age-appropriate basic language skills with evidence of higher order language processing deficiency (e.g., deficits in recognizing and using word associations, attributes, multiple meaning words, and ambiguous statements). Additionally, the student had performed poorly on a screening test of central auditory function, as well as on several measures of related auditory-language function. Following the basic audiologic evaluation, which indicated normal peripheral hearing function, a central auditory evaluation was completed, which indicated normal performance for degraded speech and auditory patterning tasks, but bilaterally poor scores for three tests of dichotic listening. Taken together, auditory and language test results and presence of functional difficulties when asked to *apply* the rules of language across contexts (e.g., tended to answer *yes* initially to questions such as *Which do you want, A or B?*; displayed poor topic maintenance in conversation; and tended to respond to literal meaning of statements where response to implied meaning was required, such as responding *yes* to questions that began: *Didn't I tell you yesterday . . .*), resulted in diagnoses of (C)APD-associative profile, and comorbid language processing disorder.

This student's IEP (Individualized Education Plan) included a 30-week therapy program to improve dichotic listening, metalinguistic, and metacognitive skills, language processing, and social/pragmatic language skills. Recommended modifica-

tions and compensations for this student included: rephrasing using concrete language; clarification and demonstration of abstract concepts; avoidance of ambiguous and/or misleading language by parents and teachers (e.g., *Don't park your bike in the driveway* instead of *How many times have I told you not to park your bike in the driveway?*); preteaching new vocabulary, especially in science classes; waiver of middle school second language requirement; use of books on tape, study guides, and *Cliffs Notes*™[1]; and academic tests administered by speech-language pathologist with questions read to student and clarified as needed.

The student's family was encouraged to play games at home that could build auditory-language proficiency including Password®, Taboo®, Catch-Phrase®, Scattergories®, Plexers® (word puzzles), and Quizzles®[2] (logic puzzles). Reevaluation of auditory skills at 10-week intervals during therapy and 12 weeks after termination of therapy indicated steady improvement in dichotic listening skills with age-appropriate levels noted at final evaluation (12 weeks post-therapy). Speech-language evaluation conducted at the beginning of 9th grade indicated significant improvement in language processing and related functional communication skills. Therapy was discontinued and environmental modifications and compensations were maintained as needed through high school to minimize residual effects on day-to-day functioning. In this case, differential diagnosis and intervention with a motivated student created successful functional outcomes in a relatively short period of time.

---

[1]*Cliffs Notes* is a registered trademark of Hungry Minds, Inc.

[2]*Scattergories, Catch Phrase,* and *Taboo* are registered trademarks of Hasbro, Inc; *Password* is a registered trademark of Mark Goodson Productions, LLC; *Plexers* is a registered trademark of Plexers, Inc.; *Quizzles* is a registered trademark of Dale Seymour Publications, Inc.

Brooke—Management of (C)APD and ADHD

This 10-year-old student was referred for evaluation upon arrival from another school district. Parents reported that previous evaluation had indicated (C)APD and the need for computer-assisted auditory perceptual training and classroom use of an assistive listening device; however, no documentation was available. As a new student to the district, the case study team recommended re-evaluation prior to the implementation of what was considered an intensive and costly intervention plan.

The student reported difficulty sustaining attention and neuropsychologic evaluation could not rule out ADHD as a contributing factor. Parents were reluctant to initiate a medication trial based on available diagnostic information. Central auditory evaluation confirmed presence of deficits in auditory closure and discrimination with poor performance noted on degraded speech and temporal discrimination tasks. Behavioral characteristics exhibited by the student were consistent with an auditory decoding deficit profile, but also could be accounted for by presence of ADHD. Intervention team concurred with the original reported recommendations of trial use of an assistive listening device (personal FM system) and participation in the Fast ForWord auditory perceptual training program.

Use of a personal FM system was terminated after 3 weeks based on reports by the teacher of minimal noticeable change in classroom listening behaviors and the student's negative response to the device. Auditory re-evaluation 3 months *after* conclusion of intensive (daily) computer-assisted therapy revealed normal performance on all tests of central auditory function. However, observational and self-assessment checklists indicated only modest improvement in day-to-day listening skills despite the apparent resolution of the auditory deficits and implementation of a customized classroom management plan. Although treatment outcome was excellent with respect to specific, discrete auditory performance (as measured by central auditory function tests), overall intervention effectiveness was judged to be unsatisfactory. Additional consultation with parents led to trial use of nonstimulant medication to control symptoms of (apparent) ADHD. Student, parents, and teachers noted significant change in listening and daily communication skills within 30 days of addition of medication to the intervention plan.

This case illustrates the importance of diagnosing comorbid conditions and addressing those conditions concurrently. Although diagnosis of ADHD was inconclusive and parents were reluctant to pursue pharmacologic intervention options, limited treatment success led to review and revision of the intervention plan.

Summary

(C)APD can affect adversely academic achievement, communication proficiency, and life skills and can coexist with deficits in learning, language, or listening. The differential diagnosis of (C)APD and related, often comorbid disorders leads to differential intervention that is essential to efficacy. Intervention recommendations should be deficit- and listener-specific. Treatment programs should be chosen to target deficient auditory and related skills, and this customized plan should be extended and expanded throughout the day and across listening environments. In so doing, resources, both personal and financial, available for assessment and intervention, are used effectively to create positive outcomes for the listener.

References

Americans with Disabilities Act, Public Law 336. (1990). Retrieved January 10, 2006, from http://www.usdoj.gov/crt/ada/publi cat.htm.

American Psychiatric Association. (2000). *Diagnostic criteria from the DSM-IV-TR®.* Arlington, VA: Author.

American Speech-Language-Hearing Association. (1996). Central auditory processing: current status of research and implications for clinical practice. *American Journal of Audiology, 5,* 41–54.

American Speech-Language-Hearing Association. (2005). *Technical report: (Central) auditory processing disorders.* Rockville, MD: Author.

Ayers, M. (1994). *Sensory integration and the child.* Los Angeles: Western Psychological Services.

Bellis, T. (2002). Developing deficit-specific intervention plans for individuals with auditory processing disorders. *Seminars in Hearing, 23,* 287–295.

Bellis, T. (2003). *Assessment and management of central auditory processing disorders in the educational setting* (2nd ed.). Clifton Park, NY: Thomson Delmar Learning.

Bellis, T. (2006). Interpretation of APD test results. In T. K. Parthasarathy (Ed.), *An introduction to auditory processing disorders in children* (pp.145–160). Mahwah, NJ: Lawrence Erlbaum Associates.

Bellis, T., & Ferre, J. (1999). Multidimensional approach to differential diagnosis of central auditory processing disorders in children. *Journal of the American Academy of Audiology, 10,* 319–328.

Carrow-Woodfolk, E. (1999). *Comprehensive assessment of spoken language.* Circle Pines, MN: American Guidance Service, Inc.

Chermak, G. D. (1998). Metacognitive approaches to managing central auditory processing disorders. In M. Masters, N. Stecker, & J. Katz. (Eds.), *Central auditory processing disorders: Mostly management* (pp. 49–61). Boston: Allyn & Bacon.

Chermak, G. D., Curtis, L., & Seikel, J. (1996). The effectiveness of an interactive hearing conservation program for elementary school children. *Language Speech and Hearing Services in the Schools, 27,* 29–39.

Chermak, G. D., & Musiek, F. E. (1997). *Central auditory processing disorders: New perspectives.* San Diego, CA: Singular Publishing Group.

Chermak, G. D., & Musiek, F. E. (2002). Auditory training principles and approaches for remediating and managing auditory processing disorders. *Seminars in Hearing, 23,* 297–308.

Duesenberg, D. (2006). ADHD: Diagnosis and current treatment options to improve functional outcomes. In T. Parthasarathy (Ed.), *An introduction to auditory processing disorders in children* (pp. 187–201). Mahwah, NJ: Lawrence Erlbaum Associates.

Ferre, J. (1997). *Processing power: A guide to CAPD assessment and management.* San Antonio, TX: The Psychological Corporation.

Ferre, J. (1998). The M3 model for treating central auditory processing disorders. In M. Masters, Stecker, & J. Katz (Eds.), *Central auditory processing disorders: Mostly management* (pp. 103–116). Boston: Allyn & Bacon.

Ferre J. (2002a). Behavioral therapeutic approaches for central auditory problems. In J. Katz (Ed.), *Handbook of clinical audiology* (5th ed., pp. 525-531). Philadelphia: Lippincott Williams & Wilkins.

Ferre, J. (2002b). Managing children's auditory processing deficits in the real world: What teachers and parents want to know. *Seminars in Hearing, 23*, 319-326.

Ferre, J. (2006). Management strategies for APD. In T. K. Parthasarathy (Ed.), *An introduction to auditory processing disorders in children* (pp. 161-183). Mahwah, NJ: Lawrence Erlbaum Associates.

Flowers, A. (1983). *Auditory perception, speech, language, and learning.* Dearborn, MI: Perceptual Learning Systems.

Gerber, A. (1993). *Language-related learning disabilities: Their nature and treatment.* Baltimore: Paul H. Brookes Publishing Co.

Goldstein, H. (1990). Assessing clinical significance. In L. Olswang, C. Thompson, S. Warren, & N. Minghetti (Eds.), *Treatment efficacy research in communication disorders* (pp. 91-98). Rockville, MD: ASHA.

Horn, S., & Horn, D. (2005). *ADHD and dyslexia: Choosing effective interventions.* Paper presented at the annual meeting of the International Dyslexia Association. Denver, CO.

Hunter, S. (2005). *Working memory as an executive function: Implications for education.* Paper presented at the annual meeting of the Illinois Branch of the International Dyslexia Association, Oakbrook Terrace, IL.

Individuals with Disabilities in Education Act Amendments of 1997. (1997). Retrieved January 9, 2006, from http://www.kidstogether.org/idea/htm

Ingersoll, B., & Goldstein, S. (1993). *Attention deficit disorder and learning disabilities: Realities, myths, and controversial treatments.* New York: Doubleday Dell Publishing Group.

Jirsa, R. (2002). Clinical efficacy of electrophysiologic measures in auditory processing disorders management programs. *Seminars in Hearing, 23*, 349-356.

Johnson, D. (1983). Design for individualization of language intervention programs. In J. Miller, D. Yoder, & R. Schiefelbusch (Eds.), *Contemporary issues in language intervention. ASHA Reports 12* (pp. 165-176). Rockville, MD: ASHA.

Kelly, D. (1995). *Central auditory processing disorders: Strategies for use with children and adolescents.* San Antonio, TX: The Psychological Corporation.

Kraus, N., McGee, T., Carrell, T., King, C., Tremblay, K., & Nicol, T. (1995). Central auditory system plasticity associated with speech discrimination training. *Journal of Cognitive Neuroscience, 7*, 25-32.

Kraus, N., McGee, T., Ferre, J., Hoeppner, J., Carrell, T., Sharma, A., & Nicol, T. (1993). Mismatch negativity in the neurophysiologic/behavioral evaluation of auditory processing disorders: A case study. *Ear and Hearing, 14*, 223-234.

Luria, A. (1973). *The working brain.* London: Penguin Press.

Masters, G. (1998). Speech and language management of central auditory processing disorders. In M. Masters, N. Stecker, & J. Katz (Eds.), *Central auditory processing disorders: Mostly management* (pp. 117-129). Boston: Allyn & Bacon.

Mosby's medical, nursing, and allied health dictionary (6th ed.). (2002). St. Louis, MO: Mosby.

Musiek, F. (2004). Hearing and the brain: Audiological consequences of neurobiological Disorders. *Journal of the American Academy of Audiology,15*(Special issue).

Musiek, F. (2005, September). *Advances in CAPD diagnosis and management.* Seminar presented at the annual meeting of the Massachusetts Speech-Hearing Language Association, Worcester, MA.

Myklebust, H. (1954). *Auditory disorders in children* (p. 8). New York: Grune & Stratton.

Palombo, J. (2001). *Learning disorders and disorders of the self in children and adolescents.* New York: W.W. Norton & Co., Inc.

Phillips-Keeley, S. (2003). *The source for executive function disorders.* East Moline, IL: LinguiSystems, Inc.

Putter-Katz, H., Said, A., Feldman, I., Miran, D., Kushnir, D., Muchnik, C., & Hildesheimer, M. (2002). Treatment and evaluation indices of auditory processing disorders. *Seminars in Hearing, 23,* 357–364.

Richard, G. (2001). *The source for processing disorders.* East Moline, IL: LinguiSystems, Inc.

Richard, G., & Fahey, J. (2005). *The source for development of executive function disorders.* East Moline, IL: LinguiSystems, Inc.

Seats, T. (1998, November). *Treatment efficacy of temporal exercises in habilitating children with central auditory processing disorders.* Paper presented at annual meeting of the American Speech-Language-Hearing Association, San Antonio, TX.

Shapiro, A., & Mistal, G. (1985). ITE-aid auditory training for reading and spelling-disabled children: Clinical case studies. *Hearing Journal, 38,* 14–16.

Shapiro, A., & Mistal, G. (1986). ITE-aid auditory training for reading and spelling-disabled children: A longitudinal study of matched groups. *Hearing Journal, 39,* 14–16.

Shapiro, H., & Balthazar, C. (2004, February). *A study of treatment effectiveness for two children learning reading skills.* Paper presented at the annual meeting of the Illinois Speech-Language-Hearing Association. Arlington Heights, IL.

Sloan, C. (1995). *Treating auditory processing difficulties in children.* San Diego, CA: Singular Publishing Group.

Smoski, W., Brunt, M., & Tannahill, C. (1998). *Children's Auditory Performance Scale.* Tampa, FL: Educational Audiology Association.

Tallal, P., & Merzenich, M. (1997, November). *Fast ForWord training for children with language-learning problems. National field test results.* Paper presented at the annual meeting of the American Speech-Language-Hearing Association, Boston.

Tanguay, P. (2001). *Nonverbal learning disabilities at home: A parent's guide.* London: Jessica Kingsley Publishers.

Thompson, S. (1997). *The source for nonverbal learning disorders.* East Moline, IL: LinguiSystems, Inc.

Tremblay, K., & Kraus, N. (2002). Auditory training induces asymmetrical changes in cortical activity. *Journal of Speech, Language, Hearing research, 45,* 564–572.

Tremblay, K., Kraus, N., Carrell, T., & McGee, T. (1997). Central auditory system plasticity: Generalization to novel stimulation following listening training. *Journal of the Acoustical Society of America, 102,* 3762–3773.

Tremblay, K., Kraus, N., McGee, T., Picton, C., & Otis, B. (2001). Central auditory plasticity: Changes in the N1-P2 complex after speech-sound training. *Ear and Hearing, 22,* 79–90.

Tyler, A. (1997). Evidence of linguistic interactions in intervention. *Topics in Language Disorders, 17,* 23–40.

CHAPTER 11

INTERVENTION FOR COGNITIVE-COMMUNICATIVE AND LANGUAGE FACTORS ASSOCIATED WITH (C)APD

A Speech-Language Perspective

GAIL J. RICHARD

Role of Differential Diagnosis

The term "auditory processing" encompasses a wide range of functional skills. The ability to attach meaning to an auditory stimulus to then mediate an appropriate response (Richard, 2001) entails integrated neurological coordination of multiple structures within the auditory sensory system. The effectiveness and efficiency of the auditory system can be compromised by a variety of deficits that occur at different neurological sites (Noback, 1985, Protti, 1983). Diagnosis must carefully differentiate the various components of auditory processing if intervention efforts are to be successful.

Early debate within the profession attempted to differentiate the nature of processing as an auditory phenomenon (Katz, 1978; Keith, 1981; Tallal, Stark, Kallman, & Mellits, 1981), versus a language phenomena (Gerber & Bryen, 1981; Kamhi, 1981, Rice & Kemper, 1984), or a combination of both auditory and language factors (Butler, 1981; Duchan & Katz, 1983; Rees, 1973, 1981). Lubert (1981) completed a comprehensive review of the current literature at the time, and cited several studies that documented impairments in phonemic hearing, discrimination of rapid sound sequences, and dysfunction in the acoustic feature-detection aspects of speech as the crux of problems in higher level language tasks. However, the issue of whether language processing disorders are a result of auditory processing deficits, a contributing factor, or stand-alone disorders continues to be debated (ASHA, 1996, 2005a; Friel-Patti, 1994; Schow & Chermak, 1999).

Consequently, consensus has been lacking among audiologists as to what constitutes an auditory processing disorder. As a result, a mixed group of deficits have been historically identified and diagnosed as auditory processing disorders. The deficits can range from impairment in the central auditory nervous system (CANS) (Keith, 1981) to problems in executive function skills necessary for organizing a motor response to indicate reception and interpretation of an auditory signal (Rees, 1981). It is not unusual for linguistic aspects to factor into the perceived auditory processing deficits (Friel-Patti, 1994). However, the recent task force reports (ASHA, 2005a, 2005b) have begun to promote a professional consensus among audiologists.

Although audiologists are responsible for diagnosis of central auditory processing disorder ([C]APD), speech-language pathologists often are the professionals who assume primary responsibility for treatment of the disorder. Discrete aspects of auditory processing need to be differentiated within the diagnostic process by the audiologist. This entails delineating discrete aspects of auditory processing that can be evaluated along a continuum of abilities, beginning with the peripheral auditory system and continuing through the brainstem into the cortex. Tasks in binaural integration and pitch pattern discrimination might be examples of skills evaluated. The speech-language pathologist assumes responsibility for assessing the cognitive–communicative

factors associated with (C)APD, which are the functional application skills of auditory processing. Tasks might include phoneme discrimination, sound-symbol correspondence, or word segmentation. Higher level assessment by the speech-language pathologist would probe the linguistic attachment of meaning through tasks evaluating comprehension of vocabulary or concepts.

The delineation of functional skills encompassed within auditory processing has significant clinical implications for treatment objectives. A clinical approach necessitates an operational definition of the major aspects of auditory processing. The symptomatic characteristics along the continuum of auditory processing (see Figure 11–1) become the behavioral aspects that need to be targeted in therapy. A functional division of auditory processing can be derived by presenting auditory processing on a continuum that moves through a neurological hierarchy in the central nervous system and brain (Richard, 2001). It should be noted that:

> Although abilities such as phonological awareness, attention to and memory for auditory information, auditory synthesis, comprehension and interpretation of auditorily presented information, and similar skills may be reliant on or associated with intact central auditory function, they are considered higher order cognitive-communicative and/or language-related functions and, thus, are not included in the definition of (C)AP (ASHA, 2005a, p. 2).

The initial section on the auditory processing continuum (i.e., acoustic processing) is the responsibility of an audiologist to assess and determine deficits. The peripheral system receives the

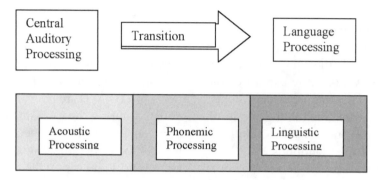

Figure 11–1. Continuum of auditory processing.

acoustic stimulus and conducts it to the CANS. Transmitting auditory information from the cochlea through the central auditory nervous system requires that elements of the signal (e.g., timing, frequency, intensity) be coded and retained (Bhatnagar & Korabic, 2006). This component of the auditory processing continuum is primarily discrimination of the acoustic features of the auditory signal, or feature detection.

The acoustic stimulus is transferred through the brainstem to the upper cortex. The temporal lobe is the primary acoustic center in the cortex, where discrimination of the acoustic aspects of the signal occurs (Gaddes, 1980; Protti, 1983). Research has suggested that the temporal lobe is of vital importance in recognition and discrimination of sound patterns that are important to accurate perception of human speech (Bhatnagar & Korabic, 2006). It is this stage of the auditory processing continuum (i.e., phonemic processing) that entails a transition from acoustic feature detection to discrimination of speech segments within the signal. The phonemic processing stage of the auditory processing continuum is also a transition within assessment

responsibilities. Both the audiologist and speech-language pathologist conduct assessment procedures that evaluate this stage of the continuum (Richard, 2006). The individual must recognize phonemes of language as discrete sound units that are combined to form syllables, words, and sentences. If difficulty is encountered in recognizing sounds of a language, then additional problems are likely when an individual must subsequently match sounds to their alphabetic/orthographic symbol (McAndrews, 2006). It is also important to realize that phonological processing is critical for developing literacy skills, even in non-English-speaking individuals. Research has established that phonological awareness and phonological coding are core aspects of literacy (Troia, 2004).

The linguistic processing stage on the continuum is primarily the responsibility of the speech-language pathologist. Meaning is attached once the acoustic characteristics are decoded, using the phonemic sound-symbol system associated with a specific linguistic system. Meaning cannot be attached to the signal without language knowledge (Richard, 2001). Once the auditory task has transitioned to interpretation of the acoustic signal to derive the encoded message and formulate a response, then the processing demand is within the purview of language processing. A more extensive discussion of the speech-language pathologist's assessment responsibilities along the continuum is included in Chapter 16, Volume I, of this Handbook.

The continuum of auditory processing illustrated in Figure 11–1 facilitates a more defined differentiation of abilities encompassed within the disorder area. The audiologist conducting an evaluation should include procedures in the assessment battery that will discriminate strengths and weaknesses throughout the neurological hierarchy represented in the acoustic and phonemic processing levels. The speech-language pathologist should supplement the audiologic procedures that evaluated the phonemic level of processing, and add assessment procedures to evaluate linguistic processing. The shared assessment responsibilities become important when attempting to create an accurate diagnostic picture to then plan an encompassing multidisciplinary intervention program for implementation.

Recommendations for treatment of (C)APD at one time were fairly scripted by practicing audiologists, with little deviation or individualization in treatment objectives. Most audiologists' treatment recommendations tend to focus on assistive listening technology and environmental modifications to enhance the signal-to-noise ratio in an attempt to maximize the auditory stimulus. In some cases, this manipulation will facilitate better signal reception and compensate for acoustic deficits. However, these intervention strategies do not comprehensively address the range of deficits associated with a (C)APD (Chermak & Musiek,

1997), especially the deficits that are more phonemic or linguistic in nature.

The complexity of auditory processing creates a challenge for the professional responsible for intervention. When aspects of a (C)APD are not carefully differentiated during the assessment process, intervention becomes ineffective because it lacks focus. By grouping all brainstem and cortical auditory skills together, the professional responsible for treatment must engage in functional evaluation tasks to determine the level of breakdown before specific treatment goals can be generated. Treatment goals need to address specific functional skills in the processing continuum, rather than generic all-encompassing goals.

The assessment report should include discussion of performance and interpretation of various test results. Reporting scores alone does not effectively present the nature of an individual's performance deficits at a functional level. In communicating diagnostic findings to speech-language pathologists, it is helpful for audiologists to include the clinical implications of poor performance on a specific diagnostic measure. Goals and therapy activities can be designed more specifically if a report provides some interpretative detail.

Effective treatment is always dependent on effective diagnosis. If the evaluation procedures provide specific and differential information, a treatment program can be generated to address individual needs. If the assessment results are general, then treatment becomes a "hit and miss" proposition of trying various techniques until something results in progress. The audiologist is key to facilitating a customized treatment program for individuals diagnosed with processing disorders.

Selecting Intervention Goals

"Auditory processing disorder" can refer to a deficiency in a variety of functional skills, ranging from very discrete to fairly integrated and complex (Ferre, 2006). More comprehensive intervention models include three major aspects in intervention—signal enhancement via assistive listening systems and environmental modifications, direct skills intervention, or auditory training, and compensatory strategies (e.g., central resources training) (ASHA 2005a; Bellis, 2003; Chermak & Musiek, 1997).

Environmental modifications focus on signal enhancement. The signal can be enhanced through addressing the signal-to-noise ratio, using assistive listening devices, or supplementing the auditory signal with input from other sensory modalities, or modification of room acoustics (Chermak & Musiek, 1997). Direct skills intervention involves working with the individual to develop stronger auditory pathways through intense practice on specific functional tasks (Chermak & Musiek, 2002). Certain behavioral responses are modified through focused instruction in specific auditory abilities (e.g., auditory discrimination, temporal ordering, etc.). Compensatory strategies focus on a variety of components, but most are indirect. (See Chapters 4, 5, and 7 in this volume for discussion of auditory training, central resources training, and signal enhancement.)

For intervention to be effective, the professional must first discriminate the level in the auditory processing continuum that needs to be addressed. Although more than one area could be impacted (e.g., acoustic and phonemic process-

ing), it is usually beneficial not to address all aspects of the disorder simultaneously (Gaddes, 1980). Discrete skills should be developed first; then those skills used to build strategies to address more integrated aspects of the deficit.

Table 11-1 summarizes example goals in the three major aspects of the auditory processing continuum. Compensatory (and signal enhancement) and direct intervention goals included in the table are explained in the following section. It is important to understand that the examples included in the table are not inclusive; there are many other strategies and skills that could be addressed in treatment. Rather, they are considered to be illustrative of the type of goals that could be addressed, depending on the client's functional deficit profile.

Acoustic Processing Goals

The identification of a (C)APD at the acoustic level implies that the individual is receiving a compromised auditory stimulus (Richard, 2001). There could be a variety of reasons that account for the compromised signal. The signal itself could be fine; the individual's auditory system is not able to transfer the stimulus, resulting in a compromised signal received at the cortical level. Another possibility could be that the signal was modified due to interference by a loud environmental noise. Attention deficit disorder could also contribute to only parts of a presented auditory stimulus being received and transferred to the cortex.

Intervention should be designed to minimize the adverse effects of the disorder through compensatory techniques, and develop skills to overcome some of the acoustic challenges (Ferre, 2006).

Table 11–1. Sample Goals Within Levels of the Auditory Processing Continuum

Processing Level	Sample Compensatory Goals	Sample Direct Intervention Goals
Acoustic Processing	Assistive listening devices Preferential seating Noise reduction procedures Tape recording Speech-reading	Pitch discrimination Sound /word discrimination Auditory sequencing/pattern recognition Figure ground Sound localization
Phonemic Processing	Visual imaging supplements Verbal modifications Tactile supplements	Phonemic analysis/ segmentation Phonemic synthesis/blending Sound-symbol correspondence Alliteration Rhyme Phoneme manipulation
Linguistic Processing	Cues/prompts Scaffolding Schemas/context Mnemonic devices	Vocabulary development Conceptual meaning Multiple meaning Inferences Prosodic feature detection

The audiologist diagnosing the (C)APD should project what impact the deficit could have on the individual's ability to function successfully in everyday life. The symptoms present in the client's auditory profile will assist in determining the treatment direction. The goals, both compensatory and direct skill-based, will require active participation on the individual's part to overcome the compromised auditory stimulus. Given the range of compensatory and direct intervention goals encompassed at the acoustic processing stage, collaborative efforts between the audiologist and the speech-language pathologist are preferable, if not crucial.

Compensatory strategies at the level of acoustic processing could include the following:

■ **Assistive listening devices:** FM systems are intended to enhance the signal-to-noise ratio within an individual's immediate environment. The general principle is to amplify the auditory signal being sent so it is more dominant to the listener within the acoustic background. Technology continues to improve in this area, becoming less cumbersome and more fine-tuned in signal enhancement.

- **Preferential seating:** The goal in preferential seating is to place an individual in close proximity to the primary auditory signal. In other words, a child should sit close to the instructor so background noise encoded with the signal is minimized. It is important to explain that preferential seating does not necessarily mean placing a child in the front of the room. The seating preference might change, based on the location of the instructional source. Access to visual signals is also enhanced in preferential seating. It is imperative that the teacher, parent, or consultant maintain the principles of preferential seating throughout the school day and in various settings.
- **Noise reduction procedures:** Limiting or minimizing background noise present in an acoustic environment is the goal in noise reduction strategies. Competing auditory signals are problematic for students with (C)APD. Closing doors and windows to reduce hallway or street noise are examples of strategies to accomplish noise reduction. Acoustic enhancements in the structural environment can also accomplish this, such as installing acoustic ceiling tiles, drapes or fabric dividers, and other sound absorbing materials.
- **Tape recording:** Providing a permanent record of the auditory signal is one technique to compensate for (C)APD. A child who cannot process an auditory message accurately or quickly could use a tape recorder to listen and replay the verbal instructional content, providing signal redundancy. However, it

is important that the tape recorder be close to the speaker so the quality of the recording is not compromised.
- **Speech-reading:** The ability to perceive speech by observing the speaker's mouth, facial expressions, and gestures can often facilitate better reception of the auditory signal. An individual can be taught to pay attention and watch a speaker to supplement the acoustic stimuli with visual stimuli.

Direct intervention goals at the level of acoustic processing could include the following:

- **Pitch discrimination:** The ability to identify changes in frequency of the acoustic signal is the goal within pitch discrimination tasks. Usually the task involves discrimination of low versus high pitch, rather than more subtle pitch changes. This can be done with a piano, pitch pipe, keyboard, or by simply singing or humming different tones.
- **Sound/word discrimination:** The ability to discriminate phonemes is addressed in sound discrimination. The individual learns to hear the difference between sound units in isolation or sequences, i.e., words. At this level, the words do not need to be meaningful or part of the language code; they can be nonsensical. Linguistic variables should be minimized when working on this skill.
- **Auditory sequencing/pattern recognition:** The ability to recognize the order of sound units is addressed in auditory sequencing tasks. The

individual might need to recognize the pattern in a sequence of different pitches/tones, sounds, or words. Rhythmic motor patterns, such as clapping, could also be used to work on this auditory skill.

■ **Figure-ground:** The ability to discriminate the primary auditory signal from other competing acoustic stimuli is addressed in figure-ground tasks. Different types of competing stimuli can be used to develop discrimination of the primary signal, such as white noise, instrumental music, environmental noise, and competing voices.

■ **Sound localization:** The ability to identify the source of sound being generated is addressed in sound localization tasks. Environmental noises and speech can be used as the auditory stimulus to develop this skill. The individual works on developing the ability to attenuate directionally toward the source of the acoustic signal.

Phonemic Processing Goals

The phonemic processing level in the auditory processing continuum represents a transition from discrimination of specific acoustic features of an auditory signal (e.g., pitch, loudness, rate), to discrimination of the sound segments that comprise speech (e.g., specific phonemes). An individual must develop awareness of discrete phonemes for the association between sounds and letters to evolve (Troia, 2004). Phonological awareness is the ability to identify and manipulate the discrete sound units of a language (Apel, Masterson, & Niessen, 2004) to transition from speech to print literacy. This awareness of phonemic sound segments occurs independent of semantic meaning (Justice & Schuele, 2004). Collaborative efforts at this stage of the continuum should include teachers and the speech-language pathologist.

Compensatory strategies at the level of phonemic processing could include the following:

■ **Visual imaging:** Many of the phonological awareness programs pair a character with a specific sound to facilitate the sound-symbol correspondence. Introducing a visual image of Granny Gray Goose with the "g" sound, for example, helps a child associate the phoneme with the grapheme representation.

■ **Verbal modifications:** A classroom teacher could speak slower to enhance clarity in verbal articulation. Exaggerated emphasis or stress could be used to enhance specific phonemes in words.

■ **Tactile supplements:** Incorporating motor movements can facilitate recognition of acoustic features. For example, when teaching awareness of phonemes that are continuants, the child can be encouraged to run a finger down their arm, illustrating the elongated feature of the sound when produced.

Direct intervention goals at the level of phonemic processing could include the following:

■ **Phonemic analysis/segmentation:** The ability to isolate specific sound segments in a phonetic unit is emphasized in phonemic analysis tasks. A student learns to separate the individual phoneme segments that comprise a syllable or word. For example, a child might be asked how many sounds are in the word "cake."

■ **Phonemic synthesis/blending:** The ability to combine isolated sound segments and blend them into a syllable or word is taught in phonemic synthesis tasks. Co-articulation aspects of language are addressed when a child is asked to put individual phonemes together to form a connected unit. For example, a student might be asked to put /k/ . . . /a/ . . . /t/ . . . together to form a word.

■ **Phoneme manipulation:** The ability to modify a sound unit by adding, deleting, or changing phonemes within it is entailed in phoneme manipulation tasks. For example, a child might be asked to delete the /s/ in "stop" and change the /t/ to /h/. This skill cannot be addressed until the previous two (i.e., phonemic analysis and synthesis) are developed.

■ **Alliteration:** The ability to recognize a common acoustic feature in sound units is encompassed in alliteration. Tasks could include discriminating words that all start with /p/ or identifying what the similar sound feature could be in "dog, dish, deep." Alliteration tasks usually include both discrimination and generation/production tasks.

■ **Rhyme:** The ability to recognize a similar sound pattern among words is addressed in rhyming tasks. As in alliteration, the child needs to learn to recognize similar sound sequenced words, as well as generate words with the same sound sequence. For example, the child might be asked which word rhymes with "hat"—"cap, cat, or catch." Then the child might be asked to make another word that rhymes with "hat".

■ **Sound-symbol correspondence:** The ability to represent an acoustic sound with a printed letter will transition a child into the phonic basis for spelling, reading, and written language. The child could be asked to match acoustic sounds to the corresponding letter or write the letter that represents a sound heard.

Linguistic Processing Goals

The linguistic level of the auditory processing continuum transitions into the semantic aspect of language. This type of processing is concerned primarily with attaching meaning to the auditory signal. Once an auditory stimulus has been decoded and the message interpreted, then the information must be stored for later access (Friel-Patti, 1994).

The compensatory strategies within this phase of auditory processing primarily facilitate organization of new materials as they are being stored, and accurate and efficient retrieval of previously stored information. The direct intervention goals are very semantic in nature, starting with acquisition of discrete language skills, and progressing to more integrated, complex language skills. The direct intervention goals are extremely diverse, based on the language expectations by developmental age. When deficits at this stage of the continuum are identified, it usually signals the presence of a language processing disorder, which can certainly occur comorbidly with a (C)APD. The linguistic processing goals are the responsibility of the speech-language pathologist and should be diagnosed as a language processing disorder, not auditory processing disorder, to ensure more focused treatment.

Compensatory techniques at the level of linguistic processing could include the following:

- **Cues/prompts:** A variety of verbal, visual, or motor prompts can be used to facilitate retrieval of learned information. For example, a teacher might test the capitals of states by providing the first letter of each city's name; a person might remember their telephone number by pressing the motor pattern on the phone; a student might remember something by visualizing where they saw it.
- **Scaffolding:** Retrieving stored information to then add new information to it is the premise of scaffolding. The individual takes learned information and builds additional knowledge on top of it. For example, a child might know what a cat is. Then they learn what a cat says, what it eats, and how it feels to pet a cat.
- **Schemata:** Using personal experiences to comprehend and remember new semantic information is entailed within schema strategies. The context in which the language terms are functionally applicable is used to facilitate comprehension and future retrieval. For example, the experience of going to the doctor is used to understand aspects of going to the dentist.
- **Mnemonic devices:** Strategies to facilitate learning and remember

new semantic material are encompassed under the use of mnemonic devices. Rehearsal, elaboration, inference, categorization, are also aspects of attempting to organize concepts for subsequent retrieval. An example is the use of the phrase "Every good boy does fine" to remember the notes of the musical scale or the word "HOMES" to remember the first letter of the five Great Lakes in the United States.

Direct intervention goals for the level of linguistic processing could include the following:

- **Vocabulary development:** The ability to connect a phonetic sequence with the actual object represented by the word builds the lexicon within a specific language. Meaning should be derived from an auditory signal by triggering a visual image or comprehension of the message encoded within the stimulus.
- **Conceptual development:** The ability to abstract meaning from a term representing a specific relationship is involved in conceptual development. Concept categories include spatial relationships (e.g., over, below, behind), quantity (e.g., few, many, most) and quality (e.g., size, shape, color terms). Conceptual language requires a solid concrete vocabulary foundation as prerequisite to abstract processing.
- **Multiple meanings:** The ability to alter a word's meaning based on the context in which it is used is taught in multiple meanings. An individual learns that a phonetic sequence of letters can be used to

represent different meanings. For example, "bat" can represent the stick used to hit a baseball or the flying mammal that lives in a cave.

- **Inference:** The ability to use situational context to "fill in" unspoken aspects of a verbal message is required for competence in inferencing. The individual must recognize shared information that is not directly included in the auditory signal received. For example, while standing in line at the school cafeteria, a peer might ask a student what he wants. The inference is what the boy wants to eat for lunch, not what he hopes to get for his birthday next week.

- **Prosodic feature detection:** The ability to alter a verbal message based on the manner in which it is delivered is a skill addressed when focusing on prosody. A child might verbalize that he or she is fine, but if they are crying with blood on the knee, then the message is not sincere. Recognizing subtle acoustic characteristics encompassed within prosody (e.g., rate, inflection, emphasis, pause) requires the listener to process the suprasegmental aspects of speech. This skill is usually not acquired until one demonstrates competence in segmental processing (i.e., units of speech). The typical meaning embedded in literal interpretation of words can be significantly changed by the prosodic features used as the utterance is spoken.

Intervention goals for (C)APD must be tailored to specifically address the type of deficits that are symptomatically evident in diagnostic and assessment proce-

dures. The audiologist who diagnoses a (C)APD must carefully analyze results when generating intervention goals. A generic list of suggestions that include preferential seating, FM system in the classroom, visual supplements, and so forth should not routinely be added to every report. These recommendations only pertain to the acoustic aspect of the processing continuum. Although these recommendations certainly pertain to the classic definition of a (C)APD, limiting recommendations to these standard approaches does not provide the comprehensive intervention needed to address the range of auditory, language, communication, and learning problems so frequently associated with (C)APD (ASHA 2005a; Chermak & Musiek, 1997). Amplification and strategies to enhance the signal-to-noise ratio, for example, will not effectively target phonemic processing deficits. Treatment goals must be related to the deficits evident in the diagnostic battery, but addressing the related issues requires more focus on intervention at the levels of phonemic and linguistic processing.

Developing Customized Intervention Programs for Cognitive-Communicative and Language Factors Associated with (C)APD

(C)APD encompasses a wide variety of discrete and integrated skills. Earlier in this chapter, the importance of differential diagnosis to determine more specifically the neurological level of difficulty was emphasized. A differentiation of strengths and weaknesses along the auditory processing continuum allows the professional responsible for intervention to appropriately focus goals to address individual needs.

The audiologist responsible for diagnosis of a (C)APD also is responsible for generating appropriate recommendations that will address the specific deficits identified in the evaluation process. Although a similar battery of tests might be used in the assessment process, interpretation of results is always individualized. The recommendations also should be individualized. A broad list of generic recommendations is ethically irresponsible. The audiologist should carefully evaluate results to determine what specific areas would be beneficial for the individual in a treatment program.

A Sample of Specific Intervention Programs

Treatment programs to address (C)APD are becoming more available on the commercial market. The professional providing treatment needs to discern the theoretical foundation of the various treatment programs to determine if the approach will address the specific deficits symptomatic of an individual client. Marketing techniques tend to blur the details of an intervention program by attempting to appeal to a broader group of consumers. It becomes imperative for the professional designing intervention to carefully scrutinize the treatment program objectives and methodology to ensure efficacy in service delivery. Although no endorsement is suggested or implied, a few examples of commercially available treatment programs are provided to illustrate the importance of carefully analyzing marketed products.

The sample commercial programs presented here are designed, purportedly, to address the acoustic and/or phonemic levels on the auditory processing continuum. These two levels are the primary focus for recommendations made by an audiologist diagnosing (C)APD.

Earobics

Earobics is published by a computer software company to assist professionals in developing learning skills for success in language and reading. The program uses digitized naturally produced, but acoustically altered speech (Ferre, 2006). Disorder areas for which Earobics has been recommended have included dyslexia, peripheral hearing impairment, (C)APD, attention deficit hyperactivity disorder (ADHD), and speech-language impairments (Cognitive Concepts, 1998).

The software is designed to develop phonological awareness skills through a series of game activities that target processing syllables, sound blending, segmentation, rhyming, sound discrimination, and an introduction to phonics. The stepped series includes games for ages four years to adult. An advantage in Earobics is that the professional controls the learning process by determining the level of difficulty and length of time spent on the computer game activities. No special training or certification is required to access the program.

Fast ForWord

Dr. Paula Tallal's extensive research record focused primarily on the smallest unit of auditory processing and temporal aspects of signal detection. Her conclusion over time was that individuals with language impairment struggle to process acoustic stimuli at the typical rate of presentation, resulting in poor performance in response to acoustic signals (Richard, 2001). She teamed with Dr. Michael Merzenich, whose research focused on brain plasticity in learning, to develop the Fast ForWord (Scientific Learning Corporation) program.

Fast ForWord is a computer program that provides exercises in temporal processing and phoneme identification using acoustically modified speech. The purpose is to develop the auditory skills necessary for success in language and reading in ages 4 through 14 years. Individuals play a series of games which target discrimination of minimal pairs, phoneme identification, temporal acoustic differences in phonemes, tone sequences, following directions, and word recognition skills. The methodology has been marketed for a wide variety of deficits, including language disorders, (C)APD, hyperlexia, and dyslexia, among others. The specific skills addressed include signal detection, recognition, discrimination, working memory, sequencing, and executive function.

It is suggested that the acoustic and phonemic aspects incorporated into the games provide a foundation for language and reading, addressed through the perspective of modified temporal processing. Sounds presented are acoustically manipulated to slow down until the child can detect the acoustic features accurately. With success, the rate of presentation is gradually increased until a normal timing pattern is reached.

Certification and training is required to administer the Fast ForWord program. It requires Internet access and a financial commitment to purchase a license for the program. It is intensive, recommended to be used for approximately 100 minutes,

five days per week for 6 to 8 weeks. Individual modifications are difficult to accomplish within the regimented program sequence.

Lindamood Bell Phoneme Sequencing Program (LiPS)

Pat and Phyllis Lindamood with Nancy Bell developed a program designed to address phonemic awareness and comprehension essential to success in reading, spelling, and speech. Their research and clinical experience showed that children gradually improve in the ability to represent words as discrete phonemic segments (Justice & Schuele, 2004).

The methodology utilized in the LiPS program is to develop phonological awareness through multisensory input, allowing children to manipulate materials as they develop a feedback system for developing speech, reading, and spelling skills. The authors require clinicians to train in the program, but do not actually certify participants for use of their program. The LiPS program is almost exclusively geared toward the phonemic processing level of the auditory processing continuum, although some temporal patterning is included through the phoneme sequencing and speech-sound discrimination skills (Ferre, 2006).

Auditory Integration Training (AIT)

Auditory Integration Training is marketed as addressing (C)APD, as well as ADHD, learning disabilities, autism, and a host of behavioral symptoms. It is a technique designed to expose individuals to electronically modulated sound by filtering certain frequencies to reduce hypersensitive reactions to auditory stimuli. It is a global methodology that is focused at the level of acoustic processing on the continuum.

One of the most well-known AIT programs was developed by Guy Berard, an otolaryngologist in France. The intent was to assist children who had difficulty learning in school due to hypersensitive hearing that resulted in avoidance of acoustic stimuli or distortion in the signal received. Specific auditory frequencies were filtered out electronically as children listened to music under headphone conditions. The objective was to build a threshold of tolerance for auditory signals, resulting in a decrease in the distorted auditory perceptions that led to social, language, and learning difficulties (Richard, 2000). The methodology was called the Ear Education and Retraining System (EERS).

The French Audiokinetron developed by Dr. Berard led to the development of a similar machine in the United States called the Audio Tone Enhancer/Trainer by the BGC Company. The inspiration for Dr. Berard was another AIT methodology developed by French physician Alfred Tomatis called the Tomatis Audio-Psycho-Phonology approach, which actually preceded the Berard method but was not as refined.

Professional certification and ethical questions were raised in the United States in regard to the AIT methodologies. The American Academic of Audiology (1993) and American Speech-Language-Hearing Association (1994) both adopted position statements reiterating the need for empirical research before engaging in AIT as part of one's professional practice. Research continues to produce mixed results in regard to the effectives of the methodology (Edelson et al., 1999; Madell, 1999; Tharpe, 1999). The diagnosing audiologist should carefully consider the advantages and disadvantages of recom-

mending AIT, to ensure that the potential benefits are consistent with the concerns present in an individual's auditory profile. The reader is referred to Chapter 4 in this volume for a review of auditory training efficacy and procedures.

Limitations of Commercial Programs to Deficit-Specific Intervention

Commercial products are generally designed to target a wide audience, resulting in a more general treatment approach. As a result, it is difficult to address specific deficits that have been identified during diagnostic procedures. This two-volume Handbook is testament to the complexity of auditory processes. For example, assessment batteries for (C)APD include evaluation of dichotic listening, yet there are no commercial products which target this auditory skill. (See Chapter 4 in this volume, however, for presentation of techniques to train dichotic listening.) Careful delineation of deficit symptoms within auditory processing has been emphasized repeatedly. Treatment programs need to more directly address the specific symptoms identified, rather than approach therapy in a generic methodology that encompasses multiple aspects.

Studies have been conducted on specific commercial programs, such as Earobics, Fast ForWord, LiPS, and AIT, producing some encouraging results with most of these programs. Developers of the commercial programs have a vested interest in positive results and conduct their own research projects, which can lead to biased results. The studies completed often used evaluation measures that were consistent with the program methodologies, positively skewing the results (McFarland & Cacace, 2006; Richard, 2000). (See Chapter 6 in this volume for discussion of computer-assisted intervention. Also, see Chapter 4 of Volume I of the Handbook for review of some studies of Earobics.)

Ferre (2006) provides a model for approaching the question of treatment effectiveness. She advocates asking three questions when trying to make methodology decisions in regard to treatment for auditory processing disorders:

- Does it work?
- Should it work?
- Does it make sense?

The first question is answered by determining if any efficacy data exist on the treatment methodology being considered. The professional should carefully evaluate the research studies, considering the age of the client and type of disorder identified. Generalization of data from research studies can be problematic when extrapolating from one clinical population to another.

The second question requires that the professional consider the theoretical constructs upon which the treatment methodology is founded. If the intervention approach makes clinical sense from a neuroscientific perspective, then it may be worth considering, despite a lack of empirical evidence (Ferre, 2006).

The final question is in relation to the differential aspect of (C)APD. Test results should be evaluated to determine which level(s) on the continuum are deficient and if the aspect in question is addressed in the treatment program. If a child has difficulty with figure-ground and background noise, then a recommendation for Fast ForWord is questionable. The treatment program needs to be attuned to the deficits evidenced in the evaluation.

There are a number of treatment options that have been advocated by var-

ious specialists in the area of auditory processing. These approaches are more informal than the commercially sequenced and programmed methodologies discussed in the previous section. However, the ability to customize a treatment program to the individual's presented deficits is critical to effective intervention. For example, deficits in binaural integration (e.g., dichotic listening) should be targeted more directly in treatment than would be accomplished in the general commercial programs. Exercises in figure-ground or sound localization can be generated using treatment guidelines from various sources that more specifically meet an individuals needs (e.g., Katz & Fletcher, 1982; Kelly, 1995; Masters et al.,1998; Richard, 2001; Sloan, 1986). In the absence of a commercially appropriate program, audiologists and speech-language pathologists must design programs and exercises using the guidance provided by a number of contributors to this Handbook.

As the audiologist might not be the professional responsible for treatment, a specific discussion of strengths and weaknesses derived from assessment results would be beneficial to include in the diagnostic report. A diagnosis of (C)APD and a generic list of environmental modifications is not particularly helpful to a parent or professional attempting to address the deficits evidenced during the evaluation. In addition, it is irresponsible to recommend a commercially expensive program that requires specific clinician training (e.g., Fast ForWord, LiPS), without justification of the auditory skills that need to be targeted. A generic approach is not the most effective way to approach intervention for any disorder, including (C)APD. (See Chapters 1 and 10 in this volume for additional discussion of deficit-specific intervention.

Treatment Effectiveness and Efficacy

Treatment efficacy refers to the effectiveness and efficiency of treatment. It requires documentation that a particular treatment produces the intended behavioral or physiological change in an efficient manner (e.g., cost- and time-effective) (Singh & Kent, 2000). Both concepts are important when addressing intervention. (See Chapter 2 in this volume for a discussion of evidence-based practice and efficacy.)

Good treatment can be poorly delivered and an excellent service delivery system can provide weak treatment. This statement is very powerful in addressing the concepts of treatment effectiveness and efficacy. An excellent treatment program that is commercially marketed and empirically researched can be applied to an individual in a manner that will render it ineffective. For example, the treatment program might be very worthwhile, but if it does not target the individual's deficits, then the program's benefit may be minimal and valuable treatment time will have been lost. On the other hand, an individual might be enrolled for private therapy every day, but if the professional providing service does not know what to work on, treatment will not be effective. Time and intensity of service do not guarantee results.

Summary

The term "auditory processing" encompasses an array of skills. (C)APD can occur in isolation or in association with other disorders, such as autism, ADHD, mental impairment, and cognitive disorders. The primary comorbid disorder can have a significant impact on the prognosis for treatment of the (C)APD. (C)APD presents some unique challenges for the professionals responsible for diagnosis, assessment, and intervention. The clinical implications of a (C)APD on academic performance are undeniable. The ASHA 2005 position paper on (C)APD emphasized the importance of an interdisciplinary approach to intervention. The ASHA working group also stated that goals should be deficit-driven, based on diagnostic assessment results and treatment methodology should be consistent with the principles of neuroscience (ASHA, 2005b). In summary, collaboration between audiologists and speech-language pathologists is essential to address the issues of efficacious treatment and service delivery in (C)APD.

References

American Academy of Audiology. (1993). Position statement: Auditory integration training. *Audiology Today, 5*, 21.

American Speech-Language-Hearing Association. (1994). Technical report on Auditory Integration Training. *ASHA, 36*, 55–58.

American Speech-Language-Hearing Association, Task Force on Central Auditory Processing Consensus Development. (1996). Central auditory processing: Current status of research and implication for clinical practice. *American Journal of Audiology 5*, 41–54.

American Speech-Language-Hearing Association. (2005a). Central auditory processing disorders (Technical report). Rockville, MD: Author.

American Speech-Language-Hearing Association. (2005b). *(Central) auditory processing disorders—The role of the audiolo-*

gist [Position statement]. Rockville, MD: Author.

Apel, K., Masterson, J., & Niessen, N. (2004). Spelling assessment frameworks. In C. Stone, E. Silliman, B. Ehren, & K. Apel (Eds.), *Handbook of language and literacy* (pp. 644–660). New York: The Guilford Press.

Bellis, T. (2003). *Assessment and management of central auditory processing disorders in the educational setting: From science to practice* (2nd ed.). Clifton Park, NY: Thompson Learning.

Bhatnagar, S., & Korabic, E. (2006). Neuroanatomy and neurophysiology of the central auditory pathways. In T. K. Parthasarathy (Ed.), *An introduction to auditory processing disorders in children* (pp. 1–19). Mahwah, NJ: Lawrence Erlbaum Associates.

Butler, K. (1981). Language processing disorders: Factors in diagnosis and remediation. In R. Keith (Ed.), *Central auditory and language disorders in children* (pp. 160–174). San Diego, CA: College-Hill Press.

Chermak, G., & Musiek, F. (1997). *Central auditory processing disorders: New perspectives.* San Diego, CA: Singular Publishing Group.

Chermak, G., & Musiek, F. (2002). Auditory training: Principles and approaches for remediating and managing auditory processing disorders. *Seminars in Hearing, 23*(4), 297–308.

Cognitive Concepts, Inc. (1998). *Earobics.* Evanston, IL: Author.

Duchan, J., & Katz, J. (1983). Language and auditory processing: Top down plus bottom up. In E. Lasky & J. Katz (Eds.), *Central auditory disorders: Problems of speech, language, and learning* (pp. 31–45). Baltimore: University Park Press.

Edelson, S., Arin, D., Bauman, M., Lukas, S., Rudy, J., Sholar, M., & Rimland, B. (1999). Auditory Integration Training: A double-blind study of behavioral and electrophysiological effects in people with autism. *Focus on Autism and Other Developmental Disabilities, 14*, 73–81.

Ferre, J. (2006). Management strategies for APD. In T. K. Parthasarathy (Ed.), *An introduction to auditory processing disorders in children* (pp. 161–185). Mahwah, NJ: Lawrence Erlbaum Associates.

Friel-Patti, S. (1994). Auditory linguistic processing and language learning. In G. Wallach & K. Butler (Eds.), *Language learning disabilities in school-aged children and adolescents* (pp. 373–392). New York: Macmillan College Publishing.

Gaddes, W. H. (1980). *Learning disabilities and brain function—A neuropsychological approach.* New York: Springer-Verlag.

Gerber, A., & Bryen, D. (1981). *Language and learning disabilities.* Baltimore: University Park Press.

Justice, L., & Schuele, C. (2004). Phonological awareness: Description, assessment, and intervention. In J. Bernthal & N. Bankson (Eds.), *Articulation and phonological disorders* (5th ed., pp. 376–405). Boston: Allyn & Bacon.

Kamhi, A. (1981). Nonlinguistic symbolic and conceptual abilities of language-impaired and normally developing children. *Journal of Speech and Hearing Research, 24*, 446–453.

Katz, J. (1978). Evaluation of central dysfunction. In J. Katz (Ed.), *Handbook of clinical audiology* (2nd ed., pp. 233–243). Baltimore: Williams & Wilkins.

Katz, J., & Fletcher, C. (1982). *Phonemic synthesis: Blending sounds into words.* Vancouver, WA: Precision Acoustics.

Keith, R. (1981). *Central auditory and language disorders in children.* San Diego, CA: College-Hill Press.

Kelly, D. (1995). *Central auditory processing disorders: Strategies for use with children and adults.* San Antonio, TX: The Psychological Corporation.

Lindamood-Bell Learning Processes. (1998). *Lindamood Phoneme Sequencing Program (LiPS).* San Luis Obispo, CA.

Lubert, N. (1981). Auditory perceptual impairments in children with specific language disorders: A review of the literature.

Journal of Speech and Hearing Disorders, *46,* 3-9.

Madell, J. (1999). Auditory Integration Training: One clinician's view. *Language, Speech and Hearing Services in Schools, 30,* 371-377.

Masters, M., Stecker, N., & Katz, J. (1998). *Central auditory processing disorders: Mostly management.* Boston: Allyn & Bacon.

McAndrews, S. (2006). Linking literacy assessment to diagnostic instructional strategies for children with an APD. In T. K. Parthasarathy (Ed.), *An introduction to auditory processing disorders in children* (pp. 109-143). Mahwah, NJ: Lawrence Erlbaum Associates.

McFarland, D., & Cacace, A. (2006). Current controversies in CAPD: From Procrustes' bed to Pandora's box. In T. K. Parthasarathy (Ed.), *An introduction to auditory processing disorders in children* (pp. 247-263). Mahwah, NJ: Lawrence Erlbaum Associates.

Noback, C. (1985). Neuroanatomical correlates of central auditory function. In M. Pinheiro & F. Musiek (Eds.), *Assessment of central auditory dysfunction* (pp. 7-21). Baltimore: Williams & Wilkins.

Protti, E. (1983). Brainstem auditory pathways and auditory processing disorders. In E. Lasky & J. Katz (Eds.), *Central auditory processing disorders* (pp. 117-139). Baltimore: University Park Press.

Rees, N. (1973). Auditory processing factors in language disorders: The view from Procrustes' bed. *Journal of Speech and Hearing Disorders, 38*(3), 304-315.

Rees, N. (1981). Saying more than we know: Is auditory processing disorder a meaningful concept? In R. Keith (Ed.), *Central auditory and language disorders in children.* San Diego, CA: College-Hill Press

Rice, M., & Kemper, S. (1984). *Child language and cognition.* Baltimore: University Park Press.

Richard, G. (2000). *The source for treatment methodologies in autism.* East Moline, IL: LinguiSystems.

Richard, G. (2001). *The source for processing disorders.* East Moline, IL: LinguiSystems.

Richard, G. (2006). Language based assessment and intervention of APD. In T. K. Parthasarathy (Ed.), *An introduction to auditory processing disorders in children* (pp. 95-108). Mahwah, NJ: Lawrence Erlbaum Associates.

Schow, R., & Chermak, G. (1999). Implications from factor analysis for central auditory processing disorders. *American Journal of Audiology, 8,* 137-142.

Scientific Learning Corporation. (1997). *Fast ForWord training program for children-Procedural manual for professionals.* Berkeley, CA.

Singh, S., & Kent, R. (2000). *Pocket dictionary of speech-language pathology.* San Diego, CA: Singular Publishing Group.

Sloan, C. (1986). *Treating auditory processing difficulties in children.* San Diego, CA: College-Hill Press.

Tallal, P. Stark, R., Kallman, C., & Mellits, D. (1981). A re-examination of some nonverbal perceptual abilities of language-impaired and normal children as a function of age and sensory modality. *Journal of Speech and Hearing Research, 24,* 351-357.

Tharpe, A. (1999). Auditory Integration Therapy: The magical mystery cure. *Language, Speech, and Hearing Services in Schools, 30,* 378-382.

Troia, G. (2004). Phonological processing and its influence on literacy learning. In C. Stone, E. Silliman, B. Ehren, & K. Apel (Eds.), *Handbook of language and literacy* (pp. 271-301). New York: The Guilford Press.

CHAPTER 12

INTERVENTION FOR INDIVIDUALS WITH (C)APD AND ADHD

A Psychological Perspective

WARREN D. KELLER AND KIM L. TILLERY

The history of clinicians and researchers studying "what we do with what we hear" dates back to the 1950s when dysfunction of the central auditory nervous system (CANS) was first reported (Bocca, Colearo, & Cassinari, 1954). The terminology used to describe dysfunction of the CANS has changed over the years; however, most recently these conditions are labeled as central auditory processing disorder (C)APD. Even though there is a growing literature on intervention for (C)APD, there seems to be a need for more evidence-based research to support the efficacy and effectiveness of these interventions. In fact, one United States based third-party provider concluded that "any diagnostic tests or therapies for the management of CAPD are experimental and investigational because there is insufficient scientific evidence to support the validity of any diagnostic tests and the effectiveness of any therapies for CAPD" (Aetna, 2005, p. 1). Aetna's policy is based upon "the limited evidence for (C)APD as a distinct pathophysiologic entity, upon a lack of evidence established criteria and well validated instruments to diagnose (C)APD and reliably distinguish it from other conditions affecting listening and/ or spoken language and comprehension, and upon the lack of evidence from well designed clinical studies proving the effectiveness for treating (C)APD" (Aetna, 2005, p. 3). The policy statement further elaborated that given the frequent comorbidities of (C)APD with other disorders that might affect listening or language comprehension, they concluded that (C)APD was not a distinct entity.

In reaching these conclusions, Aetna cited Chermak's (2002) overview of the nature, diagnosis, and treatment for (C)APD in which she noted that "additional controlled case studies and single-subject and group research designs are needed to ascertain systemically the relative efficacy of various treatment and management approaches" (p. 744). Unfortunately, Aetna seems to have misused this statement to ignore research that has been accomplished prior to and since 2002 that indicates that (C)APD is in fact a distinct clinical entity (e.g., Tillery, Katz, & Keller, 2000; see ASHA, 2005 for a review) and that "a solid base of evidence documents improved psychophysical performance, neurophysiologic representation of acoustic stimuli, and listening and related function in children and adults following targeted auditory training" (Musiek, Bellis, & Chermak, 2005, p. 2). Similar to Chermak (2002), Musiek et al. (2005) remarked, however, that more studies are needed to produce the level of evidence (e.g., randomized controlled trials; meta-analysis of randomized controlled trials) to establish the efficacy of various interventions. We would expect that many of the interested readers of this volume may well take issue with some of Aetna's conclusions.

Evidence-based practice (EBP) refers to the conscientious, explicit, and purposeful use of current research evidence, integrated with individual clinical expertise, to provide the best available care to patients (Sackett, Rosenberg, Muir Gray, Haynes, & Richardson, 1996). Criticism over the concept of EBP ranges from the fear that health care treatment will evolve into a "cookbook" approach without any attention to individual differences, to concerns that third-party reimbursers will feel empowered to further reduce coverage for health care treatment, and that the clinical freedom of the practi-

tioner will be suppressed. Notwithstanding these concerns, there has been a strong movement in psychology to adopt EBP policies and guidelines in psychology (Pelham, 1999), as there has been in other areas of health care delivery. For the study of and clinical service delivery for (C)APD to continue to advance, it is necessary that the field of audiology join with other professions in emphasizing EBP guidelines, where treatment becomes more rooted in research. In fact, such movement is evident in statements by professional audiology associations and publications (see for example the special issue on EBP of the *Journal of the American Academy of Audiology* (volume 16, number 7, 2005). (See Chapter 2 for discussion of EBP and efficacy.)

Intervention for (C)APD

(C)APD involves one or more deficits in localization, lateralization, auditory discrimination, pattern recognition skills, temporal processing, and performance decrements with competing or degraded auditory signals (ASHA, 1995, 1996, 2005. As these auditory deficits are associated with a range of functional deficits in listening, communication, language, and learning, a multidisciplinary assessment and intervention team approach is needed to delineate the deficient areas of function and to determine which interventions should be employed to improve those deficiencies (ASHA, 2005; Chermak & Musiek, 1997). Detailed reviews of the range of interventions appropriate for individuals with (C)APD are provided in Chapters 4, 5, and 7.

Difficulties associated with (C)APD include hearing in noise, following directions, and understanding speech, especially in the presence of background noise or competition (Katz & Smith, 1991). Although these behaviors may be associated with (C)APD, they may also be associated with other disorders (Keller, 1992, 1998; Keller & Tillery, 2002). Indeed (C)APD often presents comorbidly with attention deficit hyperactivity disorder (ADHD), learning disability, and language impairment, among others (Chermak & Musiek, 1997; Chermak, Hall, & Musiek, 1999; Keller, 1998). Although questionnaires cannot be used to diagnose (C)APD, they can be useful in describing some of the functional behavioral limitations associated with (C)APD. Behavioral questionnaires also may be useful in determining which other professionals should be involved in multidisciplinary assessment (Tillery, 1998). The general consensus of both clinicians and researchers is that the diagnosis and treatment of (C)APD needs to assume a multidisciplinary focus, thus leading to accurate diagnosis, assessment of related deficits and functional problems, and effective therapy and management (Keller & Tillery, 2002). (See Chapters 13, 14, and 15 in Volume I of this Handbook for discussion of differential diagnosis and Chapters 10 and 11 in this volume for additional discussion of differential intervention for children with language disorders, learning disabilities, and [C]APD.)

What Should (C)APD Mean to the Psychologist?

In instructing pediatric residents about neuropsychological assessment and treatment, the first author of this chapter would often begin the lecture by pre-senting a computerized tomography (CT) scan of a brain-injured adolescent with the referring question being "Is the patient capable of driving a motor vehicle?" Although a CT scan can certainly document the existence of a brain injury, the *functional behavioral limitations* accompanying the injury remain unknown without further neuropsychological assessment. Similarly, although a greater number of errors on the left in the competing condition of dichotic tests may document a particular (C)APD subtype (Katz & Smith, 1991; Katz, 1992) or (C)APD deficit (Bellis, 1999, 2002; Bellis & Ferre, 1999), it tells us little about the *functional behavioral limitations* accompanying the (C)APD. Furthermore, neuropsychological assessment, behavioral assessment, speech and language assessment, academic assessment, as well as the observations of parents, teachers, and other caregivers are needed to determine the extent to which the inability to process an auditory signal to the left ear in a competing condition is actually impairing, limiting, and adversely affecting the quality of an individual's life.

Although there has been some discussion of the greater need to document the neurophysiologic basis for a (C)APD, it is our position that the *functional behavioral limitations* of (C)APD need to be described for the concept to have clinical validity or utility. The ASHA (1995) consensus statement recommended that an emphasis be placed on describing the functional limitations accompanying impairments in auditory processing. That statement, combined with the more recent technical report (ASHA, 2005), encourages audiologists to continue to document the underlying CANS dysfunction seen in referred clients, while seeking with other team members to fully explore their listening, communication, learning, and social issues.

A disorder is not a disorder unless it adversely affects the quality of one's life and has pervasive deleterious effects in several areas of life functioning. One cannot argue that an individual who returns home to check to see if he or she actually unplugged the coffee pot has an anxiety disorder, but if anxiety prevents the individual from developing close interpersonal relationships, prevents the person from remaining at work due to panic, leads to underachievement due to the fear of failure, induces an excessive fear of risks, then clearly the anxiety becomes debilitating and a disorder. The impairments that individuals with ADHD experience in a school setting and in their psychosocial development, along with the associated features of anxiety, depression, predisposition to substance use disorders, underachievement, and learning difficulties are well documented (Barkley, 1990, 1998).

In over 25 years of clinical practice as a neuropsychologist, the first author continues to encounter clinicians, teachers, school personnel, and other professionals who doubt the reality of (C)APD. In our judgment, these doubts stem from the need for more research to document the *associated features and functional behavioral limitations* correlated with (C)APD. To accomplish this, an audiologist should access the expertise and assessment of others to determine fully the extent to which, for example, the inability to process an auditory signal to the left ear while receiving a competing signal to the right ear is exerting functional limitations on the quality of one's life. Bamiou, Musiek, and Luxon (2001) stated that the assessment of (C)APD requires a multidisciplinary approach,

based upon a synthesis of information from medical, educational, and developmental histories, behavioral and electrophysiologic tests, as well as procedures from neuroimaging, speech and language evaluation, and psychological/cognitive evaluation. To provide the best treatment and management once a diagnosis is made, we need to determine the functional limitations associated with the disorder. If audiologic research were able to reliably and validly document particular (C)APD subtypes, and their associated comorbidities, this would enhance our understanding and improve effective treatment of (C)APD (Keller & Tillery, 2002). The authors have practiced clinically and have been involved in research during the past decade with the goal of better understanding just what (C)APD should mean to the psychologist. The inability to efficiently and correctly process auditory information can have far reaching effects on an individual's learning, attention, behavior and ultimately, quality of life. The associated features of (C)APD are becoming more clearly understood (ASHA, 2005).

Keller, Tillery, and McFadden (submitted for publication) have described some of the associated impairments of (C)APD in children with a particular subtype of learning disorder. Although there has been speculation about the prevalence of (C)APD (Chermak & Musiek, 1997), we found that the prevalence of (C)APD among a population of children with nonverbal learning disabilities (NVLD) was 65%. Ninety-one percent of the children from this sample exhibited a type of (C)APD, namely the tolerance-fading memory (TFM) subtype of (C)APD, as defined by Katz and Smith (1991). Although we still are substantiating the validity of the proposed subtypes of

(C)APD (ASHA, 2005), it is clear that a multidisciplinary approach will be helpful in this process (Keller et al., submitted). (See Chapter 5 in Volume I of the Handbook and Chapter 10 in this volume for discussion of subprofiling [C]APD.)

We have found, for example, that particular subtests from the Wechsler Intelligence Scale for Children-III (Psychological Corporation, 1989) were also associated with auditory processing disorders. Children with (C)APD exhbited greater impairments on the Information, Similarities, Arithmetic, Vocabulary, Comprehension, and Digit Span subtests of the Wechsler Scales. Finding greater difficulty on the arithmetic subtest might be explained on the basis of the reliance of this measure on "mental math," which involves auditory processing of information and working memory, the latter of which is known to support auditory processing (Marler, Champlin, & Gillam, 2002; Martinkauppi, Rama, Aronen, Korvenoja, & Carolson, 2002; Zattore, 2001). Children with auditory processing disorders from this sample also showed an inverse correlation between measured intelligence and (C)APD status, indicating that those with higher measured intelligence tended to compensate better for their auditory processing disabilities. Unfortunately, the arithmetic subtest is now an optional test on the newly reformatted Wechsler Intelligence Scale for Children (WISC-IV) (Psychological Corporation, 2003) and Digit Span performance, which did not contribute to one's overall measured intelligence, on prior versions, is now included in the overall intelligence score. Both changes may serve to penalize many children with (C)APD and may lead to an under-diagnosis of learning disorders, given the continuing emphasis on the *discrepancy model* (i.e., between intelligence and performance) used to identify children with learning disabilities. Furthermore, inclusion of a new measure of processing speed in the WISC-IV may also lead to suppressed intelligence scores for children with (C)APD.

Children with (C)APD from this sample also exhibited uniform weaknesses on standardized measures of memory functioning, the Wide Range Assessment of Memory and Learning (WRAML). In addition to the General Memory score being suppressed in children with (C)APD, their overall verbal memory scores, overall visual memory scores, and their ability to improve memory with repeated trials (i.e., the learning scale composite score) was significantly weaker in children with (C)APD. Ten of the 12 tests involving memory for recent information were suppressed in this sample, for the first time documenting the memory deficits that have been purported to accompany the TFM subtype of (C)APD (Katz & Smith, 1991). It is this type of documentation that is necessary to establish the *functional behavioral limitations* of children with (C)APD. Once again, a multidisciplinary team assists to comprehensively explore and document functional deficits, as different professionals focus on different areas of disability (e.g., the audiologist focuses on auditory processing and listening, the psychologist focuses on cognition and behavior, and the speech-language pathologist focuses on language and communication).

On further neuropsychological evaluation, the Speech Sounds Perception test (Reitan & Wolfson, 1993), an auditory perceptual measure involving sound/symbol correspondences was the only neuropsychological measure associated with (C)APD status for which performance was impaired. Although the incidence of ADHD is believed to be 4 to 6% of the population (Barkley, 1990), the incidence of ADHD among this sample of children was 18%. Clearly, (C)APD is associated with a larger range of deficits than just an inability to process auditory signals.

What Is ADHD?

Three main behaviors impulsivity, hyperactivity, and inattention, if inappropriate to the child's chronologic age, characterize one of the most common childhood disorders, ADHD (Barkley, 1990, 1998). Currently, the *Diagnostic and Statistical Manual of Mental Disorders (DSM-IV)* (American Psychiatric Association, 1994) describes ADHD as falling into three particular subtypes: (1) Hyperactive-Impulsive ADHD-HI, (2) Predominantly Inattentive (ADHD-PI), and (3) Combined (ADHD-C). Individuals with ADHD exhibit difficulties that are cross-situational, occurring in both home and school environments, when interacting with family members and with peers. Most social situations will be challenging for such individuals as they have difficulty engaging in appropriate activity levels and reducing their impulsivity and maintaining their attention. Poor self-control, lying, stealing, aggressiveness, temper outbursts, noncompliance, and weak peer relations are usually seen as associated features.

Children with ADHD are especially difficult to discipline and parents exhibit a tendency to approach these children using increased coercive parenting strategies. Socioemotional difficulties include explosive behaviors, low self-esteem, low frustration tolerance, and mood swings that most certainly challenge the individual and family, further causing children with ADHD to be disliked by peers (Pelham & Bender, 1982). The general health of an individual with ADHD is usually poor, with histories of chronic otitis media (Hagerman & Falkenstein, 1987), disturbance in sleep/wake patterns (Barkley, 1998), minor physical anomalies (Pomeroy, Sprafkin, & Gadow, 1988), and poor motor coordination (Barkley, 1998) being characteristic. Impulsivity in the classroom is seen in interactions with classmates as children with ADHD have difficulty sharing, are highly impulsive, may be the first to run to the head of the line, and have difficulty following rules and regulations. A negative cycle begins with these types of behaviors and difficulties, which results in peer rejection, conflict within the family, temper outbursts, and increased frustration and confusion for all involved.

Academic difficulties seen in ADHD include specific learning disabilities and underachievement. It also has been demonstrated that the incidence of (C)APD occurs more frequently in individuals with ADHD (Keller & Tillery, 2002; Tillery et. al., 2000). Learning disabilities occur comorbidly with the general estimate that 25 to 40% exhibit an associated learning disability (Keller, 1992). In addition, although many individuals with ADHD may experience a comorbid learning disorder, up to 90% will manifest academic underachievement due to the primary attentional and behavioral problems that affect their learning. When evaluated in a one-to-one setting, these individuals may show above-average or superior academic performance, yet often are failing in the academic setting (Barkley, 1998). Teachers often describe these children as having a short attention span as they are unable to complete assignments or stay on task, they may take inordinate amounts of time to complete basic assignments, or they may rush through the assignments causing inaccuracies.

ADHD for most is a life-long disorder with only approximately 30% of individuals with ADHD outgrowing their symptomatology over time (Barkley, 1990, 1998). Adults with ADHD make more frequent moves, experience more tumultuous interpersonal relationships, are involved in more automobile accidents, switch jobs more frequently, and are much more prone to experience problems with alcohol and substance abuse (Barkley, 1990, 1998).

ADHD also has been referred to as an arousal disorder as evidence suggests that individuals with ADHD may be experiencing an underarousal of the central nervous system (CNS) (Zametkin, Nordahl & Gross, 1990). Lou, Henrickson, and Bruhn (1984) described a hypoperfusion of blood flow in the frontal area of the brain in children and adults with ADHD. Increased slow brain wave activity seen in some individuals with ADHD has been the subject of increased interest both clinically and from a diagnostic research perspective (Monastra, Lubar, & Linde, 1998). Neuropsychologically, individuals with ADHD will often evidence functional impairments on measures of executive functioning and impaired performance on measures such as the Category Test (Reitan & Wolfson, 1993) or the Wisconsin Card Sort Test (Grant & Berg, 1981), which are executive function tasks believed to be sensitive to frontal lobe functions such as reasoning, problem-solving, and inhibiting impulsive behavior.

Diagnosing and Assessing ADHD

It is the authors' clinical judgment that ADHD cannot be reliably and validly diagnosed on the basis of standardized parental and/or teacher report measures alone. Clinically elevated scores on standardized behavioral measures only indicate the presence of symptomatology that may be characteristic of ADHD; such scores indicate nothing about the underlying causes of the reported behaviors. The DSM-IV criteria for ADHD outline specific behavioral symptoms of inattention, hyperactivity, and impulsivity required to meet the diagnosis of ADHD. Merely asking parents whether or not their child seemingly does not listen, is always "on the go," or talks excessively and interrupts or intrudes on others can lead to an improper diagnosis (Colegrove, Homayounjan, Williams, & Hanken, 2001).

A comprehensive assessment of ADHD should include not only the behavioral observations of teachers, parents, and other caregivers, but also should include objective measures of sustained attention and concentration to demonstrate that the impairments a child exhibits deviate from that which we would expect from children at a specific chronologic or mental age. The administration of the Weschler Scales, as part of a comprehensive assessment of ADHD, allows the clinician to obtain an objective assessment on tasks that load substantially on the capacity for sustained attention. Comparing cognitive competence with performance on standardized memory tests will often yield statistically significant differences that reflect difficulties sustaining attention to that which we are asking the individual to remember. One of the prerequisites to remembering information is being able to sustain attention to the information to be retained.

A comprehensive medical and developmental history, as well as standardized, normed behavioral measures should be obtained to comprehensively assess behavior that may suggest ADHD. In addition, an assessment of cognitive and memory functions may provide additional information regarding whether an individual's inattention, hyperactivity, and impulsivity, deviate significantly from what we might expect from individuals at the same chronologic age. Given the high comorbity between ADHD and specific learning disorders, psychoeducational assessments and academic measures should be obtained to rule out whether inattention may be secondary to a learning disability and not primarily ADHD. The use of continuous performance tests also allows the clinician to objectively assess an individual's capacity for sustained attention. An assessment of socioemotional and personality factors also needs to be completed to rule out whether or not factors such as anxiety and depression are the causes of the individual's inattention, hyperactivity, and impulsivity.

Evidence-Based Treatments for Children with ADHD

Increasingly in psychology and psychiatry, there has been an emphasis upon the use of treatment interventions that have empirical support for their effectiveness (Pelham, Wheeler, & Chronis,

1998). There has been some controversy among academic psychologists and clinicians, with the latter group arguing that clinical research cannot always document some of the subtle positive changes that occur as the result of psychotherapy. Increasingly, managed care companies and other third-party insurance carriers, as well as consumers of mental health care themselves, have demanded that empirical support be provided for the interventions that are used to treat a variety of mental health disorders, including ADHD (Pelham, 1999). This emphasis on evidence-based practice (EBP) is consistent with the scientist-practitioner model, or Boulder model, that has been at the core of psychological training and practice for more than 50 years, emphasizing an intimate relationship between clinical practice and science (Raimy, 1950).

As early as 1995, the American Psychological Association Task Force on Promotion and Dissemination of Psychological Procedures developed guidelines for empirically supported treatments for psychosocial interventions for childhood mental disorders (Pelham, 1999). These guidelines stipulated that to develop criteria for well-established psychosocial interventions it was necessary to have at least two well-conducted group design studies, conducted by different investigators, showing the treatment to be either superior to pill placebo or alternative treatments, or equivalent to an already established treatment. Random assignment to study comparison groups was required. Criteria could also include a large series of single-case design studies that used both good experimental design and compared the intervention to another treatment. Case studies in and of themselves, however, were deemed inadequate to demonstrate treatment efficacy and establish a treatment approach that would meet the criteria for EBP. The guidelines also indicated that it was preferable that treatment manuals be developed to provide for standardization of the treatment. The Niagara Conference (Pelham, 1999) was established so that researchers and clinicians could review the increasing documentation or evidence-based treatments for a variety of issues and disorders among children including ADHD, drugs and substance abuse, and interventions for children of divorce, depression, and other internalizing disorders.

The National Institute of Mental Health and Department of Education sponsored the well-known Multimodal Treatment Study of ADHD (MTA Study) to investigate which evidence-based treatments would be most efficacious for children with ADHD (MTA Cooperative Group, 1999). Four study groups, involving 578 children, were assigned either: (1) medication alone in a very carefully titrated fashion, (2) psychosocial treatments alone including behavioral interventions, also involving parent education, (3) community care (control group), or (4) a combination of medication and psychosocial interventions. The combination of medication and psychosocial treatments group was found to yield benefits not seen in the therapy or medication only groups. Parents expressed greater satisfaction with nonpharmacologic interventions.

ADHD has met the rigorous criteria documenting the range of empirically supported treatments, both psychosocial and pharmacologic, that are of assistance in ameliorating the symptomatology associated with this disorder. It would be advantageous for researchers and clinicians to adopt similar guidelines and research designs in the study of (C)APD to advance the validity and clinical utility of the construct, and reaffirm (C)APD as a distinct clinical entity that not only can be accurately diagnosed, but also effectively treated.

The associated features of ADHD often become the focus of treatment (Keller, 1992). A combined treatment approach utilizing stimulant medication, therapy, parent and classroom behavioral training, and educating family, teachers, and the individual regarding ADHD are essential components of evidence-based treatments for ADHD (Barkley, 1998). Most children, between 70 to 80%, respond with an immediate and positive improvement, when provided stimulant medication (Barkley, 1990, 1998). Treatment efficacy is improved when the range of available stimulant medications is considered. Behavioral functioning is improved and treatment efficacy is enhanced with the use of behavioral interventions including use of novelty, immediate feedback, and daily report cards combined with incentives (Pelham, Wheeler, & Chronis, 1998). For the small percentage of individuals who do not respond to stimulant medication, the range of psychosocial and behavioral interventions may prove effective.

Stimulant Medications

Psychosocial interventions have been described above that meet the standards for empirically supported treatments. Individualized medication management also is well established as evidence-based treatment for individuals with ADHD, with considerable research establishing its effectiveness in well-controlled studies that meet the criteria for empirically supported treatments (Barkley, 1998; MTA Cooperative Group, 1999).

Newer stimulant medications such as Adderall XR, Concerta, Focalin XR, Ritalin LA, and Metadate are longer acting medications that avoid multiple dosing throughout the day. It is expected that the Food and Drug Administration will release the use of the amphetamine patch sometime this year that will permit yet another delivery system for stimulant medication that may well be advantageous for many individuals (*Physician's Desk Reference,* 2005).

Strattera, or atomoxetine, is the first selective norepinephrine reuptake inhibitor that has been approved for treatment of ADHD (*Physician's Desk Reference,* 2005). Given the purported role of dysfunction of the norepinephrine and/or dopaminergic systems in ADHD, Straterra may be appropriate for some individuals with greater involvement of the norepinephrine system.

Provigil or modafanil is an agent used in the treatment of narcolepsy, an arousal disorder (*Physician's Desk Reference,* 2005). Although Provigil is indicated to improve the wakefulness of individuals experiencing the excessive daytime sleepiness associated with narcolepsy, its value as an efficacious pharmacologic treatment for ADHD is being investigated and the medication is already being used clinically despite limited empirical support.

As our knowledge of ADHD grows, it is expected that we will be able to gain an even greater understanding of the disorder so that the specific medication prescribed will be tailored to the specific genetic subtype of ADHD. Such specification of diagnosis will improve our capability to provide evidence-based treatments.

Evidence-Based Treatments for Children with (C)APD

Although the functional impairments associated with ADHD, and its adverse impact on academic, socioemotional, and long-term development are well documented, the associated features and the impact of (C)APD are still being documented through controlled research studies (Chermak, 2002; Musiek et al., 2005). Several recommendations for comprehensive intervention programs have been proposed (e.g., Bellis, 2003; Chermak & Musiek, 1997) and a number of commercially available software programs and print workbooks also are available. These programs generally focus on three areas: auditory training, signal enhancement, and central resources training (i.e., metacognition, metalanguage, and cognition). Remediation programs that purport to be useful in the treatment and management of (C)APD include: Earobics (Cognitive Concepts, 1997, 1998), Fast ForWord Training Program (Scientific Learning Corporation, 1997), (C)APD Strategies for Children and Adolescents (Kelly, 1995); Processing Power (Ferre, 1997), Phonemic Synthesis Training (Katz & Harmon-Fletcher, 1982); and Lindamood Phoneme Sequencing Program (LiPS) (Lindamood-Bell Learning Processes, 1998).

A number of interventions for (C)APD have been demonstrated to be effective. Most of the efficacy data have been obtained in support of auditory training (e.g., Hayes, Warrier, Nicol, Zecker, & Kraus, 2003; Jirsa, 1992; Kraus & Disterhoft, 1982; Kraus, McGee, Carrell, King, Tremblay, & Nicol, 1995; Merzenich, Grajski, Jenkins, Recanzone, & Perterson, 1991; Merzenich et al., 1996; Miller &

Knudsen, 2003; Musiek, Baran, & Pinheiro, 1992; Musiek, Baran, & Shinn, 2004; Russo, Nicol, Zecker, Hayes, & Kraus, 2005; Tallal et al., 1996; Tremblay & Kraus, 2002; Tremblay, Kraus, Carrell, & McGee, 1997; Tremblay, Kraus, & McGee, 1998; Tremblay, Kraus, McGee, Ponton, & Otis, 2001; Warrier, Johnson, Hayes, Nicol, & Kraus, 2004) and signal enhancement strategies (Blake, Field, Foster, Platt, & Wertz, 1991; Crandell, 1998; Rosenberg, 2002; Stach, Loiselle, Jerger, Mintz, & Taylor, 1987). Research also has demonstrated the value of preferential seating, visual cues (i.e., auditory-visual summation) and preteaching of information for children with (C)APD (Crandell & Smaldino, 2001; Massaro, 1987). Fewer studies have documented the efficacy of central resources training. (See Chapter 5 for a review of efficacy studies in this area.) Additional research regarding the range of (C)APD interventions meeting the strict criteria and highest standards for EBP is needed (i.e., well-designed, randomized controlled trials) as acknowledged by professional organizations representing audiology and others (ASHA, 1996; Bellis, 2002; Chermak, 2001; Cox, 2005; Ferre, 2002; Valente, 2005).

Differential Interventions for ADHD and (C)APD

Interventions designed to treat and manage children and adults with ADHD focus on the amelioration of symptomatology associated with the disorder, namely, improving sustained attention and concentration, reducing noncompliance, improving school performance, and developing improved social skills. As elaborated above, evidence-based treatments have been shown to be effective in improving performance in these deficit areas.

As we develop evidence-based treatments for individuals with (C)APD, it will be important to designate the specific symptomatology associated with (C)APD that we are attempting to address. We are still in the process of delineating the specific deficits accompanying specific types of (C)APD (ASHA, 2005). It is reasonable to assume that not all interventions employed for individuals with (C)APD will effectively address the entire range of deficits that may be experienced by this very heterogeneous group. Similar to intervention for ADHD, intervention for (C)APD will most always be multifaceted.

Keller & Tillery (2002) speculated on different treatment approaches that may be effective for individuals with comorbid ADHD and (C)APD, as well as approaches that might be helpful for individuals with (C)APD alone or only ADHD. It is without debate that medication is an effective treatment for the large majority of individuals with ADHD (although as shown in the MTA study, multiple interventions are most effective). These same medications do not appear to be effective treatment for those with (C)APD (Tillery et al., 2000). The Tillery et al. study begins to document treatment approaches that meet the stringent standards for evidence-based treatment. If an individual exhibits both disorders, they should receive the evidence-based treatments that have been shown to be effective for ADHD in combination with the evidence-based treatments that have been (and will be) shown to be effective for (C)APD (e.g., auditory and metacognitive training, preferential seating, environmental modifications, self-advocacy, pretutoring, medication management, psychosocial treatments, parent education, behavioral interventions, etc.).

Multicultural Issues

The decision to seek evaluation and treatment for either ADHD or (C)APD is in large part dependent upon an individual's knowledge about the disorder and its effects on development. There is certainly an indication that ADHD has not become a significant part of the consciousness of African-American social networks. African-American parents describe themselves as being less aware and less knowledgeable about ADHD than their Caucasian peers (Bussing, Schoenberg, & Perwien, 1998). Given that ADHD is not as well known among African-American parents, we might assume that this is also true for (C)APD. Indeed, we do not know whether the prevalence of (C)APD varies across racial and ethnic groups, although given the ethnic/racial differences in incidence of chronic otitis media, sickle cell anemia, noise-induced hearing loss, fetal alcohol syndrome, and other conditions often associated with (C)APD, one might hypothesize varying prevalence as well (Chermak & Musiek, 1997). Less knowledge about any disorder will certainly impact adversely upon accessing effective treatment. Efforts to inform and educate people of various multicultural groups need to be accomplished and services need to be provided in a manner that is sensitive to issues of cultural diversity.

Summary

ADHD was first described in the medical literature as early as the 1900s and our knowledge of the disorder has been increasing exponentially since that time. The use of stimulant medications in the treatment of ADHD has occurred at least since 1935 (Barkley, 1998). Research efforts since then have been able to delineate treatment approaches, both pharmacologic and psychosocial, that have been documented as efficacious and with empirical support. In contrast, the concept of (C)APD was given birth by Helmer Myklebust in the 1950s when he first began emphasizing that higher level auditory processes needed to be investigated rather than just peripheral hearing function (Myklebust, 1954). Katz (1962) developed one of the first dichotic tests to assess the integrity of the central auditory system and the field of (C)APD blossomed. Clearly, the science and practice of (C)APD is in its infancy when compared to ADHD. (See Chapter 5 in Volume I of the Handbook for historical perspectives.)

We are beginning to understand better the associated features and functional deficits that have an adverse impact on individuals with (C)APD. We have been studying ADHD for well over 100 years and are now beginning to describe empirically supported treatments. Certainly in the next several decades, if we model our research efforts on those utilized for the investigation of ADHD, we will develop more empirically supported customized interventions for (C)APD. For the science and practice of (C)APD to continue to evolve and mature, efforts need to focus on a multidisciplinary approach to differentiate specific profiles or subtypes of (C)APD and their associated *functional behavioral limitations*.

References

Aetna. (2005). Central auditory processing disorder (CAPD). *Clinical Policy Bulletin*. No. 0668, pp. 1–4.

American Psychiatric Association. (1994). *Diagnostic and statistical manual of mental disorders* (4th ed.). Washington DC: Author.

American Psychological Association Task Force on Promotion and Dissemination of Psychological Procedures. (1995). Training in and dissemination of empirically validated treatments. *The Clinical Psychologist, 48*, 2-3.

American Speech-Language-Hearing Association (ASHA). (1995). *Central auditory processing current status of research and implications for clinical practice.* A report from the Task Force on Central Auditory Processing. Rockville, MD: Author.

American Speech-Language- Hearing Association (ASHA) Task Force on Central Auditory Processing Consensus Development. (1996). Central auditory processing: Current status of research and implications for clinical practice. *American Journal of Audiology, 5*, 41-54.

American Speech-Language- Hearing Association (ASHA) (2005). (Central) auditory processing disorders (Technical report). Rockville, MD: Author.

Bamiou, D. E., Musiek, F. E., & Luxon, L. M. (2001). Aetiology and clinical presentations of auditory processing disorders: A review. *Archives of Disorders of Children, 85*, 361-365.

Barkley, R. A. (1990). *Attention deficit hyperactivity disorder: A handbook for diagnosis and treatment.* New York: Guilford Press.

Barkley, R. A. (1998). *Attention-deficit hyperactivity disorder: A handbook for diagnosis and treatment* (2nd ed.). New York: Guilford Press.

Bellis, T. J. (1999). Subprofiles of central auditory processing disorders. *Education Audiology Review, 2*, 9-14.

Bellis, T. J. (2002). Developing deficit-specific intervention plans for individuals with auditory processing disorders. *Seminars in Hearing, 23*(4), 287-295.

Bellis, T. J. (2003). *Assessment and management of central auditory processing disorders in the educational setting: From science to practice* (2nd ed.). Clifton Park, NY: Thompson Learning.

Bellis, T. J., & Ferre, J. M. (1999). Multidimensional approach to the differential diagnosis of central auditory processing disorders in children. *Journal of the American Academy of Audiology, 10*(6), 319-328.

Blake, R., Field, B., Foster, C., Platt, F., & Wertz, P. (1991). Effect of FM auditory trainers on attending behaviors of learning disabled children. *Language, Speech and Hearing Services in Schools, 22*, 111-114.

Bocca, E., Calearo, C., & Cassinari, V. (1954). A new method for testing hearing in temporal lobe tumor. *Acta Otolaryngologica, 44*, 219-221.

Bussing, R., Schoenberg, N. E., & Perwien, A. R. (1998). Knowledge and information about AD/HD; evidence of cultural differences among African-American and white parents. *Social Science and Medicine, 46*(7), 919-928.

Chermak, G. D. (2001). Auditory processing disorder: An overview for the clinician. *Hearing Journal, 54*(7), 10-25.

Chermak, G. D. (2002). Deciphering auditory processing disorders in children. *Otolaryngology Clinics of North America, 35*(4), 733-749.

Chermak, G. D., Hall, J. W., & Musiek, F. E. (1999). Differential diagnosis and management of central auditory processing disorder and attention deficit hyperactivity disorder. *Journal of the American Academy of Audiology, 10*, 289-303.

Chermak, G. D., & Musiek, F. E. (1997). *Central auditory processing disorders: New perspectives.* San Diego, CA: Singular Publishing Group.

Cognitive Concepts. (1997). Earobics—auditory development and phonics program. Evanston, IL: Author.

Cognitive Concepts. (1998). Earobics—step two auditory development and phonics program. Evanston, IL: Author.

Colegrove, R., Homayounjan, H., Williams, J., & Hanken, J. (2001). Reducing the over identification of childhood ADHD: A stepwise diagnostic model. *ADHD Report, 9*, 4.

Cox, R. (2005). Evidence-based practice in audiology. *Journal of the American Academy of Audiology*, *16*(7), 408–409.

Crandell, C. (1998). Page ten: Utilizing sound field FM amplication in the educational setting. *Hearing Journal*, *51*, 10–19.

Crandell, C. & Smaldino, J. (2001). Acoustical modifications for the classroom. In C. Crandell & J. Smaldino (Eds.), Classroom acoustics: Understanding barriers to learning. *Volta Review*, *101*, 33–46.

Ferre, J. M. (1997). *Processing power: A guide to CAPD assessment and management.* San Antonio, TX: Communication Skill Builders.

Ferre, J. M. (2002). Behavioral therapeutic approaches for central auditory problems. In J. Katz (Ed.), *Handbook of clinical audiology* (5th ed., pp. 525–531). Philadelphia: Lippincott Williams and Wilkins.

Grant, D., & Berg, E. (1981). *Wisconsin Card Sort Test.* Odessa, FL: Psychological Assessment Resources, Inc.

Hagerman, R., & Falkenstein, A. (1987). An association between recurrent otitis media in infancy and later hyperactivity. *Clinical Pediatrics*, *5*, 253–257.

Hayes, E. A., Warrier, C. M., Nichol, T. G., Zecker, S. G., & Kraus, N. (2003). Neural plasticity following auditory training in children with learning problems. *Clinical Neurophysiology*, *114*, 673–684.

Jirsa, R. E. (1992). The clinical utility of the P3 AERP in children with auditory processing disorders. *Journal of Speech and Hearing Research*, *35*, 903–912.

Katz, J. (1962). The use of staggered spondaic words for assessing the integrity of the central auditory system. *Journal of Auditory Research*, *2*, 327–337.

Katz, J. (1992). Classification of auditory processing disorders. In J. Katz, N. Stecker, & D. Henderson (Eds.), *Central auditory processing: A transdisciplinary view* (pp. 81–93). St. Louis, MO: Mosby Year Book.

Katz, J., & Harmon-Fletcher, C. (1982). *Phonemic Synthesis Program Training.* Vancouver, WA: Precision Acoustics.

Katz, J., & Smith, P. (1991). The Staggered Spondaic Word Test: A ten-minute look at the central nervous system through the ears. *Annals of the New York Academy of Sciences*, *620*, 233–251.

Keller, W. (1992). Auditory processing disorder or attention deficit disorder? In J. Katz, N. Stecker, & D. Henderson (Eds.), *Central auditory processing: A transdisciplinary view* (pp 107–114). St. Louis, MO: Mosby.

Keller, W. (1998). The relationship between attention deficit hyperactivity disorder, central auditory processing disorders, and specific learning disorders. In G. Masters, N. Stecker, & J. Katz (Eds.), *Central auditory processing disorders: Mostly management* (pp. 33–48). Boston: Allyn & Bacon.

Keller, W., & Tillery, K. (2002). Reliable differential diagnosis and effective management of auditory processing and attention deficit hyperactivity disorders. *Seminars in Hearing*, *23*(4), 337–348.

Keller, W., Tillery, K. L., & McFadden, S. (2006). *Auditory processing disorders in children diagnosed with nonverbal learning disorders.* Manuscript submitted for publication.

Kelly, D. A. (1995). *Central auditory processing disorder: Strategies for use with children and adolescents.* San Antonio, TX: Communication Skill Builder.

Kraus, N., & Disterhoft, J. F. (1982). Response plasticity of single neurons in rabbit auditory association cortex during tone-signalled learning. *Brain Research*, *246*(2), 205–215.

Kraus, N., McGee, T., Carrell, T., King, C., Tremblay, K. & Nicol, T. (1995). Central auditory system plasticity associated with speech discrimination training. *Journal of Cognitive Neuroscience*, *71*(1), 25–32.

Lindamood-Bell Learning Processes. (1998). LiPS. Lindamood phoneme sequencing program. San Luis Obispo, CA: Author.

Lou, H., Henrickson, L., & Bruhn, P. (1984). Focal cerebral hypoperfusion in children with dysphasia and/or attention deficit disorder. *Archives of Neurology*, *41*, 825–829.

Marler, J. A., Champlin, C. A., & Gillam, R. B. (2002). Auditory memory for backward masking signals in children with language impairment. *Psychophysiology, 39,* 767–780.

Martinkauppi, S., Rama, P., Aronen, H. J., Korvenoja, A., & Carolson, S. (2002). Working memory of auditory localization. *Cerebral Cortex, 10,* 889–898.

Massaro, D. W. (1987). *Speech perception by ear and eye: A paradigm for psychological inquiry.* Hillsdale, NJ: Lawrence Erlbaum.

Merzenich, M. M., Grajski, K., Jenkins, W., Recanzone, G., & Perterson, B. (1991). Functional cortical plasticity. Cortical network origins of representations changes. *Cold Spring Harbor Symposium on Quantitative Biology, 55,* 873–887.

Merzenich, M. M., Jenkins, W. M. Johnston, P., Schreiner, C., Miller, S. L. & Tallal, P. (1996). Temporal processing deficits of language-learning impaired children ameliorated by training. *Science, 271,* 77–80.

Miller, G. L. & Knudsen, E. I. (2003). Adaptive plasticity in the auditory thalamus of juvenile barn owls. *Journal of Neuroscience, 23*(3), 1059–1065.

Monastra, V. J., Lubar, J. F., & Linde, M. (1998). Assessing attention deficit hyperactivity disorder via quantitative electroencephalography: an initial validation study. *Neuropsychology, 13,* 424–433.

MTA Cooperative Group. (1999). A 14-month randomized clinical trial of treatment strategies for attention-deficit/hyperactive disorder. *Archives of General Psychiatry, 56,* 1073–1086.

Musiek, F. E., Baran, J. A., & Pinheiro, M. L. (1992). P300 results in patients with lesions of the auditory areas of the cerebrum. *Journal of the American Academy of Audiology, 3,* 5–15.

Musiek, F. E., Baran, J. A., & Shinn, J. (2004). Assessment and remediation of an auditory processing disorder associated with head trauma. *Journal of the American Academy of Audiology, 15*(2), 117–132.

Musiek, F. E., Bellis, T. J., & Chermak, G. D. (2005). Nonmodularity of the CANS: Implications for (central) auditory processing disorder: A critique of Cacace and McFarland's "The Importance of Modality Specificity in Diagnosing Central Auditory Processing Disorder (CAPD)." *American Journal of Audiology, 14,* 128–138.

Myklebust, H. R. (1954). *Auditory processing disorders in children: A manual for differential diagnosis.* New York: Grune and Stratton.

Pelham, W. E. (1999). Evidence based treatments for childhood disorders: Section initiatives. *Clinical Child Psychology Newsletter, 14*(1), 1–3.

Pelham, W. E., & Bender, M. (1982). Peer relationships and hyperactive children: Description and treatment. In K. Gadow & I. Bailer (Eds.), *Advances in learning and behavioral disabilities* (Vol. 1). Greenwich, CT: JAI Press.

Pellham, W. E., Wheeler, T., & Chronis, A. (1998). Empirically supported psychosocial treatments for attention deficit hyperactivity disorder. *Journal of Clinical Child Psychology, 27*(2), 190–205.

Physician's Desk Reference (55th ed.). (2005). Montvail, NJ: Medical Economics, Inc.

Pomeroy, J., Sprafkin, J., & Gadow, K. (1988). Minor physical anomalies, as a biologic marker for behavioral disorders. *Journal of the American Academy of Children and Adolescent Psychiatry, 27,* 466–473.

Psychological Corporation (1989). *The Wechsler Intelligence Scale for Children—III.* New York: Harcourt Brace Jovanovich.

Psychological Corporation (2003). *The Wechsler Intelligence Scale for Children—IV* (WISC-IV). New York: Harcourt Brace Jovanovich.

Raimy, V. C. (Ed.). (1950). *Training in clinical psychology.* Englewood Cliffs, NJ: Prentice-Hall.

Reitan, R., & Wolfson, D. (1993). *The Halstead-Reitan Neuropsychological Test Battery: Theory and clinical interpretation* (2nd ed.). Tuscon, AZ: Neuropsychology Press.

Report of the Planning Committee on the Boulder Conference on Graduate Education of Clinical Psychologists. (1949). (Shakow Papers, M1383). *Archives of the History of American Psychology*. University of Akron, Akron, Ohio.

Rosenberg, G. (2002). Classroom acoustics and personal FM technology in management of auditory processing disorders. *Seminars in Hearing, 23*(4), 309–318.

Russo, N., Nicol, T., Zecker, S., Hayes, E., & Kraus, N. (2005). Auditory training improves neural timing in the human brainstem. *Behavioral Brain Research, 156*, 95–103.

Sacket, D. L., Rosenberg, W. M., Muir Gray, J. A., Haynes, R. B., & Richardson, W. S. (1996). Evidence-based medicine: What it is and what it isn't. *British Medical Journal, 12*, 71–72.

Scientific Learning Corporation. (1997). *Fast ForWord training program for children. Procedure manual for professionals.* Berkeley, CA: Author.

Stach, B., Loiselle, L., Jerger, J. Mintz, S., & Taylor, C. (1987). Clinical experience with personal FM assistive listening devices. *Hearing Journal, 40*, 24–30.

Tallal, P., Miller, S., Bedi, G., Wang, X., Nagarajan, S. S., Schreiner, C., Jenkins, W. M. & Merzenich, M. M. (1996). Language comprehension in language-learning impaired children improved with acoustically modified speech. *Science, 271*, 81–84.

Tillery, K. L., (1998). Central auditory processing assessment and therapeutic strategies for children with attention deficit hyperactivity disorder. In G. Masters, N. Stecker, & J. Katz (Eds.), *Central auditory processing disorders: Mostly management* (pp. 175–194). Boston: Allyn & Bacon.

Tillery, K. L., Katz, J., & Keller, W. (2000). Effects of methylphenidate (Ritalin) on auditory performance in children with attention and auditory processing disorders. *Journal of Speech-Language and Hearing Research, 43*, 893–901.

Tremblay, K., & Kraus, N. (2002). Auditory training induces asymmetrical changes in cortical neural activity. *Journal of Speech, Language, and Hearing Research, 45*, 564–572.

Tremblay, K., Kraus, N., Carrell, T., & McGee, T. (1997). Central auditory system plasticity: Generalization to novel stimulation following listening training. *Journal of the Acoustical Society of America, 102*, 3762–3773.

Tremblay, K., Kraus, N., & McGee, T. (1998). The time course of auditory perceptual learning: Neurophysiological changes during speech-sound training. *NeuroReport, 9*, 3557–3560.

Tremblay, K., Kraus, N., McGee, T., Ponton, C., & Otis, B. (2001). Central auditory plasticity: Changes in the N1-P2 complex after speech-sound training. *Ear and Hearing, 22*(2), 79–90.

Valente, M. (2005). Using evidence-based principles to make clinical decisions. *Journal of the American Academy of Audiology, 16*(10), 768–769.

Warrier, C. M., Johnson, K. L., Hayes, E. A., Nicol, T. & Kraus, N. (2004). Learning impaired children exhibit timing deficits and training-related improvements in auditory cortical responses to speech in noise. *Experimental Brain Research, 157*, 431–441.

Zametkin, A. J., Nordahl, T. E., & Gross, M. (1990). Cerebral glucose metabolism in adults with hyperactivity of childhood onset. *New England Journal of Medicine, 323*, 1361–1366.

Zatorre, R. J. (2001). Neural specialization for tonal processing. *Annals of the New York Academy of Sciences, 930*, 193–210.

SECTION IV

Future Directions

CHAPTER 13

EMERGING AND FUTURE DIRECTIONS IN INTERVENTION FOR (CENTRAL) AUDITORY PROCESSING DISORDER

GAIL D. CHERMAK AND FRANK E. MUSIEK

Identification, diagnosis, and intervention for (central) auditory processing disorder ([C]APD) have improved markedly over the last 10 years due in large part to research advances in auditory neuroscience and related fields and their innovative applications to clinical practice. The intense interest in (C)APD shown by professional associations over this same time period has encouraged this translation of science into practice. The convening of task forces and consensus conferences, the publication of position papers and technical reports (e.g., ASHA, 1996, 2005a, 2005b), and featured and keynote sessions at professional conferences have raised the visibility of issues pertaining to (C)APD, promoted best clinical practices, and encouraged research into the various clinical and basic science dimensions of the disorder. Perhaps a watershed event, the consensus report of the American Speech-Language-Hearing Association's (ASHA) task force delineating the status of research and clinical practices in (C)APD (ASHA, 1996) heralded a renewed commitment to additional research, expanded professional education, and improved clinical services.

In this final chapter, we focus on emerging and projected behavioral, technologic, and pharmacologic treatment strategies and research priorities. Underlying this discussion is the recognition that collaboration between clinicians and scientists—combining the clinician's first-hand knowledge of clinical needs with the researcher's expertise in the scientific method—provides a potent approach to asking the right questions and obtaining enduring answers. It is imperative that we exploit the momentum that has taken us to our current level of understanding and delivery of clinical services, as described in the preceding chapters.

Auditory Training

Ongoing research continues to reveal the neurobiologic processes underlying auditory processing, the linkages between neural encoding of sound in the central auditory nervous system (CANS) and higher-level language skills, and learning-associated brain plasticity (e.g., Banai, Nicol, Zecker, & Kraus, 2005; Cunningham, Nicol, Zecker, Bradlow, & Kraus, 2001; King, Warrier, Hayes, & Kraus, 2002; Kraus, McGee, Carrell, Zecker, Nicol, & Koch, 1996; Purdy, Kelly, & Davies, 2002; Wible, Nicol, & Kraus, 2005). The capability to change auditory behavior through auditory training is perhaps the most exciting development in intervention for (C)APD. An extensive corpus of research has documented improved psychophysical performance, neurophysiologic representation of acoustic stimuli, and listening and related function in children and adults following targeted auditory training (e.g., Hayes, Warrier, Nicol, Zecker, & Kraus, 2003; Jirsa, 1992; Kraus & Disterhoft, 1982; Kraus, McGee, Carrell, King, Tremblay, & Nicol, 1995; Merzenich, Jenkins, Johnston, Schreiner, Miller, & Tallal, 1996; Musiek, Baran, & Pinheiro, 1992; Musiek, Baran, & Shinn, 2004; Russo, Nicol, Zecker, Hayes, & Kraus, 2005; Tallal et al., 1996; Tremblay & Kraus, 2002; Tremblay, Kraus, Carrell, & McGee, 1997; Tremblay, Kraus, & McGee, 1998; Tremblay, Kraus, McGee, Ponton, & Otis, 2001; Warrier, Johnson, Hayes, Nicol, & Kraus, 2004).

Grounded in the neurophysiology of the CANS, a number of new auditory training techniques are gaining widespread clinical use in changing auditory behavior. For example, following training employing the dichotic interaural intensity difference (DIID) paradigm, Musiek and Schochat (1998) reported improved binaural listening and academic performance. Similarly, Musiek et al. (2004) reported markedly improved dichotic listening by a client with mild head trauma following DIID training. Post-DIID training, left ear scores increased and right ear scores decreased for split-brain patients and for children with left ear deficits (Musiek, Shinn, & Hare, 2002). Interhemispheric transfer training also has emerged as an important component of auditory training. Because interhemispheric transfer of information underlies binaural hearing and binaural processing, exercises to train interhemispheric transfer using interaural offsets and intensity differences, as well as other unimodal (e.g., linking prosodic and linguistic acoustic features) and multimodal (e.g., writing to dictation, verbally describing a picture while drawing) exercises lead to improve auditory behavior (Chermak & Musiek, 1997, 2002; Musiek, Baran, & Schochat, 1999).

A number of interactive computer-based auditory training programs are now commercially available (Diehl, 1999; Kraus, 2001; Morrison, 1998; Phillips, 2002; Tallal, Merzenich, Miller, & Jenkins, 1998). Research is needed to determine the comparative efficacy of various interactive computer-based auditory training programs for individuals presenting different clinical profiles. It is important to determine for whom particular training is most useful, as well as how training alters the neural representation of sound at various levels in the CANS (Kraus, 2001; Phillips, 2002).

Appearing on the horizon soon may be new auditory training approaches involving musical training. Music offers many advantages as a vehicle for auditory training. It is an enjoyable activity that taxes timing skills and the act of singing emphasizes the sound patterns of speech (Overy, 2003). Recent reports demonstrate that musical training alters auditory cortical representations. Trainor, Shahin, and Roberts (2003) measured enhancement of the P2 auditory evoked potential in adult nonmusicians following auditory training. Gabb et al. (2005) concluded that musical training may enhance the brain's efficiency in distinguishing split-second differences between rapidly changing sounds, and thereby improve temporal processing. Other work has demonstrated that musical training enhances pitch pattern recognition and increases verbal memory and that preschool children's phonemic awareness and early reading skill are correlated with their musical training (Anvari, Trainor, Woodside, & Levy, 2002; Chan, Ho, & Cheung, 1998; Kilgour, Jakobson, & Cuddy, 2000; Lamb & Gregory, 1993). Overy (2003) reported that group music lessons, as well as more individualized passive and active music listening, may improve timing (i.e., temporal) deficits in children with dyslexia. Music training, including rhythmic games, was shown to improve phonologic and spelling skills. Using functional magnetic resonance imaging (fMRI), Bodner, Muftuler, Nalcioglu, and Shaw (2001) documented the so-called *Mozart effect*, the short-term enhancement of spatial-temporal reasoning ability following listening to Mozart's *Sonata for Two Pianos in D Major* (K.

448) (Rauscher, Shaw, & Ky, 1993, 1995). Bodner et al. (2001) reported dramatic, statistically significant activation differences in normal adults listening to the Mozart *Sonata* in areas of the brain (e.g., dorsolateral prefrontal cortex, occipital cortex, and cerebellum) important to spatial-temporal reasoning. Additional research is needed to explore further the potential of music for auditory training.

Technology

Technology to reduce noise and improve the listening environment is of high priority because difficulties understanding speech in backgrounds of noise is perhaps the number one complaint presented by individuals with (C)APD. Such technology is crucial for children since listening activities occupy approximately 75% of a typical elementary school day and poor academic performance is linked to noisy classrooms (Hubble-Dahlquist, 1998). Continuing developments in the application of active noise control technology (i.e., sound cancellation by generation of a sound field that is an exact mirror image [i.e., *anti-noise*] of the disturbing sound]) may lead to quieter classrooms and other settings where noise control is desired. Similarly, assistive listening systems (e.g., sound field amplification) offer enhanced listening experiences for all children, and particularly those at risk for listening and learning problems (Rosenberg et al., 1999). Nonetheless, neither sound field nor personal FM systems are valid alternatives to good classroom acoustics. In fact, assistive listening systems and other attempts to reduce noise through furnishings (e.g., carpet) and arrangement of furniture (e.g., reducing distance between teacher and students through circular or rectangular arrangements) are only interim steps.

Amplification is not the panacea for all classroom acoustics problems: amplification has limited benefits in excessively noisy or reverberant classrooms. Moreover, amplification does not address sound leakage caused by poorly isolated or insulated classrooms. A recent standard for classroom acoustics (i.e., ANSI S12.60, 2002) specifies acoustical performance criteria, design requirements, and guidelines for schools. However, this standard is completely voluntary and must be incorporated into building codes for widespread implementation. In the meantime, school districts should require all school construction and renovation to comply with the new standard by including it in the bidding process.

Given the importance of temporal cues as well as spectral (frequency-specific) cues for recognition of speech (Shannon, Zeng, Kamath, Wygonski, & Ekelid, 1995; Van Tassell, Soli, Kirby, & Widin, 1987), developments in real-time speech rate conversion technology are encouraging. By reducing the speed of speech delivery, while maintaining pitch and quality, and synchronizing auditory and visual cues, individuals with temporal processing deficits (as well as those with peripheral hearing impairment) may be able to follow ongoing speech (Imai, Takagi, & Takeishi, 2005). This technology incorporates an algorithm that expands speech while contracting pauses and has been shown helpful for older adults (Imai et al., 2005). Speech processing algorithms that increase the salience of the rapidly changing acoustic elements of speech offer promise for enhancing comprehension of spoken language among those with (C)APD and language impairment (Tallal et al., 1996).

Perhaps also forthcoming in the near future is software that converts ongoing speech into *clear speech*, the speech speakers reliably produce when asked to speak more clearly (Picheny, Durlach, & Braida, 1985, 1986, 1989). In contrast to speech produced in casual conversation, clear speech is more intelligible due to the marked reduction in speaking rate, increased energy in the 1000 to 3000 Hz range, enhanced temporal and amplitude modulations, and expanded voice pitch range and vowel space. The benefits of clear speech have been demonstrated in diverse populations, including those with learning disabilities, auditory neuropathy, and cochlear implants (Bradlow, Kraus, & Hayes, 2003; Kraus et al., 2000).

In addition to offering new solutions to processing problems, technologic enhancements, especially computer technology, have begun to demonstrate the potential of technology to provide more novel instructional formats, which elicit greater attention, motivation, and persistence than more traditional formats (Chermak & Musiek, 1997). Computerized delivery offers multisensory stimulation in an engaging format that provides generous feedback and reinforcement and thereby facilitates intensive training (ASHA, 2005a). Moreover, adaptive approaches that alter parameters of subsequent trials based on subject performance improve training efficiency. As discussed above under Auditory Training, a growing number of reports have documented the advantages of computer-assisted therapy for (C)APD and associated listening and language processing deficits (e.g., Hayes et al., 2003; Russo et al., 2005; Tallal et al., 1996). Despite the potential of computerized approaches, additional data are needed to demonstrate the effectiveness and efficacy of these approaches (ASHA, 2005b; Phillips, 2002).

Neuropharmacologic Treatment of (C)APD

Knowledge of the plastic changes in the CANS may open new vistas in the pharmacological treatment of (C)APD. The essential role of neurotransmitters and molecular mechanisms in facilitating auditory plasticity and central auditory processing has intensified research in pharmacologic interventions that can alter physiologic and behavioral aspects of audition, including selective auditory attention, signal detection in noise, and temporal processing (Aoki & Siekevitz, 1988; Feldman, Brainard, & Knudsen, 1996; Gleich, Hamann, Klump, Kittel, & Strutz, 2003; Gopal, Bishop, & Carney, 2004; Gopal, Daly, Daniloff, & Pennartz, 2000; Morley & Happe, 2000; Musiek & Hoffman, 1990; Sahley, Kalish, Musiek, & Hoffman, 1991; Sahley, Musiek, & Nodar, 1996; Sahley & Nodar, 1994; Syka, 2002; Wenthold, 1991). By altering, primarily, dopamine metabolism, several drugs have been shown to improve behavioral regulation and vigilance in attention deficit hyperactivity disorder (ADHD), which may lead to improved performance on a number of behaviors including auditory processing (AAP, 2001). However, no pharmacologic agent has yet been demonstrated effective specifically for (C)APD (Chermak & Musiek, 1997; Tillery, Katz, & Keller, 2000).

Pickles and Comis' (1973) early finding that injected atropine sulfate raised noise thresholds more so than quiet thresholds suggested that this drug affects the olivocochlear system, the system posited to improve neural signal-to-noise ratios and enhance the detection of signals in noise (Dewson, 1968; Dolan & Nuttall, 1988; Nieder & Nieder, 1970; Wiederhold, 1986). Other findings have suggested an even broader role for the olivocochlear system, influencing selective auditory attention, improving the clarity of sound, and modulation of auditory nerve activity, as well as signal in noise detection (Art & Fettiplace, 1984; Wiederhold, 1986).

More recent work underscores the potential of pharmacologic intervention to alter the efferent system. Gopal, Bishop, and Carney (2004) demonstrated the potential of pharmacologic intervention to alter central auditory processing by comparing electrophysiologic potentials of unmedicated and medicated patients taking selective serotonin reuptake inhibitors (SSRI) for treatment of depression. As the neurotransmitter serotonin modulates the cholinergic-mediated efferent system's inhibitory function, Gopal et al. (2004) explained their findings of shorter latencies of auditory brainstem and late latency responses in the unmedicated patients as a result of lower serotonin levels which led to reduced efferent system function and reduced inhibition.

Reported decrements in neurotransmitter levels in the auditory areas of the brains of aged animals suggest that central auditory processing deficits among older adults may respond to pharmacologic intervention (Banay-Schwartz, Laztha, & Palkovits, 1989; Caspary, Milbrandt, & Helfert, 1995; Caspary, Raza, Lawhorn-Armour, Pippin, & Arneric, 1990). For example, Gleich, Hamann, Klump, Kittel, and Strutz (2003) demonstrated improved temporal processing in *older* mice following the administration of GABA. In another study, clozapine boosted insufficient inhibitory processing in older mice as measured by the P50 auditory evoked potential (Simoski, Stevens, Adler, & Freedman, 2002).

Preliminary reports suggesting some therapeutic efficacy for a number of pharmacologic agents (e.g., adrafinil, aniracetam, modafanil, pentoxifylline, physostigmine, piracetam, propentofylline, vinpocetine) in reducing cognitive, metacognitive, learning, and communication deficits of older adults with organic brain disease and others suffering from a variety of cognitive disorders may presage the development of similar drugs for treatment of similar deficits frequently associated with (C)APD (Asthana et al., 1995; Baranski, Pigeau, Dinich, & Jacobs, 2004; Chai, Li, & Long, 2000; Derouesne et al., 2001; Devasenapathy & Hachinski, 1998; Ferraro et al., 2000; Greener, Enderby, & Whurr, 2001; Hock, 1995; Huber et al., 1993; Ikeda et al., 1992; Kemény, Molnár, Andrejkovics, Makai, & Csiba, 2005; Moller, Maurer, & Saletu, 1994; Muller, Steffenhagen, Regenthal, & Bublak, 2004; Nicholson, 1990; Parkinson, Rudolphi, & Fredholm, 1994; Saletu, Moller, Grunberger, Deutsch, & Rossner, 1990; Sano et al., 1993; Torigoe et al., 1994; Winblad, 2005). We may soon witness discoveries that will revolutionize the treatment of (C)APD and related disorders in children and adults.

Genetic Enhancement

With the completion of the Human Genome Project (HGP) in 2003, interest in genetics has soared both among the public and across the scientific community. The HGP has provided detailed information about the structure, organization and function of the complete set (approximately 30,000–40,000) of human genes. The insights provided will likely transform all aspects of health care from disease prevention, to treatment of disease and disorders, and ultimately lead to long sought after cures for the multitude of diseases and disorders that now devastate human beings.

Even prior to the completion of the HGP, researchers suggested that genetic enhancement of cognitive abilities, learning, and intelligence in mammals was feasible (Tang et al., 1999). Much of the research in this area has focused on the role of an enriched environment in promoting biochemical and structural changes in the cortex, the hippocampus, and other brain regions (Kemperman, Kuhn, & Gage, 1997; Rampon et al., 2000). Expression of a large number of genes may serve important roles in modulating learning and memory change in response to enriched environments (Rampon et al., 2000). As these changes in gene expression can be linked to neuronal structure, synaptic plasticity, and transmission, genetic enhancement may someday serve a role in intervention for (C)APD, especially in improving often associated deficits in learning. Demonstrating the specific role of genetics for (C)APD, Bamiou and colleagues reported that PAX6 mutations in humans may affect development of the anterior commissure and possibly the corpus callosum (Bamiou et al., 2004). Individuals with the PAX6 mutation presented dichotic listening deficits linked to callosal dysfunction. If this mutation is an identifiable genetic trait, genetic treatment could possibly minimize or eliminate the callosal dysfunction and the (C)APD.

Profiling (C)APD and Customizing Intervention

The varied functional deficits and clinical profiles presented by individuals diagnosed with (C)APD reflect variation in the underlying neurophysiologic sources and mechanisms responsible for the flawed auditory processing and behavioral deficits. Documented links, both behavioral and electrophysiologic, between inefficient auditory processing and language and learning problems (e.g., Bellis & Ferre, 1999; Kraus et al, 1996; Moncrieff & Musiek, 2002; Wible et al., 2005) may lead to subprofiles of (C)APD characterized by patterns or clusters of functional symptoms, central auditory test findings, and associated neurophysiologic bases.

With a firm understanding of (C)APD gained from auditory and cognitive neuroscience, it now may be possible to develop functional deficit profiles that reflect patterns of central auditory deficits and functional cognitive, language, learning, and communication sequelae (Bellis, 2002; Bellis & Ferre, 1999). These deficit profiles, which should conform to well-established neuroscience tenets that demonstrate the presence of brain-behavior relationships across a wide variety of functional areas, could be used to guide development of comprehensive intervention programs that address efficiently and effectively the specific cluster of central auditory and functional symptoms. Such subprofiles should lead to more customized and deficit-focused intervention and, therefore, to more effective intervention (King et al., 2002).

An example of a subprofiling model was provided by Bellis and Ferre (1999). In their model, for example, they inferred that the corpus callosum is the neurophysiologic source of their integration subprofile. Additional research demonstrating different neurochemical or neurotransmitter responses underlying the presumed (C)APD subprofiles would strengthen the position that different neurobiologic mechanisms underlie these subprofiles.

Regarding the potential of subprofiling for treatment effectiveness, King et al. (2002) demonstrated how subtyping individuals as a function of the neurophysiologic source of auditory dysfunction can lead to specific and customized treatment decisions that might not be as effective for other subgroups. In the King et al. (2002) study, subjects with learning disabilities (LD) with abnormal brainstem timing benefitted more from listening training than did LD subjects not presenting the abnormal brainstem response. Banai et al. (2005) extended these findings demonstrating that LD individuals with abnormal brainstem timing were more likely to show reduced processing of acoustic change at the cortical level and more depressed reading, listening comprehension, and general cognitive ability compared with LD individuals with normal brainstem timing.

Measuring Efficacy and Outcomes of Intervention

Establishing the efficacy of our treatments is among the highest research priorities in the intervention arena. Although studies generating the highest levels of evidence (e.g., randomized controlled trials; meta-analysis of randomized controlled trials) may be lacking (Musiek, Bellis, & Chermak, 2005), there is a solid base of evidence documenting improved auditory and listening behavior following auditory training (see Auditory Training above). The benefits of sound field amplification, particularly for children at risk for listening and learning problems, are well documented (Rosenberg, 1998; Rosenberg et al., 1999), although only limited data have been published demonstrating the efficacy of personal FM amplification for individuals with (C)APD (Bellis, 1996; Rosenberg, 2002; Stach, Loiselle, Jerger, Mintz, & Taylor (1987). A growing body of research continues to demonstrate the effectiveness of central resources training strategies (as reviewed in Chapter 5).

Nevertheless, additional carefully designed clinical studies, controlling threats to internal validity and incorporating appropriate outcome measures, are needed to firmly establish the efficacy of a number of treatments currently recommended for (C)APD. Research is needed in the area of treatment effectiveness and efficacy to enhance the selection and customization of deficit-focused remediation approaches and to guide recommendations regarding necessary and sufficient frequency, intensiveness, and duration of treatment programs and treatment termination (ASHA, 2005a, 2005b). Controlling subject selection and precisely defining subject characteristics are necessary given the comorbidity and possible linkage among a number of related disorders (e.g., (C)APD, attention deficit hyperactivity disorder, learning disability). Such controls should lead to clarification regarding the relationships among the spectrum of conditions manifesting central auditory processing deficits, and will enable us to determine how treatment programs affect well-defined (C)APD, including which treatment strategies and programs are most efficacious in meeting the needs of clients with particular (C)APD subprofiles at particular life stages (Chermak & Musiek, 1997).

Additional research is needed as well to develop customized, deficit-focused intervention plans to address particular clinical subprofiles. For example, a left-ear deficit related to corpus callosum transfer problems would suggest training using interhemispheric transfer and dichotics exercises (Bellis & Ferre, 1999). In contrast, temporal patterning, pragmatics, and prosody training might be more appropriate for a patient with a left-ear deficit that reflects right hemisphere involvement (Bellis & Ferre, 1999). Finally, outcome measures must be carefully selected and sufficiently broad (e.g., improved spoken language comprehension) to demonstrate significant change in central auditory processing as well as listening in functionally relevant contexts (e.g., school, home, work). Outcome measures should include probes of specific central auditory processes previously determined to be deficient (e.g., gap detection or pitch pattern recognition), as well as more expansive measures (e.g., listening comprehension and spoken language processing).

The use of auditory brainstem and cortical potentials to document treatment outcomes is especially promising. Electrophysiolgic measures may be more sensitive than comparable behavioral indices and are less influenced by extraneous variables (i.e., confounds) (Hendler, Squires, & Emmerich, 1990; Jerger et al., 2002; McPherson & Salamat 2004; Tremblay et al., 1998). At the same time, they are more time consuming and more expensive to administer, some are difficult to observe in young children (e.g., middle-latency response), some are highly variable (e.g., P300), and some are difficult to identify and present poor correlation with behavioral measures (e.g., MMN) (Dalebout & Fox, 2001). Recent findings suggesting that the auditory brainstem response to speech may reflect the subcortical source of deficient temporal processing of speech sound onset ultimately may provide for a reliable, objective marker of auditory processing (Banai et al., 2005). Other applications of this finding include the potential for differentiating among cortical and brainstem sources of (C)APD and better customizing intervention, as discussed above in Profiling (C)APD and Customizing Intervention.

Professional Issues

Recent ASHA position papers, technical reports, and statements of preferred practice patterns affirm the need for a team approach to the diagnosis, assessment, and intervention for children and adults with (C)APD (ASHA, 2004, 2005a, 2005b). Specifically, the audiologist diagnoses (C)APD, whereas the speech-language pathologist (SLP) is responsible for assessing "aspects of auditory processing involved in language development and use . . . including determining if an auditory-related cognitive-communication and/or language disorder is present . . . " (ASHA, 2004). Professional collaboration also is pivotal to intervention. The audiologist is responsible for enhancing the acoustic signal and the listening environment using assistive technology and noise/reverberation reduction techniques. The SLP provides intervention services for the cognitive-communication and/or

language impairments associated with (C)APD (ASHA, 2004). Both professionals should be engaged in auditory training: the audiologist in more formal auditory training techniques and the SLP in the more informal approaches to auditory training (Chermak & Musiek, 2002; also see Chapter 4).

Collaboration is consistent with the systems (i.e., ecologic) approach to intervention that we have advocated throughout this volume. Individuals cannot be evaluated without an analysis of the contexts in which they interact because environmental factors influence development, learning, and performance (Barkley, 1996; Bartoli & Botel, 1988; Palincsar, Brown, & Campione, 1994; Poplin, 1988a, 1988b; Sameroff, 1983). Although performance deficits noted on a battery of central auditory processing tests may justify a diagnosis of (C)APD, comprehensive assessment of (C)APD demands evaluation of functional deficits in the variety of contexts in which the individual operates. Information regarding home, school, and employment settings, as well as interactions with family, teachers, peer group, and coworkers should be obtained through case history and/or systematic observation to appropriately evaluate the client and plan effective treatments. The presence of central auditory processing deficits in association with language and/or cognitive deficits (e.g., aphasia, traumatic head injury, learning disabilities) underscores the need for collaboration among audiologists, SLPs, and other professionals responsible for assessment and intervention.

Reimbursement is a professional issue of vital importance to the continued improvement of the quality of clinical services for (C)APD. Although recent additions and changes to procedure codes (CPT) improve reimbursement for diagnosis, assessment, and treatment services related to (C)APD, additional changes are needed to fairly reimburse professionals for their service contributions (ASHA, 2005b). Based on findings of a follow-up survey conducted recently, we found as we did in 1998 that audiologists continue to cite poor reimbursement as a major deterrent to becoming involved in the evaluation of (C)APD (Chermak, Silva, & Musiek, unpublished manuscript; Chermak, Traynham, Seikel, & Musiek, 1998). The survey also revealed a continuing shortage of SLPs to whom audiologists can refer clients diagnosed with (C)APD for intervention. The shortage of SLPs involved in intervention may be more related to professional education issues than to reimbursement issues, as discussed below.

Professional Education

The quality of clinical services provided by practitioners determines society's valuation of their clinical specialty. Several key studies have demonstrated the underpreparation of both speech-language pathology and audiology graduates in the area of central auditory processing, confirming the urgency to improve graduate education in this area and to develop guidelines for knowledge and skill competencies in diagnosis, assessment, and treatment of (C)APD (Chermak et al., unpublished manuscript; Chermak et al., 1998; Henri, 1994). The guidelines should be developed by university educators and clinicians to reflect the demands of the workplace while recognizing the resource constraints of today's graduate education programs. With the move to doctoral level education in audiology, inclusion of appropriate basic science (e.g., anatomy, physiology, and pharmacology of the CANS; psychoacoustics) and applied coursework and clinical experiences in diagnosis, treatment, and management of (C)APD is anticipated. Moreover, integration of evidence-based practice (EBP) into undergraduate and graduate audiology curricula will teach students how to incorporate clinical research into clinical decisions. Future graduates will be better prepared to formulate focused clinical questions, efficiently locate and appraise available evidence, and apply their findings to improve clinical services for individual patients (Oppenheimer, Self, & Sieff, 2005). (See Chapter 2 in this volume of the Handbook for discussion of EBP.) Perhaps most important, university faculty and clinical supervisors must conceptualize audiologic evaluation and rehabilitation more broadly, teaching students that comprehensive evaluation and effective intervention require careful attention to both the peripheral and central auditory systems.

Summary

Accumulating scientific and clinical advances have expanded our understanding of (C)APD, resulting in improved diagnostic and intervention services. The neurobiologic, genetic, technologic, and professional practice frontiers reviewed in this chapter may soon transform clinical practice, perhaps even revolutionizing diagnostic and treatment procedures. Our research priorities are attainable and intertwined: dramatic improvements in clinical care will continue to unfold rapidly as long as the commitment to the twin engines of basic research and clinical trials that drive these improvements are nourished. More efficient diagnostic test batteries and assessment tools will lead to greater treatment efficacy by more precisely subprofiling and customizing intervention. Technologic advances will minimize the impact of (C)APD on individuals' lives. Finally, multidisciplinary collaboration among clinicians, researchers, educators, and families will incite new questions and fuel research that will accelerate the pace of clinical advances.

References

American Academy of Pediatrics Subcommittee on Attention-Deficit/Hyperactivity Disorder Committee on Quality Improvement. (2001). Clinical practice guideline: Treatment of the school-aged child with attention-deficit/hyperactivity disorder. *Pediatrics, 108*(4), 1033–1044.

American National Standards Institute. (2002). *Acoustical performance criteria, design requirements, and guidelines for schools.* (ANSI Standard S12.60). New York: Author.

American Speech-Language-Hearing Association Task Force on Central Auditory Processing Consensus Development. (1996). Central auditory processing: Current status of research and implications for clinical practice. *American Journal of Audiology, 5*(2), 41–54.

American Speech-Language-Hearing Association. (2004). *Speech-language pathology (SLP) preferred practice patterns.* Available at http://www.asha.org/members/deskref-journals/deskref/default.

American Speech-Language-Hearing Association. (2005a). *(Central) auditory processing disorders.* Available at http://www.asha.org/members/deskref-journals/deskref/default.

American Speech-Language-Hearing Association. (2005b). *(Central) auditory processing disorders—The role of the audiologist* [Position statement]. Available at http://www.asha.org/members/deskref-journals/deskref/default.

Anvari, S., Trainor, L. J., Woodside, J., & Levy, B. A. (2002). Relations among musical skills, phonological processing, and early reading ability in preschool children. *Journal of Experimental Child Psychology, 83,* 111–130.

Aoki, C., & Siekevitz, P. (1988). Plasticity in brain development. *Scientific American, 259*(6), 56–64.

Art, J. J., & Fettiplace, R. (1984). Efferent desensitization of auditory nerve fibre responses in the cochlea of the turtle *Pseudemys scripta elegans. Journal of Physiology, 356,* 507–523.

Asthana, S., Greig, N. H., Hegedus, L., Holloway, H. H., Raffaele, K.C., Schapiro, M. B., & Soncrant, T. T. (1995). Clinical pharmacokinetics of physostigmine in patients with Alzheimer's disease. *Clinical Pharmacology and Therapeutics, 58,* 299–309.

Bamiou, D.E., Musiek, F.E., Sisodiya, S. M., Free, S. L. Davies, R. A., Moore, A., Van Heyningen, V., & Luxon, L. M. (2004). Deficient auditory interhemispheric transfer in patients with PAX6 mutations. *Annals of Neurology, 56*(4), 503–509.

Banai, K., Nicol, T., Zecker, S., & Kraus, N. (2005). Brainstem timing: Implications for cortical processing and literacy. *The Journal of Neuroscience, 25*(43), 9850–9857.

Banay-Schwartz, M., Laztha, A., & Palkovits, M. (1989). Changes with aging in the levels of amino acids in rat CNS structural elements: I. Glutamate and related amino acids. *Neurochemical Research, 14,* 555–562.

Baranski, J., Pigeau, R., Dinich, P., & Jacobs, I. (2004). Effects of modafinil on cognitive and meta-cognitive performance. *Human Psychopharmacology, 19*(5), 323–332

Barkley, R. A. (1996). Linkages between attention and executive functions. In G. R. Lyon & N. A. Krasnegor (Eds.), *Attention, memory, and executive function* (pp. 307–326). Baltimore: Paul H. Brookes.

Bartoli, J., & Botel, M. (1988). *Reading/learning disability: An ecological approach.* New York: Teachers College Press.

Bellis, T. (1996). *Assessment and management of central auditory processing disorders in the educational setting: From science to practice.* San Diego, CA: Singular Publishing Group.

Bellis, T. J. (2002). Developing deficit-specific intervention plans for individuals with auditory processing disorders. *Seminars in Hearing, 23*(4), 287–295.

Bellis, T. J., & Ferre, J. M. (1999). Multidimensional approach to the differential diagnosis of central auditory processing disorders in children. *Journal of the American Academy of Audiology, 10,* 319–328.

Bodner, M., Muftuler, L., Nalcioglu, O., & Shaw, G. (2001). fMRI study relevant to the Mozart effect: Brain areas involved in spatial-temporal processing. *Neurology Research, 23,* 683–690.

Bradlow, A., Kraus, N., & Hayes, E. (2003). Speaking clearly for children with learning disabilities: Sentence perception in noise. *Journal of Speech, Language, and Hearing Research, 46*(1), 80–97.

Caspary, D. M., Milbrandt, J. C., & Helfert, R. H. (1995). Central auditory aging: GABA changes in the inferior colliculus. *Experimental Gerontology, 30,* 349–360.

Caspary, D. M., Raza, A., Lawhorn-Armour, B., Pippin, J, & Arneric, S. (1990). Immunocytochemical and neurochemical evidence for age-related loss of GABA in the inferior colliclus: Implications for neural presbycusis. *Journal of Neuroscience, 10*(7), 2363–2372.

Chai, B., Li, J., & Long, J. (2000). Therapeutic effects of aniracetam and piracetam in treatment of hypomnesis. *Chinese Pharmaceutical Journal, 35*(4), 272–273.

Chan, A. S., Ho, Y. C., & Cheung, M. C. (1998). Music training improves verbal memory. *Nature, 396*(6707), 128.

Chermak, G. & Musiek, F. (1997). *Central auditory processing disorders: New per-*spectives. San Diego, CA: Singular Publishing Group.

Chermak, G. D., & Musiek, F. E. (2002). Auditory training: Principles and approaches for remediating and managing auditory processing disorders. *Seminars in Hearing, 23*(4), 297–308.

Chermak, G. D., Silva, M. & Musiek, F. E. *Professional education and clinical practices in central auditory processing disorders.* Unpublished manuscript. Washington State University, Pullman, Washington.

Chermak, G. D., Traynham, W. A., Seikel, J. A., & Musiek, F. E. (1998). Professional education and assessment practices in central auditory processing. *Journal of the American Academy of Audiology, 9*(6), 452–465.

Cunningham, J., Nicol, T., Zecker, S. G., Bradlow, A., & Kraus, N. (2001). Neurobiologic responses to speech in noise in children with learning problems: Deficits and strategies for improvement. *Clinical Neurophysiology, 112,* 758–767.

Dalebout, S., & Fox, L. (2001). Reliability of the mismatched negativity in the response of individual listeners. *Journal of the American Academy of Audiology, 12,* 245–253.

Derouesne, C., Cailler, I., Kohler, F., Piette, F., Boyer, P., Sauron, B., & Lubin, S. (2001). Effectiveness of adrafinil on the memory complaint in the adult over fifty years of age: Results of a controlled double blind therapeutic trial of adrafinil versus placebo. *Revue de Geriatrie, 26*(10 S), 851–858.

Devasenapathy, A., & Hachinski, V.C. (1998). Cognitive impairment poststroke. *Physical Medicine and Rehabilitation, 12*(3), 543–555.

Dewson, J. H. (1968) Efferent olivocochlear bundle: Some relationship to stimulus discrimination in noise. *Journal of Neurophysiology, 31,* 122–130.

Diehl, S. (1999). Listen learn? A software review of Earobics. *Language, Speech, and Hearing Services in Schools, 30,* 108–116.

Dolan, D. F., & Nuttall, A. L. (1988). Masked cochlear whole-nerve response intensity functions altered by electrical stimulation of the crossed olivocochlear bundle. *Journal of the Acoustical Society of America*, *83*, 1081–1086.

Feldman, D. E., Brainard, M. S., & Knudsen, E. I. (1996). Newly learned auditory responses mediated by NMDA receptors in the owl inferior colliculus. *Science, 271*, 525–528.

Ferraro, L., Fuxe, K., Tanganelli, S., Fernandez, M., Rambert, F., & Antonelli, T. (2000). Amplification of cortical serotonin release: A further neurochemical action of the vigilance-promoting drug modafinil. *Neuropharmacology, 39*(11), 1974–1983.

Gabb, N., Tallal, P., Kim, H., Lakshminarayanan, K., Archie, J., Glover, G., & J. Gabrieli (2005). Neural correlates of rapid spectrotemporal processing in musicians and non-musicians. *Annals of the New York Academy of Sciences, 1060*, 82–88.

Gleich, O., Hamann, I., Klump, G., Kittel, M., & Strutz, J. (2003). Boosting GABA improves auditory temporal resolution in the gerbil. *NeuroReport, 14*, 1877–1880.

Gopal, K., Bishop, C., & Carney, L. (2004). Auditory measures in clinically depressed individuals. II. Auditory evoked potentials and behavioral speech tests. *International Journal of Audiology, 43*, 499–505.

Gopal, K. V., Daly, D. M., Daniloff, R. G., & Pennartz, L. (2000). Effects of selective serotonin reuptake inhibitors on auditory processing: Case study. *Journal of the American Academy of Audiology, 11*, 454–463.

Greener, J., Enderby, P., & Whurr, R. (2001). Pharmacological treatment for aphasia following stroke. *The Cochrane Database of Systematic Reviews*, Issue 4. Art. No.: CD000424. DOI: 10.1002/14651858. CD000424.

Hayes, E. A., Warrier, C. M., Nichol, T. G., Zecker, S. G., & Kraus, N. (2003). Neural plasticity following auditory training in children with learning problems. *Clinical Neurophysiology, 114*, 673–684.

Hendler, T., Squires, N., & Emmerich, D. (1990). Psychophysical measures of central auditory dysfunction in multiple sclerosis: Neurophysiological and neuroanatomical correlates. *Ear and Hearing, 11*(6), 403–416.

Henri, B. P. (1994). Graduate student preparation: Tomorrow's challenge. *Asha, 36*, 43–46.

Hock, F. J. (1995). Therapeutic approaches for memory impairments. *Behavioral Brain Research, 66*, 143–150.

Hubble-Dahlquist, L. (1998). Classroom amplification: Not just for the hearing impaired anymore. *CSUN '98 Papers*. Available from http://www.dimf.ne.jp/doc/english/Us_Eu/conf/csun_98/csun98_124.htm.

Huber, M., Kittner, B., Hojer, C., Fink, G. R., Neveling, M., & Heiss, W. D. (1993). Effect of propentofylline on regional cerebral glucose metabolism in acute ischemic stroke. *Journal of Cerebral Blood Flow and Metabolism, 13*(3), 526–530.

Ikeda, T., Yamamoto, K., Takahashi, K., Kahu, Y., Uchiyama, M., Sugiyama, K., & Yamada, M. (1992). Treatment of Alzheimer-type dementia with intravenous mecobalamin. *Clinical Therapeutics, 14*(3), 426–427.

Imai, A., Takagi, T., & Takeishi, H. (2005). Development of radio and television receiver with functions to assist hearing of elderly people. *IEEE Transactions on Consumer Electronics, 51*(1), 268–272.

Jerger, J., Thibodeau, L., Martin, J., Mehta, J., Tillman, G., Greenwald, R., Britt, L., Scott, J., & Overson, G. (2002). Behavioral and electrophysiologic evidence of auditory processing disorder: A twin study. *Journal of the American Academy of Audiology, 13*, 438–460.

Jirsa, R. E. (1992). The clinical utility of the P3 AERP in children with auditory processing disorders. *Journal of Speech and Hearing Research, 35*, 903–912.

Kemény, V., Molnár, S., Andrejkovics, M., Makai, A., & Csiba, L. (2005). Acute and chronic effects of vinpocetine on cerebral hemodynamics and neuropsychological performance in multi-infarct patients. *The Journal of Clinical Pharmacology, 45*(9), 1048–1054.

Kemperman, G., Kuhn, H., & Gage, F. (1997). More hippocampal neurons in adult mice living in an enriched environment. *Nature, 386*(3), 493-495.

Kilgour, A. R., Jakobson, L. S., & Cuddy, L. L. (2000). Music training and rate of presentation as mediators of text and song recall. *Memory and Cognition., 28*, 700-710.

King, C., Warrier, C. M., Hayes, E., & Kraus, N. (2002). Deficits in auditory brainstem encoding of speech sounds in children with learning problems. *Neuroscience Letters, 319*, 111-115.

Kraus, N. (2001). Auditory pathway encoding and neural plasticity in children with learning problems. *Audiology Neuro-otology, 6*, 221-227.

Kraus, N., Bradlow, A., Cheatham. M., Cunningham, J., King, C., Koch, D., Nicol, T., McGee, T., Stein, L., & Wright, B. (2000). Consequences of neural asynchrony: A case of auditory neuropathy. *The Journal of the Association for Research in Otolaryngology, 1*(1), 33-45.

Kraus, N., & Disterhoff, J.F. (1982). Response plasticity of single neurons in rabbit auditory association cortex during tone-signalled learning. *Brain Research, 246*(2), 205-215.

Kraus, N., McGee, T., Carrell, T., King, C., Tremblay, K., & Nicol, T. (1995). Central auditory system plasticity associated with speech discrimination training. *Journal of Cognitive Neuroscience, 7*(1), 25-32.

Kraus, N., McGee, T. J., Carrell, T. D., Zecker, S. G., Nicol, T. G., & Koch, D. B. (1996). Auditory neurophysiologic responses and discrimination deficits in children with learning problems. *Science, 273*, 971-973.

Lamb, S. J., & Gregory, A. H. (1993). The relationship between music and reading in beginning readers. *Journal of Educational Psychology, 13*, 13-27.

McPherson, D. L., & Salamat, M. T. (2004). Interactions among variables in the P_{300} response to a continuous performance task in normal and ADHD adults. *Journal of the American Academy of Audiology, 15*, 666-677.

Merzenich, M., Jenkins, W. M., Johnston, P., Schreiner, C., Miller, S. L., & Tallal, P. (1996). Temporal processing deficits of language-learning impaired children ameliorated by training. *Science, 271*, 77-80.

Moller, H. J., Maurer, I., & Saletu, B. (1994). Placebo controlled trial of the xanthine derivative propentofylline in dementia. *Psychopharmacology, 101*(2), 147-159.

Moncrieff, D. & Musiek, F. (2002). Interaural asymmetries revealed by dichotic listening tests in normal and dyslexic children. *Journal of the American Academy of Audiology, 13*, 428-437.

Morley, B. J., & Happe, H. K. (2000). Cholinergic receptors: Dual roles in transduction and plasticity. *Hearing Research, 147*, 104-112.

Morrison, S. (1998). Computer applications: Earobics. *Child Language Teaching and Therapy, 14*, 279-284.

Muller, U., Steffenhagen, N., Regenthal, R., & Bublak, P. (2004). Effects of modafinil on working memory processes in humans. *Psychopharmacology, 177*(1-2), 161-169.

Musiek, F. E., Baran, J. A., & Pinheiro, M. L. (1992). P300 results in patients with lesions of the auditory areas of the cerebrum. *Journal of the American Academy of Audiology, 3*, 5-15.

Musiek, F. E., Baran, J., & Schochat, E. (1999). Selected management approaches to central auditory processing disorders. *Scandinavian Audiology, 51*, 63-76.

Musiek, F. E., Baran, J. A. & Shinn, J. (2004). Assessment and remediation of an auditory processing disorder associated with head trauma. *Journal of the American Academy of Audiology, 15*(2), 117-132.

Musiek, F. E., Bellis, T. J., & Chermak, G. D. (2005). Nonmodularity of the CANS: Implications for (central) auditory processing disorder. *American Journal of Audiology, 14*, 128-138.

Musiek, F. E., & Hoffman, D. W. (1990). An introduction to the functional neurochemistry of the auditory system. *Ear and Hearing, 11*(6), 395-402.

Musiek, F. E., & Schochat, E. (1998). Auditory training and central auditory processing disorders: A case study. *Seminars in Hearing, 19,* 357-366.

Musiek, F. E., Shinn, J., & Hare, C. (2002). Plasticity, auditory training, and auditory processing disorders. *Seminars in Hearing, 23*(4), 263-275.

Nicholson, C. D. (1990). Pharmacology of nootropics and metabolically active comounds in relation to their use in dementia. *Psychopharmacology, 101*(2), 147-159.

Nieder, P. C., & Nieder, I. (1970). Antimasking effect of crossed olivocochlear bundle stimulation with loud clicks in guinea pigs. *Experimental Neurology, 28,* 179-188.

Oppenheimer, B., Self, T., & Sieff, S. (2005). *Integration of clinical practice and research: Successful curriculum models.* Rockville, MD: American Speech-Language-Hearing Association.

Overy, K. (2003). Dyslexia and music: From timing deficits to musical intervention. *Annals of the New York Academy of Sciences, 999,* 497-505.

Palincsar, A. S., Brown, A. L., & Campione, J. C. (1994). Models and practices of dynamic assessment. In G. P. Wallach & K. G. Butler (Eds.), *Language learning disabilities in school-age children and adolescents* (pp. 132-144). New York: Charles E. Merrill.

Parkinson, F. E., Rudolphi, K. A., & Fredholm, B. B. (1994). Propentofylline: A nucleoside transport inhibitor with neuroprotective effects in cerebral ischemia. *General Pharmacology, 25*(6), 1053-1058.

Phillips, D. P. (2002). Central auditory system and central auditory processing disorders: Some conceptual issues. *Seminars in Hearing, 23*(4), 251-261.

Pichney, M. A., Durlach, N. I., & Braida, L. D. (1985). Speaking clearly for the hard of hearing. I: Intelligibility differences between clear and conversational speech. *Journal of Speech and Hearing Research, 28,* 96-103.

Pichney, M. A., Durlach, N. I., & Braida, L. D. (1986). Speaking clearly for the hard of hearing. II: Acoustic characteristics of clear and conversational speech. *Journal of Speech and Hearing Research, 29,* 434-446.

Picheny, M. A., Durlach, N. I., & Braida, L. D. (1989). Speaking clearly for the hard of hearing: III. An attempt to determine the contribution of speaking rates to differences in intelligibility between clear and conversational speech. *Journal of Speech and Hearing Research, 32,* 600-603.

Pickles, J. O., & Comis, S. D. (1973). Role of centrifugal pathways to cochlear nucleus in detection of signals in noise. *Journal of Neurophysiology, 36*(6), 1131-1137.

Poplin, M. S. (1988a). Holistic/constructivist principles of the teaching/learning process: Implications for the field of learning disabilities. *Journal of Learning Disabilities, 21,* 401-416.

Poplin, M. S. (1988b). The reductionist fallacy in learning disabilities: Replicating the past by reducing the present. *Journal of Learning Disabilities, 21,* 389-400.

Purdy, S., Kelly, A., & Davies, M. (2002). Auditory brainstem response, middle latency response, and late cortical evoked potentials in children with learning disabilities. *Journal of the American Academy of Audiology, 13,* 367-382.

Rampon, C., Jiang, C., Dong, H., Tang, Y., Lockhart, D., Schultz, P., Tsien, J., & Hu, Y. (2000). Effects of environmental enrichment on gene expression in the brain. *Proceedings of the National Academy of Sciences, 97*(23), 12880-12884.

Rauscher, F. H., Shaw, G. L., Ky, K. N. (1993). Music and spatial task performance. *Nature, 365,* 611.

Rauscher, F. H., Shaw, G. L., Ky, K. N. (1995). Listening to Mozart enhances spatial-temporal reasoning: Towards a neurophysiological basis. *Neuroscience Letters, 185,* 44-47.

Rosenberg, G., (1998, Summer). FM sounds field research identifies benefits for students and teachers. *Educational Audiology Review, 3,* 6-8.

Rosenberg, G. (2002). Classroom acoustics and personal FM technology in management of auditory processing disorder. *Seminars in Hearing, 23*(4), 309–318.

Rosenberg, G., Blake-Rahter, P., Heavner, J., Allen, L., Redmond, B., Phillips, J., & Stigers, K. (1999). Improving classroom acoustics (ICA): A three-year FM sound field classroom amplification study. *Journal of Educational Audiology, 7*, 8–28.

Russo, N., Nicol, T., Zecker, S., Hayes, E., & Kraus, N. (2005). Auditory training improves neural timing in the human brainstem. *Behavioural Brain Research, 156*, 95–103.

Sahley, T. L., Kalish, R. B., Musiek, F. E., & Hoffman, D. (1991). Effects of opioid drugs on auditory evoked potentials suggest a role of lateral efferent olivocochlear dynorphins in auditory function. *Hearing Research, 55*, 133–142.

Sahley, T. L., Musiek, F. E., & Nodar, R. H. (1996). Naloxone blockage of (–)pentazocine-induced changes in auditory function. *Ear and Hearing, 17*(4), 341–353.

Sahley, T. L., & Nodar, R. H. (1994). Improvement in auditory function following pentazocine suggests a role for dynorphins in auditory sensitivity. *Ear and Hearing, 15*(6), 422–431.

Saletu, B., Moller, H. J., Grunberger, J., Deutsch, H., & Rossner, M. (1990). Propentofylline in adult-onset cognitive disorders: Double-blind, placebo-controlled, clinical, psychometric and brain mapping studies. *Neuropsychobiology, 24*(4), 173–184.

Sameroff, A. J. (1983). Developmental systems: Contexts and evolution. In W. Kessen (Ed.), History, theory, and methods (Vol. 1). In P. H. Mussen (Ed.), *Handbook of child psychology* (4th ed., pp. 237–294). New York: John Wiley.

Sano, M., Bell, K., Marder, K., Stricks, L., Stern, Y., & Mayeux, R. (1993). Safety and efficacy of oral physostigmine in the treatment of Alzheimer disease. *Clinical Neuropharmacology, 16*(1), 61–69.

Shannon, R. V., Zeng, F. G., Kamath, V., Wygonski, J., & Ekelid, M. (1995). Speech recognition with primarily temporal cues. *Science, 270*, 303–304.

Simoski, J., Stevens, K., Adler, L., Freedman, P. (2002). Clozapine improves deficient inhibitory auditory processing in DBA/2 mice, via a nicotinic cholinergic mechanism. *Psychopharmacology, 165*, 386–396.

Stach, B. A., Loiselle, L. H., Jerger, J. F., Mintz, S. L., & Taylor, C. D. (1987). Clinical experience with personal FM assistive listening devices. *Hearing Journal, 10*(5), 24–30.

Syka, J. (2002). Plastic changes in the central auditory system after hearing loss, restoration of function, and duration learning. *Physiological Reviews, 82*, 601–636.

Tallal, P., Merzenich, M., Miller, S., & Jenkins, W. (1998). Language learning impairment: Integrating basic science, technology, and remediation. *Experimental Brain Research, 123*, 210–219.

Tallal, P., Miller, S., Bedi, G., Byma, G., Wang, X., Nagarajan, S. S., Schreiner, C., Jenkins, W. M., & Merzenich, M. M. (1996). Language comprehension in language-learning impaired children improved with acoustically modified speech. *Science, 271*, 81–84.

Tang, Y., Shimizu, E., Dube, G., Rampon, C., Kerchner. G., Zhuo, M., Liu, G., & Tsien, J. (1999). Genetic enhancement of learning and memory in mice. *Nature, 401*, 63–69.

Tillery, K. L., Katz, J., & Keller, W. D. (2000). Effects of methylphenidate (Ritalin) on auditory performance in children with attention and auditory processing disorders. *Journal of Speech, Language, and Hearing Research, 43*, 893–901.

Torigoe, R., Hayashi, T., Anegawa, S., Harada, K., Toda, K., Maeda, K., & Katsuragi, M. (1994). The effect of propentofylline and pentoxifylline on cerebral blood flow using 123I-IMP SPECT in patients with cerebral arteriosclerosis. *Clinical Therapeutics, 16*(1), 65–73.

Trainor, L., Shahin, A., & Roberts, L. (2003). Effects of musical training on the auditory cortex in children. *Annals of the New York Academy of Sciences, 999*, 506–513.

Tremblay, K., & Kraus, N. (2002). Auditory training induces asymmetrical changes in cortical neural activity. *Journal of Speech, Language, and Hearing Research, 45,* 564-572.

Tremblay, K., Kraus, N., Carrell, T., & McGee, T. (1997). Central auditory system plasticity: Generalization to novel stimulation following listening training. *Journal of the Acoustical Society of America, 102,* 3762-3773.

Tremblay, K., Kraus, N., & McGee, T. (1998). The time course of auditory perceptual learning: Neurophysiological changes during speech-sound training. *NeuroReport, 9,* 3557-3560.

Tremblay, K., Kraus, N., McGee, T., Ponton, C., & Otis, B. (2001). Central auditory plasticity: Changes in the N1-P2 complex after speech-sound training. *Ear and Hearing, 22*(2), 79-90.

Van Tasell, D. J., Soli, S. D., Kirby, V. M., & Widin, G. P. (1987). Speech waveform envelope cues for consonant recognition. *Journal of the Acoustical Society of America, 82*(4), 1152-1161.

Warrier, C. M., Johnson, K. L., Hayes, E. A., Nicol, T., & Kraus, N. (2004). Learning impaired children exhibit timing deficits and training-related improvements in auditory cortical responses to speech in noise. *Experimental Brain Research, 157,* 431-441.

Wenthold, R. (1991). Neurotransmitters of brainstem auditory nuclei. In R. A. Altshuler, B. M. Clopton, R. P. Bobbin, & D. W. Hoffman (Eds.), *Neurobiology of hearing: The central auditory system* (pp. 121-139). New York: Raven Press.

Wible, B., Nicol, T., & Kraus, N. (2005). Correlation between brainstem and cortical auditory processes in normal and language-impaired children. *Brain, 128,* 417-423.

Wiederhold, M. L. (1986). Physiology of the olivocochlear system. In R. A. Altschuler, D. W. Hoffman, & R. P. Bobbin (Eds.), *Neurobiology of hearing: The cochlea* (pp. 349-370). New York: Raven Press.

Winblad, B. (2005). Piracetam: A review of pharmacological properties and clinical uses. *CNS Drug Reviews, 11*(2), 169-182.

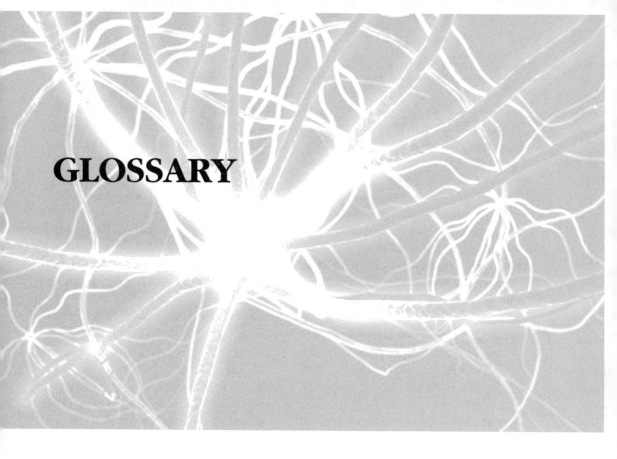

GLOSSARY

Absorption. Property of a material or an object whereby sound energy is converted into heat by propagation in a medium or when sound strikes the boundary between two media. It is determined for a specified frequency or for a stated frequency band.

Accommodation. Making facilities and programs accessible to and usable by persons with disabilities through appropriate modifications, including policy modifications, task restructuring, modified schedules, equipment acquisition or modification, training, or provision of qualified readers or interpreters, and other similar accommodations.

Acoustic access. Access through the auditory channel, either unaided or aided, to acoustic information.

Acoustic saliency. An acoustically salient phoneme (speech sound) or word is one that is obvious and prominent in an utterance. In a sentence context, acoustically nonsalient morphemes are shorter in duration and softer than louder phonemes in adjacent portions of the utterance.

Afferent. Used to refer to neurons carrying information to the brain, such as those in the ascending auditory pathways.

Amplitude modulation (AM). Variation in the envelope of a sound over time.

Analog. Refers to a signal that varies continuously over time.

Assessment. Formal and informal procedures to collect data and gather evidence; delineation of functional areas of strength or weakness and/or determination of ability or capacity in associated areas.

Assistive listening system. A device that delivers sound to individuals with

345

peripheral or central auditory deficits to mitigate listening problems (e.g., frequency modulated [FM] systems, personal amplifiers, infrared systems).

Association area. Areas of the cerebral cortex not believed to receive direct sensory inputs or send outputs to motor neurons, but communicate with other cerebrocortical areas.

Attention. Gateway to conscious experience; maintains primacy of certain information in ongoing information processing.

Selective (focused) attention. Ability to focus on relevant stimuli while ignoring simultaneously presented, but irrelevant stimuli (i.e., distractors).

Divided attention. Ability to attend to multiple stimuli simultaneously.

Sustained attention (vigilance). Ability to inhibit interference; requires sustained focus for a period of time while awaiting the occurrence of a target stimulus.

Attention deficit hyperactivity disorder (ADHD). Persistent pattern of inattention and/or hyperactivity-impulsivity that is more frequent and severe than is typically observed in individuals at a comparable level of development; manifested in at least two settings; interferes with developmentally appropriate social, academic, or occupational functions; and has been present before age 7 years.

Combined type. Attention deficit characterized by hyperactivity-impulsivity and inattention.

Predominantly inattentive type. Presents primary symptoms of inattention.

Predominantly hyperactive-impulsive type. Behavioral regulation disorder.

Attenuation. Reduction in magnitude of a physical quantity such as sound, either by electronic means (e.g., by an attenuator), or by a physical barrier, including various absorptive materials. It is usually measured in decibels.

Auditory cortex. Area of the cerebral cortex that is the final destination of auditory inputs; located in the floor of the lateral sulcus in the superior temporal gyrus; *see also* Primary auditory area.

Auditory discrimination. Differentiating similar acoustic stimuli that differ in frequency, intensity, and/or temporal parameters.

Backward masking. The presence of one sound renders a previously presented sound less detectable.

Binaural interaction. Central auditory processing of intensity or time differences of acoustic stimuli presented diotically to the two ears.

Binaural masking level difference. A measure of the advantage in signal detection that can result from the use of binaural cues; the difference in signal threshold between a situation in which the masker and signal have the same interaural time difference and interaural level difference, and a situation in which the interaural time and/or level differences for the masker and the signal differ.

Bottom-up processing. Information processing that is data driven; properties of the data are primary determinants of higher level representations and constructions.

Brain imaging. Procedures used to map the structure and metabolic and electrophysiologic properties of the brain; includes computed tomography, magnetic resonance imaging, positron emission topography, regional cerebral blood flow, and brain electrical activity mapping.

Central auditory nervous system (CANS). The auditory brainstem, subcortical pathways, auditory cortex, and corpus callosum.

Central auditory processes. Auditory system mechanisms and processes that underlie the following abilities or skills: sound localization and lateralization; auditory discrimination; auditory pattern recognition; temporal aspects of audition including, temporal integration, temporal discrimination (e.g., temporal gap detection), temporal ordering, and temporal masking; auditory performance with competing acoustic signals (including dichotic listening); and auditory performance with degraded acoustic signals.

(Central) auditory processing disorder ([C]APD). Difficulties in the perceptual processing of auditory information in the central nervous system, that cannot be *attributed to* higher order language, cognitive, or related supramodal confounds, and manifest as poor performance in one or more of the central auditory processes, with associated changes in the neurobiologic activity underlying those processes that give rise to the auditory evoked potentials.

Characteristic frequency. The pure tone frequency to which a given place on the basilar membrane, or a given neuron in the auditory system, is most sensitive at low stimulation levels.

Clear speech. Speech produced by a speaker who has been instructed to speak as clearly as possible, as if trying to communicate in a noisy background.

Closure. The ability to subjectively complete and make whole an incomplete form. Listeners use language knowledge and inductive and deductive reasoning, as well as auditory and grammatic closure to derive the meaning of words and messages.

Auditory closure. The ability to recognize a whole word despite the absence of certain elements.

Grammatic closure. The ability to complete phrases or sentences despite missing words or morphemes (e.g., filling in the verb form *are* versus *is* to conjugate with the subject *they*).

Verbal auditory closure. The ability to use spoken contextual information to facilitate speech recognition.

Cognition. Activity of knowing, encompassing the acquisition, organization, and use of knowledge; automatic and unconscious processes that transform, reduce, elaborate, store, recover, and use sensory input; processes involved in knowing, including perceiving, recognizing, conceiving, judging, sensing, and reasoning; primary phase in the development of knowledge.

Cognitive style. An individual's approach to processing information, problem-solving, and cognitive tasks (e.g., bottom-up/top-down, impulsive/reflective, field dependent/field independent).

Commissure. A group of axons of neurons passing from one side of the brain, usually, to a similar structure on the opposite side of the brain.

Commissurotomy. The medical term for surgical sectioning of a brain commissure, usually the corpus callosum.

Comorbidity. Existence of two or more disorders, diseases, or pathologic processes in an individual that are not necessarily related.

Compensation. Rehabilitative approach directed toward reducing the negative impact of a disorder or disease not amenable to complete recovery through treatment.

Consonant-vowel (CV) Syllable. Nonsense syllable comprised of a consonant followed by a vowel (e.g., ba, da, ga).

Corpus callosum. Principal commissure of the cerebral hemispheres.

Critical distance. Distance from a sound source at which direct sound level and reverberant sound level are equal.

Damping. Dissipation of energy with time or distance; loss of energy in a system resulting from friction (internal or external) or other resistance.

Deductive inferencing. Reasoning from the general to the specific.

Depolarization. An increase in the electric potential of a hair cell or neuron from a negative resting potential.

Diagnosis. Identification and categorization of impairment/dysfunction; determination of presence and nature of a disorder.

Dichotic. Simultaneous presentation of two different acoustic events, one to each ear.

Difference limen (DL). Just noticeable difference or smallest detectable change in a stimulus, usually pertaining to frequency, intensity, or duration; the difference in a quantity that a listener can just detect at some criterion level of performance.

Differential diagnosis. Distinguishing between two or more conditions presenting with similar symptoms or attributes.

Diffraction. Bending of sound waves around obstacles whose dimensions are smaller than the wavelength of the sound; the spreading out of waves beyond openings that are smaller than the wavelength of the sound. Diffraction involves a change in direction of a wave as it passes through a small opening or around a barrier in its path.

Diffusion. Process of spreading or dispersing radiated energy so that it is less direct or coherent. In acoustics, diffusion is caused by sound waves reflected from an uneven surface.

Distortion. Undesired change of a waveform resulting in the presence of some frequency components in the output signal that are not present in the input signal.

Dynamic assessment. Approach to evaluation focused on the different ways by which an individual achieves a score rather than the score achieved; approach is characterized by guided learning to determine an individual's potential for change.

Effectiveness. Effects of treatment; how well a treatment works in real-world settings.

Effect size. Calculated measure used to determine the extent of practical significance for particular research results.

Efferent system. The portion of the auditory system, also called the descending system, that courses from the brain down to the cochlea following a similar pathway as the afferent system.

Efficacy. Effects of treatment; how well a treatment can work under ideal circumstances and adequate control; documenting treatment efficacy requires demonstrating that a particular treatment produces the desired outcomes or behavior change in an efficient manner (e.g., cost effective) as a result of the treatment.

Efficiency. A measure of a test's combined sensitivity and specificity; ability of a test to identify correctly those individuals who have the dysfunction and correctly identify those individuals who do not have the dysfunction.

Electroacoustic measures. Recordings of acoustic signals from within the ear canal that are generated spontaneously or in response to acoustic stimuli (e.g., otoacoustic emissions, acoustic reflexes).

Electrophysiologic measures. Recordings of electrical potentials that reflect synchronous activity generated by the central nervous system in response to a wide variety of acoustic events (e.g., auditory brainstem response, steady-state evoked potentials, auditory middle-latency response, frequency following response, cortical auditory event-related potentials [P1, N1, P2, P300]).

Endogenous. Refers to evoked potentials (e.g., P300) that are relatively invariant to changes in the eliciting physical stimulus, but are highly influenced by subject state and require an internal or mental activity (e.g., perceptual or cognitive process) to generate the potential.

Evaluation. Interpretation of assessment data, evidence, and related information.

Evidence-based practice. Explicit and judicious use of current best evidence in making decisions about the care of individual patients by integrating individual clinical expertise with the best available external clinical evidence from systematic research; a systematic method to evaluate and implement best practices for assessment and treatment in clinical fields.

Executive function. Component of metacognition; set of general control processes that coordinate knowledge (i.e., cognition) and metacognitive knowledge, transforming such knowledge into behavioral strategies, which ensure that an individual's behavior is adaptive, consistent with some goal, and beneficial to the individual; self-directed actions of an individual that are used to self-regulate so as to accomplish self-control, goal-directed behavior, and maximize future outcomes.

Exogenous. Refers to evoked potentials that are highly dependent on acoustic features of the stimulus.

Extra-axial. Lesions of the brainstem that do not arise from within the brainstem, but from near structures that encroach upon the brainstem.

Forward masking. The presence of one sound renders a subsequent sound less detectable.

Free field. A sound environment in which there are no significant effects on sound propagation from boundaries and the medium (air) is homogeneous and motionless; under free field conditions, the loss of energy with distance may be predicted by the inverse square law.

Gyrus (pl. gyri). Bulge on the surface of the cerebral cortex consisting of gray matter with an inner core of white matter.

Impedance. Quotient of a dynamic field quantity (e.g., sound pressure) by a kinematic field quantity (e.g., particle velocity), at a specified frequency; total opposition to energy flow expressed in ohms.

Individuals with Disabilities Education Act (IDEA). A federal education act that guarantees special education and related services to children with disabilities.

Induction learning. Discovery learning; a three-step process through which a learner recognizes a pattern or relationship, explains the pattern or relationship, and hypothesizes the rule governing the pattern or relationship.

Inductive inferencing. Reasoning from the particular facts to a general conclusion.

Inferencing. Reaching a conclusion on the basis of facts or evidence.

Information processing. Assigning meaning to sensory input based on the extraction of cues or constraints through various processes or stages of cognition, including encoding, organizing, storing, retrieving, comparing, and generating or reconstructing information; these stages involve the interaction between sensory (e.g., auditory processes) and central processes (e.g., cognitive and linguistic processes) through feedback and feedforward loops.

Interaural timing. Refers to a behavioral task requiring the subject to determine the order of two acoustic events presented to each ear separately at slightly different times.

Intervention. Comprehensive, therapeutic treatment and management of a disorder.

Intra-axial. Refers to lesions of the brainstem that evolve from the brainstem tissue itself, as opposed to extra-axial lesions that arise from nonbrainstem tissue. Extra-axial lesions often are in contact with the brainstem.

Inverse square law. Principle whereby under free field conditions, sound intensity varies inversely with the square of the distance from the source; sound intensity I (in W/m^2) measured at distance r (in m) from the source producing the power P (in W) is described as $I = P/(4\pi r^2)$. Thus, if distance is doubled, sound intensity decreases by a factor of four. When expressed in decibels, level decreases by 6 dB for each doubling of the distance from the source to the point of measurement.

Isolation point. A real-time word recognition processing event, which occurs at the gate when the listener initially identifies the target word.

Latency. The time between occurrence of a physiologic event, usually a spike or evoked potential, and a stimulus.

Learning disabilities. A heterogeneous group of disorders, presumed to be due to central nervous system dysfunction, manifested by significant difficulties in the acquisition and use of listening, speaking, reading, writing, reasoning, or mathematical abilities.

Learning style. An individual's characteristic cognitive, affective, modality, and physiologic behaviors and preferences employed in perceiving, interacting with, and responding to the learning environment.

Lexical access. A spoken language processing event in which a percept comes in contact with various features of stored lexical representations.

Lexical activation. Some change in status of a subset of word candidates contained in the mental lexicon.

Linguistic-contextual information. Anything that influences the a priori probability of an upcoming utterance or the post hoc, retroactive recognition of an ongoing utterance.

Management. Procedures (e.g., compensatory strategies, environmental modifications) targeted toward reducing the effects of a disorder and minimizing the impact of the deficits that are resistant to remediation.

Masking. Process by which the threshold of one sound is raised by the presence of another (masking) sound; presence of one sound renders a subsequent sound less detectable.

Memory. Capacity to encode, process, and retrieve events, knowledge, feelings, and decisions of the past.

Short-term memory. Brief storage of limited capacity with minimal processing requirements.

Working memory. Temporary storage of information used during reasoning and planning; involves both storage and executive processing and manipulation of information.

Long-term memory. Declarative or explicit memory and procedural or implicit memory; long-term storage of unlimited capacity; involves both storage and processing of information.

Declarative or explicit memory. Conscious awareness or recollection of previously acquired information, retrieved on demand.

Procedural or implicit memory. Use of previous experience or knowledge, in the absence of conscious awareness or recollection, to support learning and guide performance.

Mesencephalic. Referring to the midbrain, just rostral to the pons.

Meta-analysis. Synthesis of treatment efficacy literature (randomized controlled trials) on a given topic using mathematical procedures to integrate results from multiple studies.

Metacognition. Awareness and appropriate use of knowledge; awareness of the task and strategy variables that affect performance and the use of that knowledge to plan, monitor, and regulate performance, including attention, learning, and the use of language; second phase (following cognition) in the development of knowledge which is active and involves conscious control over knowledge.

Metalinguistics. Aspects of language competence that extend beyond unconscious usage for comprehension and production; involves ability to think about language in its abstract form—to reflect on aspects of language apart from its content, analyze it, and make judgments about it; metalinguistic knowledge underlies performance on a number of tasks, including phonologic awareness (e.g., segmentation, rhyming), organization and storage of words (e.g., multiple meaning words), and figurative language (e.g., metaphor, idiom, humor); may be considered a subset of metacognition as using language is one of the goals of metacognitive processes.

Metamemory. Knowledge and awareness of one's own memory systems and strategies.

Minimum audible angle. The smallest detectable angular separation between two sound sources relative to the head.

Mnemonics. Artificial or contrived memory aids for organizing information (e.g., acronyms, rhymes, verbal mediators, visual imagery, drawing).

Myogenic. A response that is generated by muscle contractions.

Neural synchrony. Pattern of neural activity in which large populations of neurons fire simultaneously; this type of neural activity generates the electric activity giving rise to auditory evoked potentials.

Neurobiology. Encompasses neuroanatomy, physiology, neurochemistry, and neuropharmacology.

Neuropharmacology. Effects of drugs on neuronal tissue.

Neurotransmitter. Chemical agent released by vesicles of a nerve cell that permits synaptic transmission between neurons, between sensory cells and neurons, and between neurons and muscle cells.

No Child Left Behind Act (NCLB). A federally mandated statute enacted in 2002 designed to improve student achievement in the public schools.

Otoacoustic emissions. Subaudible sounds generated by the cochlea either spontaneously or evoked by sound stimulation.

Pansensory. Referring to higher level mechanisms that are common to and that support processing across all modalities.

Perceptual training. Regimens in which basic perceptual attributes (e.g., sound frequency or duration) are trained through repeated exposure to a task (typically discrimination or identification).

Pharmacology. Sources, chemistry, actions, and uses of drugs.

Phase. Proportion of a period through which the waveform of a sound has advanced relative to a given time.

Phase-locking. Tendency of an auditory neuron to fire at a particular time (or phase) during each cycle of vibration on the basilar membrane.

Phonemic analysis. Separating words or syllables into a sequence of phonemes.

Phonemic synthesis. Blending of discrete phonemes into the correctly sequenced, coarticulated sound patterns.

Phonologic awareness. Explicit awareness of the sound structure of language, including the recognition that words are composed of syllables and phonemes.

Plasticity. Reorganization of the cortex by experience, often reflected in behavioral change (i.e., learning); alter-

ation of neurons to conform better to immediate environmental influences, often associated with a change in behavior; changes in the properties of individual neurons or neuronal assemblies following specific use, pattern of stimulation, injury or during development; neural reorganization may be possible to some extent across the life span, as well as following injury (compensatory plasticity), and in response to learning.

Precedence effect. Refers to the dominance of information from the leading sound (as opposed to delayed or reflected versions of that sound) for the purpose of sound localization; the effect occurs for stimulus time delays varying from fractions of a millisecond to the upper limit for auditory fusion, after which separate sounds are perceived.

Prevalence. Total number of cases of a specific disease or disorder existing in a given population at a certain time.

Prevention. Procedures targeted toward reducing the likelihood that impairment will develop.

Primary auditory area (or cortex). The main auditory area of the brain, typically considered to be Heschl's gyrus.

Problem-solving. Generating a variety of potentially effective responses to a situation and recognizing and implementing the most effective response.

Prosody. Suprasegmental aspects of spoken language; the dynamic melody, timing, rhythm, and amplitude fluctuations of fluent speech.

Psychoacoustics. The study of the relation between sound (i.e., physical parameters) and perception (i.e., psychological correlates) using behavioral measurement techniques.

Real-time speech. The transitory, ephemeral nature of an ongoing speech signal; when speech is presented in a real-time manner, listeners must quickly recognize phonemes, syllables, and words based on preceding linguistic-contextual cues and ongoing acoustic-phonetic information.

Reasoning. Evaluation of arguments, drawing of inferences and conclusions, and generation and testing of hypotheses.

Reciprocal teaching. Alternating roles between the client and clinician, allowing the client to assume the role of teacher as well as learner.

Reflection. Acoustical phenomenon that occurs whenever sound strikes a surface; reflected sound is the portion of the sound energy striking the surface that bounces off the surface.

Reliability. The consistency, dependability, reproducibility, or stability of a measure.

Remediation (or treatment). Procedures targeted toward resolving an impairment.

Reverberation. Persistence or prolongation of sound in an enclosed space, resulting from multiple reflections of sound waves off hard surfaces after the source of the sound has ceased. Reverberation time (RT_{60}) refers to the time required for a steady-state sound to decay 60 dB from its initial peak amplitude offset.

Schema. Structured cluster of concepts and expectations; an abstract and generic knowledge structure stored in memory that preserves the relations among constituent concepts and generalized knowledge about a text, event, message, situation, or object.

Formal schema. Linguistic form that organizes, integrates, and predicts relationships across propositions (e.g., additives [*and, furthermore*], adversative [*although, nevertheless, however*], causal [*because, therefore, accordingly*], disjunctive [*but, instead, on the contrary*], and temporal connectives [*before, after, subsequently*], as well as patterns of parallelism and correlative pairs [*not only/but also; neither/nor*]).

Content or contextual schema. Provides a generalized interpretation of the content of experience; organizes facts and establishes a framework that imposes certain structures on events, precepts, situations, and objects and facilitates interpretation.

Screening. Procedures used to identify individuals who are *at risk* for an impairment.

Segmentation. Parsing spoken language into its constituent and successive segments; parsing sentences, words, or syllables into their constituent phonetic units; the manner in which listeners demarcate the ongoing spoken utterance into units of lexical access.

Self-regulation. Encompasses metacognitive knowledge and skills, as well as affective/emotional, motivational, and behavioral monitoring and self-control processes.

Semantic network. Construct representing a mental system of nodes and links connecting lexical units; vocabulary building in such a network involves adding new nodes and links, as well as changing activation values of the links between nodes (e.g., building synonymy by strengthening the relationships between nodes).

Sensitivity. The ability of a test to yield positive findings when the person tested truly has the dysfunction; ability of a test to identify correctly those individuals who have the dysfunction.

Signal-to-noise ratio. Relationship between the sound levels of the signal and the noise at the listener's ear, commonly reported as the difference in decibels between the intensity of the signal and the intensity of the background noise (e.g., if the speech signal is measured at 70 dB and the noise is 64 dB, the signal-to-noise ratio is +6 dB).

Sound field. The area and/or pattern of air pressure disturbance caused by the compression and rarefaction of energy in the audio frequency range.

Specificity. Ability of a test to identify correctly those individuals who do not have the dysfunction.

Spectrum level. Level of sound contained in a 1-Hz wide band; a measure of spectral density.

Speech intelligibility. Percentage of words, sentences or phonemes correctly received out of those transmitted; an important measure of the effectiveness or adequacy of a communication system or of the ability of people to communicate in noisy environments.

Spoken language processing. An interactive system of peripheral and central functions used to recognize and understand real-world transitory utterances as meaningful speech.

Standing wave. Phenomenon resulting from the interference of sound waves of the same frequency and kind traveling in opposite directions; characterized by the absence of propagation and the existence of nodes and antinodes that are fixed in space.

Sulcus. Infoldings on the cerebral surface separating gyri.

Synapse. Junction where information is transmitted between two neurons.

Synaptic transmission. Passage of an electrical impulse across a synapse through transduction to a chemical neurotransmitter presynaptically and transduction back to an electrical signal postsynaptically.

Systems theory. Study of systems as an entity rather than a conglomeration of parts; provides a conceptual framework for understanding the organization, interaction, and dynamic nature of elements comprising systems.

Temporal integration. Refers to the relationship between stimulus duration and intensity within a time frame of less than one-half second; integration of energy sampled within a time frame of approximately 200 milliseconds; sensitivity improves as signal duration increases up to approximately 200 to 300 milliseconds, after which thresholds remain essentially constant; also known as temporal summation.

Temporal masking. Masking that occurs when the signal and the masker do not overlap in time; also known as nonsimultaneous masking.

Temporal ordering. *See* Temporal sequencing.

Temporal processing. Auditory mechanisms and processes responsible for temporal patterning (e.g., phase locking, synchronization) of neural discharges and the following behavioral phenomena: temporal resolution (i.e., detection of changes in durations of auditory stimuli and time intervals between auditory stimuli over time), temporal ordering (i.e., detection of sequence of sounds over time), temporal integration (i.e., summation of power over durations less than 200 milliseconds), and temporal masking (i.e., obscuring of probe by pre- or post-stimulatory presentation of masker).

Temporal resolution. Refers to the shortest time period over which the ear can discriminate two signals; also known as temporal discrimination.

Temporal sequencing. The ability to discern the correct order of rapid acoustic events as they occur over time.

Temporal summation. *See* Temporal integration.

Tonotopic. Organization of auditory neurons in a particular structure according to their responsiveness to specific frequencies; a system of sound frequency representation in which the frequency determines the place (for example, in a neural array) of activation.

Top-down processing. Information processing that is knowledge or concept driven such that higher level constraints guide data processing, leading to data interpretation consistent with these constraints.

TORCH+S complex. A group of perinatal medical problems often linked to hearing loss. T = toxoplasmosis; O = other (e.g., associated ophthalmologic disease); R = rubella; C = cytomegalovirus; H = herpes; S = syphilis.

Total acceptance point. A late event in the real-time word recognition process when a listener recognizes the target word with a high level of confidence.

Treatment (remediation). Procedures targeted toward resolving an impairment.

Treatment outcomes. General term to denote change on measurements from pre- to postintervention.

Tuning curve. A graph depicting the response of a neuron, plotted as a function of stimulus intensity and frequency. The lowest sound level to which the neuron responds is represented by the tip of the tuning curve (i.e., characteristic frequency).

Validity. The degree to which a test measures what it is intended to measure.

Wernicke's area. The receptive auditory-language associational area of the cortex that may include part of the planum temporale and the posterosuperior temporal gyrus.

Word predictability. Amount of *fill-in-the blank* meaningfulness in a preceding spoken context. In predictability-high (PH) sentences, preceding semantic-contextual information is presented in the form of clue words; no such clue words are available in predictability-low (PL) sentences.

Word recognition. A spoken language processing event marking the conclusion of the word selection phase; also refers to a listener's ability to perceive and correctly identify a set of words usually presented at suprathreshold hearing level.

INDEX

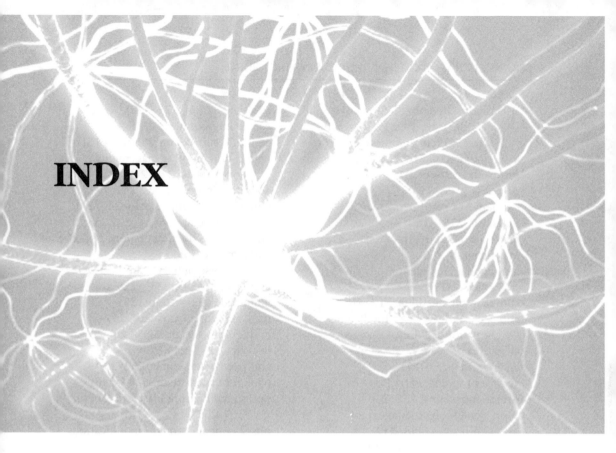